ORTHOPEDIC CLINICS OF NORTH AMERICA

www.orthopedic.theclinics.com

Infection

April 2017 • Volume 48 • Number 2

Editor-in-Chief

FREDERICK M. AZAR

Editorial Board

JAMES H. CALANDRUCCIO
BENJAMIN J. GREAR
BENJAMIN M. MAUCK
JEFFREY R. SAWYER
PATRICK C. TOY
JOHN C. WEINLEIN

ELSEVIER

1600 John F. Kennedy Boulevard • Suite 1800 • Philadelphia, Pennsylvania, 19103-2899.

http://www.orthopedic.theclinics.com

ORTHOPEDIC CLINICS OF NORTH AMERICA Volume 48, Number 2
April 2017 ISSN 0030-5898, ISBN-13: 978-0-323-52417-9

Editor: Lauren Boyle
Developmental Editor: Kristen Helm

Orthopedic Clinics of North America (ISSN 0030-5898) is published quarterly by Elsevier Inc., 360 Park Avenue South, New York, NY 10010-1710. Months of issue are January, April, July, and October. Business and Editorial Offices: 1600 John F. Kennedy Blvd., Suite 1800, Philadelphia, PA 19103-2899. Customer Service Office: 3251 Riverport Lane, Maryland Heights, MO 63043. Periodicals postage paid at New York, NY and additional mailing offices. Subscription prices are $319.00 per year for (US individuals), $686.00 per year for (US institutions), $376.00 per year (Canadian individuals), $837.00 per year (Canadian institutions), $464.00 per year (international individuals), $837.00 per year (international institutions), $100.00 per year (US students), $220.00 per year (Canadian and international students). Foreign air speed delivery is included in all *Clinics* subscription prices. All prices are subject to change without notice. **POSTMASTER: Send change of address to** *Orthopedic Clinics of North America*, **Elsevier Health Sciences Division, Subscription Customer Service, 3251 Riverport Lane, Maryland Heights, MO 63043. Customer Service (orders, claims, online, change of address): Elsevier Health Sciences Division, Subscription Customer Service, 3251 Riverport Lane, Maryland Heights, MO 63043. Tel: 1-800-654-2452 (U.S. and Canada); 314-447-8871 (outside U.S. and Canada). Fax: 314-447-8029. E-mail:** journalscustomerservice-usa@elsevier.com **(for print support);** journalsonlinesupport-usa@elsevier.com **(for online support).**

Reprints. For copies of 100 or more, of articles in this publication, please contact the Commercial Reprints Department, Elsevier Inc., 360 Park Avenue South, New York, NY 10010-1710. Tel.: 212-633-3874; Fax: 212-633-3820; E-mail: reprints@elsevier.com.

Orthopedic Clinics of North America is covered in *MEDLINE/PubMed* (*Index Medicus*), *Cinahl, Excerpta Medica, and Cumulative Index to Nursing and Allied Health Literature.*

PROGRAM OBJECTIVE

Orthopedic Clinics of North America offers clinical review articles on the most cutting-edge technologies and techniques in the field, including adult reconstruction, the upper extremity, pediatrics, trauma, oncology, and sports medicine.

TARGET AUDIENCE

Practicing orthopedic surgeons, orthopedic residents, and other healthcare professionals who specialize in orthopedic technologies and techniques for adult reconstruction, the upper extremity, pediatrics, trauma, oncology, and sports medicine.

LEARNING OBJECTIVES

Upon completion of this activity, participants will be able to:
1. Review the diagnosis and management of infections related to orthopedic injuries and surgeries.
2. Discuss orthopedic infections in pediatric populations.
3. Recognize strategies in the evaluation and management of specific orthopedic infections of the upper and lower extremities, such as flexor tenosynovitis and active infections in the foot and ankle, among others.

ACCREDITATION

The Elsevier Office of Continuing Medical Education (EOCME) is accredited by the Accreditation Council for Continuing Medical Education (ACCME) to provide continuing medical education for physicians.

The EOCME designates this enduring material for a maximum of 15 *AMA PRA Category 1 Credit*(s)™. Physicians should claim only the credit commensurate with the extent of their participation in the activity.

All other health care professionals requesting continuing education credit for this enduring material will be issued a certificate of participation.

DISCLOSURE OF CONFLICTS OF INTEREST

The EOCME assesses conflict of interest with its instructors, faculty, planners, and other individuals who are in a position to control the content of CME activities. All relevant conflicts of interest that are identified are thoroughly vetted by EOCME for fair balance, scientific objectivity, and patient care recommendations. EOCME is committed to providing its learners with CME activities that promote improvements or quality in healthcare and not a specific proprietary business or a commercial interest.

The planning committee, staff, authors and editors listed below have identified no financial relationships or relationships to products or devices they or their spouse/life partner have with commercial interest related to the content of this CME activity:

Emilie Amaro, BS; Thomas An, MD; Michael W. Aversano, MD; Frederick M. Azar, MD; Mark R. Bagg, MD; Michael Benvenuti, MD; Joseph Bosco, MD; Lauren Boyle; James H. Calandruccio, MD; David C. Carver, MD; Edward Chan, MD; Lawson A.B. Copley, MD; Erin Dean, MD; Mouhanad M. El-Othmani, MD; Howard R. Epps, MD; Perry J. Evangelista, MD; Anjali Fortna; Shawn S. Funk, MD; Benjamin J. Grear, MD; James G. Gurney, PhD; Lorraine Hutzler, BA; John S. Hwang, MD; Brad T. Hyatt, MD; Ifeoma Inneh, MPH, MBA; Richard Iorio, MD; Brandon Jonard, MD; Emmanuel Koli, MD; Kenneth L. Koury, MD; Sean B. Kuehn, MD; Mark Loftin, PhD; Steven Lovejoy, MD; Jeffrey Martus, MD; Gregory Mencio, MD; Megan Mignemi, MD; William M. Mihalko, MD, PhD; Nicole I. Montgomery, MD; Premkumar Nandhakumar; Jasmine Saleh, MD; Michael Sirkin, MD; Webb A. Smith, PhD; Patrick C. Toy, MD; Katie Widmeier; Amy Williams; Michael Williams, PT, OCS; John Womack, MD; Audrey Zucker-Levin, PhD, PT, MBA, GCS Emeritus.

The planning committee, staff, authors and editors listed below have identified financial relationships or relationships to products or devices they or their spouse/life partner have with commercial interest related to the content of this CME activity:

Benjamin M. Mauck, MD is a consultant/advisor for Olympus America.
Khaled J. Saleh, MD, MSc, FRCS(C), MHCM, CPE is on the speakers' bureau for, a consultant/advisor for, and receives royalties/patents from Aesculap, Inc. and B. Braun Medical Inc., and receives royalties/patents from Elsevier.
Jeffrey R. Sawyer, MD is on the speakers' bureau for and is a consultant/advisor for Johnson & Johnson Services, Inc, and receives royalties/patents from Elsevier.
Jonathan Schoenecker, MD, PhD is on the speakers' bureau for, a consultant/advisor for, and has research support from, OrthoPediatrics Corp., and has research support from Ionis Pharmaceuticals.
Lawrence X. Webb, MD is a consultant/advisor for Biocomposites.
John C. Weinlein, MD receives royalties/patents from Elsevier.

UNAPPROVED/OFF-LABEL USE DISCLOSURE

The EOCME requires CME faculty to disclose to the participants:
1. When products or procedures being discussed are off-label, unlabelled, experimental, and/or investigational (not US Food and Drug Administration [FDA] approved); and
2. Any limitations on the information presented, such as data that are preliminary or that represent ongoing research, interim analyses, and/or unsupported opinions. Faculty may discuss information about pharmaceutical agents that is outside of FDA-approved labelling. This information is intended solely for CME and is not intended to promote off-label use of these medications. If you have any questions, contact the medical affairs department of the manufacturer for the most recent prescribing information.

TO ENROLL

To enroll in the *Orthopedic Clinics of North America* Continuing Medical Education program, call customer service at 1-800-654-2452 or sign up online at http://www.theclinics.com/home/cme. The CME program is available to subscribers for an additional annual fee of USD 215.

METHOD OF PARTICIPATION

In order to claim credit, participants must complete the following:

1. Complete enrolment as indicated above.
2. Read the activity.
3. Complete the CME Test and Evaluation. Participants must achieve a score of 70% on the test. All CME Tests and Evaluations must be completed online.

CME INQUIRIES/SPECIAL NEEDS

For all CME inquiries or special needs, please contact elsevierCME@elsevier.com.

EDITORIAL BOARD

CONTRIBUTORS

AUTHORS

EMILIE AMARO, BS
Vanderbilt University School of Medicine,
Nashville, Tennessee

THOMAS AN, MD
Vanderbilt University School of Medicine,
Nashville, Tennessee

MICHAEL W. AVERSANO, MD
NYULMC Hospital for Joint Diseases,
New York, New York

MARK R. BAGG, MD
Attending Surgeon, Department of Hand
Surgery, The Hand Center of San Antonio,
San Antonio, Texas

MICHAEL BENVENUTI, MD
Vanderbilt University School of Medicine,
Nashville, Tennessee

JOSEPH BOSCO, MD
NYULMC Hospital for Joint Diseases,
New York, New York

DAVID C. CARVER, MD
Resident, Department of Orthopaedic
Surgery, University of Tennessee-Campbell
Clinic, Memphis, Tennessee

EDWARD CHAN, MD
Department of Hand Surgery, The Hand
Center of San Antonio, San Antonio, Texas

LAWSON A.B. COPLEY, MD
Department of Orthopaedic Surgery,
Children's Medical Center of Dallas; Professor
of Pediatric Orthopaedic Surgery, University
of Texas Southwestern, Dallas, Texas

ERIN DEAN, MD
Crystal Clinic Orthopedic Center, Hudson,
Ohio

MOUHANAD M. EL-OTHMANI, MD
Clinical Research Assistant, Department of
Orthopaedics and Sports Medicine, Detroit
Medical Center, University Health Center
(UHC), Detroit, Michigan

HOWARD R. EPPS, MD
Associate Professor, Orthopedic
Surgery, Baylor College of Medicine,
Houston, Texas

PERRY J. EVANGELISTA, MD
NYULMC Hospital for Joint Diseases,
New York, New York

SHAWN S. FUNK, MD
Department of Orthopaedic Surgery,
The Children's Hospital of San Antonio;
Assistant Professor, Baylor College of
Medicine, San Antonio, Texas

JAMES G. GURNEY, PhD
Hardin Professor and Associate Dean,
Director, Division of Epidemiology,
Biostatistics & Environmental Health, School
of Public Health, University of Memphis,
Memphis, Tennessee

LORRAINE HUTZLER, BA
NYULMC Hospital for Joint Diseases,
New York, New York

JOHN S. HWANG, MD
Department of Orthopaedics,
New Jersey Medical School, Rutgers,
The State University of New Jersey,
Newark, New Jersey

BRAD T. HYATT, MD
Fellow, Department of Hand Surgery,
The Hand Center of San Antonio,
San Antonio, Texas

IFEOMA INNEH, MPH, MBA
NYULMC Hospital for Joint Diseases,
New York, New York

RICHARD IORIO, MD
NYULMC Hospital for Joint Diseases,
New York, New York

BRANDON JONARD, MD
Summa Health System, Department of
Orthopedic Surgery, Akron, Ohio

EMMANUEL KOLI, MD
NYULMC Hospital for Joint Diseases,
New York, New York; Department of
Orthopaedic Surgery, Howard University,
Washington, DC

KENNETH L. KOURY, MD
Department of Orthopaedics, Complex
Fractures, Nonunions and Osteomyelitis,
University Physician Associates, North Jersey
Orthopaedic Institute, New Jersey Medical
School, Rutgers, The State University of
New Jersey, Newark, New Jersey

SEAN B. KUEHN, MD
Fellow, Department of Orthopaedic Surgery,
University of Tennessee-Campbell Clinic,
Memphis, Tennessee

MARK LOFTIN, PhD
Associate Dean, School of Applied Sciences,
Professor of Exercise Science, University of
Mississippi, University, Mississippi

STEVEN LOVEJOY, MD
Department of Orthopaedics, Vanderbilt
University Medical Center, Nashville,
Tennessee

JEFFREY MARTUS, MD
Department of Orthopaedics, Vanderbilt
University Medical Center, Nashville,
Tennessee

GREGORY MENCIO, MD
Department of Orthopaedics, Vanderbilt
University Medical Center, Nashville,
Tennessee

MEGAN MIGNEMI, MD
Department of Orthopaedics, Vanderbilt
University Medical Center, Nashville,
Tennessee

WILLIAM M. MIHALKO, MD, PhD
Professor & JR Hyde Chair; Chair, Joint
Graduate Program in Biomedical Engineering,
Campbell Clinic Department of Orthopaedic
Surgery & Biomedical Engineering, Director of
Adult Reconstructive Fellowship Program,
University of Tennessee Health Science
Center, Memphis, Tennessee

NICOLE I. MONTGOMERY, MD
Fellow, Pediatric Orthopedics, Baylor
College of Medicine, Houston,
Texas

JASMINE SALEH, MD
Research Fellow, National Institute of Health,
Bethesda, Maryland

KHALED J. SALEH, MD, MSc, FRCS(C),
MHCM, CPE
Executive-In-Chief, Department of
Orthopaedics and Sports Medicine, Detroit
Medical Center, University Health Center
(UHC), Detroit, Michigan

JONATHAN G. SCHOENECKER, MD, PhD
Departments of Orthopaedics,
Pharmacology, and Pathology, Microbiology
and Immunology, Vanderbilt University
Medical Center, Nashville,
Tennessee

MICHAEL SIRKIN, MD
Vice Chairman and Professor,
Department of Orthopaedics, Complex
Fractures, Nonunions and Osteomyelitis,
President, University Physician Associates,
North Jersey Orthopaedic Institute,
New Jersey Medical School, Rutgers,
The State University of New Jersey,
Newark, New Jersey

WEBB A. SMITH, PhD
Assistant Professor, Department of Pediatrics,
University of Tennessee Health Science
Center, Memphis, Tennessee

LAWRENCE X. WEBB, MD
Chairman, Department of Orthopaedic
Trauma, Medical Center Navicent Health,
Macon, Georgia, Professor, Department
of Surgery, Wake Forest University, Mercer
University School of Medicine, Macon,
Georgia; Emeritus Professor, Department
of Orthopaedic Surgery, Medical Center,
Wake Forest University, Winston-Salem,
North Carolina

JOHN C. WEINLEIN, MD
Assistant Professor, Department of
Orthopaedic Surgery, University of
Tennessee-Campbell Clinic, Memphis,
Tennessee

MICHAEL WILLIAMS, PT, OCS
Director, Department of Physical Therapy,
Campbell Clinic Orthopaedics, Germantown,
Tennessee

JOHN WOMACK, MD
Piedmont Orthopaedic Associates, Greenville,
South Carolina

AUDREY ZUCKER-LEVIN, PhD, PT, MBA,
GCS Emeritus
Professor, Department of Physical Therapy,
Assistant Dean of Research, College of Health
Professions, University of Tennessee Health
Science Center, Memphis,
Tennessee

MICHAEL WILLIAMS, PT, DCS
Director, Department of Physical Therapy,
Campbell Clinic Orthopaedics, Germantown,
Tennessee

JOHN WOMS, Sr., MD
Teckham Orthopaedic Association, Cleveland,
North Carolina

AUDREY ZUCKER LEVIN, PhD, PT, MBA,
GCS Emeritus
Professor, Department of Physical Therapy,
Assistant Dean of Research, College of Health
Professions, University of Tennessee Health
Science Center, Memphis,
Tennessee

CONTENTS

Preface: Infection   **xvii**
Frederick M. Azar

Adult Reconstruction
Patrick C. Toy

Effect of Tranexamic Acid on Transfusion Rates Following Total Joint   **109**
Arthroplasty: A Cost and Comparative Effectiveness Analysis
Perry J. Evangelista, Michael W. Aversano, Emmanuel Koli, Lorraine Hutzler,
Ifeoma Inneh, Joseph Bosco, and Richard Iorio

Tranexamic acid (TXA) is used to reduce blood loss in orthopedic total joint arthroplasty (TJA). This study evaluates the effectiveness of TXA in reducing transfusions and hospital cost in TJA. Participants undergoing elective TJA were stratified into 2 cohorts: those not receiving and those receiving intravenous TXA. TXA decreased total hip arthroplasty (THA) transfusions from 22.7% to 11.9%, and total knee arthroplasty (TKA) from 19.4% to 7.0%. The average direct hospital cost reduction for THA and TKA was $3083 and $2582, respectively. Implementation of a TJA TXA protocol significantly reduced transfusions in a safe and cost-effective manner.

Physical Function and Physical Activity in Obese Adults After Total Knee   **117**
Arthroplasty
Webb A. Smith, Audrey Zucker-Levin, William M. Mihalko, Michael Williams,
Mark Loftin, and James G. Gurney

Obese patients are more likely to have osteoarthritis and total knee arthroplasty (TKA). This investigation sought to evaluate physical function, activity level, and quality of life (QOL). Obese participants near 1-year postsurgical follow-up appointment were recruited. Evaluation included QOL and activity questionnaire, medical histories, anthropometrics, strength, and aerobic capacity. Sixty participants completed assessments. Obese TKA patients have physical performance limitations and low physical activity levels 1 year after surgery and completion of postoperative rehabilitation.

Deep Vein Thrombosis and Pulmonary Embolism Considerations in Orthopedic   **127**
Surgery
Jasmine Saleh, Mouhanad M. El-Othmani, and Khaled J. Saleh

Patients undergoing orthopedic surgery have an increased risk for deep venous thrombosis (DVT) and pulmonary embolism (PE). These complications are considered detrimental, as they cause major postoperative morbidity and mortality and lead to a substantial health care burden. Because of the high incidence and serious nature of these complications, it is essential for orthopedic surgeons to have a comprehensive knowledge of the risk factors, diagnosis, and treatment of acute DVT and PE. Perioperative management of orthopedic patients to prevent postoperative DVT and PE and optimize postoperative outcomes is also discussed in this review.

Trauma
John C. Weinlein

Role of Systemic and Local Antibiotics in the Treatment of Open Fractures   137
David C. Carver, Sean B. Kuehn, and John C. Weinlein

> The orthopedic community has learned much about the treatment of open fractures from the tremendous work of Ramon Gustilo, Michael Patzakis, and others; however, open fractures continue to be very difficult challenges. Type III open fractures continue to be associated with high infection rates. Some combination of systemic and local antibiotics may be most appropriate in these high-grade open fractures. Further research is still necessary in determining optimal systemic antibiotic regimens as well as the role of local antibiotics. Any new discoveries related to novel systemic antibiotics or local antibiotic carriers will need to be evaluated related to cost.

The Antibiotic Nail in the Treatment of Long Bone Infection: Technique and   155
Results
Kenneth L. Koury, John S. Hwang, and Michael Sirkin

> Antibiotic cement nails provide a useful and relatively simple technique to treat intramedullary osteomyelitis of the long bones. These devices provide stability as well as local, targeted antibiotics, which are both critical aspects of osteomyelitis management. Additionally, the use of a threaded core is a critical component of successful cement nail assembly. With adherence to the simple principles outlined in this review, surgeons can expect reliably good results using these drug-delivery implants.

The Impact of Negative Pressure Wound Therapy on Orthopaedic Infection   167
Lawrence X. Webb

> By hastening the resolution of edema and improving local microcirculation, topical negative pressure wound therapy (TNP) aids the establishment of early wound coverage. Its use in the setting of type III open fractures is reviewed. The author's initial use of TNP for closed surgical incisions and how it morphed its way into being applied to closed surgical wounds with heightened likelihood for infection is presented. Several case studies are presented to illustrate the role and the technique for management of acute or subacute infections involving bone and implant.

Pediatrics
Jeffrey R. Sawyer

Double-Edged Sword: Musculoskeletal Infection Provoked Acute Phase   181
Response in Children
Michael Benvenuti, Thomas An, Emilie Amaro, Steven Lovejoy, Gregory Mencio,
Jeffrey Martus, Megan Mignemi, and Jonathan G. Schoenecker

> The acute phase response has a crucial role in mounting the body's response to tissue injury. Excessive activation of the acute phase response is responsible for many complications that occur in orthopedic patients. Given that infection may be considered continuous tissue injury that persistently activates the acute phase response, children with musculoskeletal infections are at markedly increased risk for serious complications. Future strategies that modulate the acute phase response have the potential to improve treatment and prevent complications associated with musculoskeletal infection.

Acute Hematogenous Osteomyelitis in Children: Pathogenesis, Diagnosis, and   **199**
Treatment
Shawn S. Funk and Lawson A.B. Copley

Acute hematogenous osteomyelitis (AHO) in children is an ideal condition to study due to its representation of a wide spectrum of disorders that comprise pediatric musculoskeletal infection. Proper care for children with AHO is multidisciplinary and collaborative. AHO continues to present a significant clinical challenge due to evolving epidemiology and complex pathogenesis. A guideline-driven, multidisciplinary approach has been introduced and shown to effectively reduce hospital stay, improve the timing and selection of empirical antibiotic administration, reduce delay to initial MRI, reduce the rate of readmission, and shorten antibiotic duration.

Pediatric Septic Arthritis   **209**
Nicole I. Montgomery and Howard R. Epps

Acute septic arthritis is a condition with the potential for joint destruction, physeal damage, and osteonecrosis, which warrants urgent identification and treatment. The organism most frequently responsible is *Staphylococcus aureus*; however, our understanding of pathogens continues to evolve as detection methods continue to improve. MRI has improved our ability to detect concurrent infections and is a useful clinical tool where available. The treatment course involves intravenous antibiotics followed by transition to oral antibiotics when clinically appropriate. The recommended surgical treatment of septic arthritis is open arthrotomy with decompression of the joint, irrigation, and debridement and treatment of concurrent infections.

Upper Extremity
Benjamin M. Mauck and James H. Calandruccio

Flexor Tenosynovitis   **217**
Brad T. Hyatt and Mark R. Bagg

For patients with suspected flexor tenosynovitis, the mainstay of diagnosis is a thorough history and physical examination. The examination is guided by evaluating the patient for Kanavel's four cardinal signs. Empiric antibiotics should be started immediately on diagnosis covering skin flora and gram-negative bacteria. Typically, surgery is required. Appropriate exposure is required for adequate treatment and incisions should be tailored to preserve areas of skin compromised from draining sinuses and abscess pressure. Diabetes mellitus and peripheral vascular disease place patients at higher risk of poor outcomes including stiffness and amputation; early administration of antibiotics is the intervention that correlates most closely with good outcomes.

Atypical Hand Infections   **229**
Edward Chan and Mark R. Bagg

Atypical infections of the hand are caused by organisms such as *Mycobacterium*, fungi, and viruses, and often do not respond to conventional management. They exist within a wide spectrum of presentations, ranging from cutaneous lesions to deep infections such as tenosynovitis and osteomyelitis. Having a high clinical suspicion for atypical hand infections is vital because diagnosis often requires special tests and/or cultures. Obtaining a detailed medical, work, and travel history is extremely important. An indolent clinical course, late diagnosis, and delayed treatment are common. In addition to medical therapies, surgical debridement is often required to effectively treat these infections.

Foot and Ankle
Benjamin J. Grear

Charcot Arthropathy Versus Osteomyelitis: Evaluation and Management   **241**
John Womack

Charcot arthropathy of the foot and ankle is a severe complication of peripheral neuropathy and is most commonly seen in the developed world in association with diabetes mellitus. Correct diagnosis and differentiation from osteomyelitis of the foot and ankle are critical to guide treatment. It can exist concomitantly with osteomyelitis, typically in the setting of an advanced midfoot ulcer. Simple plain radiographs and contrasted MRI studies often yield inconclusive or confusing data. Correct use of imaging studies and a clinical algorithm can be effective tools to help make accurate and early diagnoses and guide clinical interventions for these conditions.

Posttraumatic Reconstruction of the Foot and Ankle in the Face of Active   **249**
Infection
Brandon Jonard and Erin Dean

Posttraumatic infection of the foot and ankle is a challenging issue for orthopedic surgeons. Making the diagnosis often requires combining laboratory and radiologic testing, patient examination, and history. Patient comorbidities should be identified and optimized whenever possible. Treatment must combine effective antibiotic therapy with thorough debridement of the infected zone. Reconstruction often requires a 2-staged approach using antibiotic spacers and temporary external fixation, with the goal of obtaining a functional, pain-free limb that is free of infection.

Index   **259**

INFECTION

FORTHCOMING ISSUES

July 2017
Orthobiologics
Frederick M. Azar, James H. Calandruccio,
Benjamin J. Grear, Benjamin M. Mauck,
Jeffrey R. Sawyer, Patrick C. Toy, and
John C. Weinlein, *Editors*

October 2017
Perioperative Pain Management
Frederick M. Azar, Clayton C. Bettin,
James H. Calandruccio, Benjamin J. Grear,
Benjamin M. Mauck, Jeffrey R. Sawyer,
Patrick C. Toy, and John C. Weinlein, *Editors*

January 2018
Outpatient Surgery
Frederick M. Azar, Clayton C. Bettin,
James H. Calandruccio, Benjamin J. Grear,
Benjamin M. Mauck, Jeffrey R. Sawyer,
Thomas Q. Throckmorton, Patrick C. Toy, and
John C. Weinlein, *Editors*

RECENT ISSUES

January 2017
Controversies in Fracture Care
James H. Calandruccio, Benjamin J. Grear,
Benjamin M. Mauck, Jeffrey R. Sawyer,
Patrick C. Toy, and John C. Weinlein, *Editors*

October 2016
Sports-Related Injuries
James H. Calandruccio, Benjamin J. Grear,
Benjamin M. Mauck, Jeffrey R. Sawyer,
Patrick C. Toy, and John C. Weinlein, *Editors*

July 2016
Orthopedic Urgencies and Emergencies
James H. Calandruccio, Benjamin J. Grear,
Benjamin M. Mauck, Jeffrey R. Sawyer,
Patrick C. Toy, and John C. Weinlein, *Editors*

THE CLINICS ARE AVAILABLE ONLINE!

Access your subscription at:
www.theclinics.com

PREFACE

Infection

Despite advances in operative techniques, infection prevention protocols, and antibiotic therapies, infection continues to be a difficult problem in all areas of orthopedic surgery, from pediatrics to geriatrics. This issue of *Orthopedic Clinics of North America* presents information on current diagnostic and treatment methods for infection-related complications in orthopedic patients.

Three articles, however, deal with other possible complications in orthopedic surgery. Evangelista and colleagues describe the use of tranexamic acid to reduce blood loss in total joint arthroplasty and evaluate its effectiveness in reducing transfusions and decreasing hospital costs. Smith and colleagues evaluated the physical function and activity after total knee arthroplasty in 60 obese patients and report low activity levels at 1 year. Saleh and colleagues present a comprehensive review of the risks of deep venous thrombosis and pulmonary embolism in orthopedic patients and discuss preventative measures.

Carver and colleagues review the latest information on systemic and local antibiotics used with open fractures and describe combinations of systemic and local antibiotics that may be most appropriate for high-grade (type III) open fractures. One relatively new "local" antibiotic delivery method is the antibiotic cement intramedullary nail. Koury and colleagues describe the technique for insertion of these nails and give some tips and tricks to improve outcomes. Another method of treatment of type III open fractures is negative pressure wound therapy, which is reported by Webb to be successful in acute and subacute infections involving bone and implant. He presents several case studies to illustrate the technique.

Orthopaedic-related infections are especially concerning in children because of the possibility of life-long disability that may result. Benvenuti and colleagues highlight a rarely considered factor in infection—the acute phase response. Evidence has shown that excessive activation of this response leads to many complications, indicating that close monitoring of this phase is important to avoid these. The authors discuss potential methods for modulating the acute phase response in patients with infections to reduce or prevent complications.

Funk and Copley emphasize the importance of a multidisciplinary approach to the treatment of acute hematogenous osteomyelitis in children and present a guideline-driven protocol for evaluation and treatment. They also recommend careful monitoring of regional trends in microbiologic epidemiology to help in formulating a treatment plan. Pediatric septic arthritis can result in a variety of musculoskeletal sequelae, including joint destruction, physeal damage, and osteonecrosis. Montgomery and Epps describe the diagnostic modalities, antibiotic treatment course, and surgical treatment of septic arthritis in children and present guidelines for decision making.

Infections of the hand can range from the common—such as tenosynovitis, as described by Hyatt and Bagg—to the very unusual—such as the atypical infections described by Chan and Bagg. Hyatt and Bagg discuss the diagnosis, physical examination, antibiotic treatment, and surgical treatment of flexor tenosynovitis and describe comorbidities, such as diabetes and peripheral vascular disease, that put patients at higher risk of poor outcomes. In their discussion of atypical hand infections, Chan and Bagg emphasize the wide spectrum of presentations of these infections as well as the many mycobacterium, fungi, and viruses that may be involved.

Womack points out the difficulty of differentiating Charcot arthropathy from osteomyelitis in the foot and ankle and describes correct use of imaging studies as well as a clinical algorithm. Dean and Jonard discuss the difficulty of reconstructing a traumatic foot or ankle injury in the setting of an active infection.

The authors and I hope the information in these articles will be useful in your practice and will help you deliver the best possible treatment to your patients.

Frederick M. Azar, MD
Department of Orthopaedic Surgery
and Biomedical Engineering
University of Tennessee–Campbell Clinic
1211 Union Avenue, Suite 510
Memphis, TN 38104, USA
E-mail address:
fazar@campbellclinic.com

Orthop Clin N Am 48 (2017) xvii
http://dx.doi.org/10.1016/j.ocl.2017.01.001
0030-5898/17/© 2017 Published by Elsevier Inc.

Adult Reconstruction

Effect of Tranexamic Acid on Transfusion Rates Following Total Joint Arthroplasty

A Cost and Comparative Effectiveness Analysis

Perry J. Evangelista, MD[a],*, Michael W. Aversano, MD[a],
Emmanuel Koli, MD[a,b], Lorraine Hutzler, BA[a],
Ifeoma Inneh, MPH, MBA[a], Joseph Bosco, MD[a],
Richard Iorio, MD[a]

KEYWORDS

• Tranexamic acid • Primary joint arthroplasty • Cost comparative analysis • Blood transfusion

---

KEY POINTS

• Tranexamic acid (TXA) is useful in total joint arthroplasty to reduce blood loss and minimizes postoperative blood transfusions.
• Cost-containment is crucial, especially in regard to elective arthroplasty cases. TXA use helps decrease costs in total joint arthroplasty.
• TXA is safe and did not result in complications in this cohort.

INTRODUCTION

Bleeding is a major contributor to intraoperative and postoperative complications for total hip arthroplasty (THA) and total knee arthroplasty (TKA). Tranexamic acid (TXA) is a synthetic amino acid derivative of lysine that works by reversibly binding to plasminogen, thereby enhancing coagulation through prevention of fibrin degradation.[1,2] Several studies have demonstrated the safety and efficacy of TXA in reducing blood loss after primary and revision total joint arthroplasty (TJA),[3,4] and others have reported the potential risks of red blood cell (RBC) transfusions after surgical procedures.[5,6] However, these studies have all been in small participant populations. To understand the clinical effects of TXA therapy and its influence on comparative cost, safety, and effectiveness, a large cohort study using a standardized treatment protocol in primary TJA participants is necessary.

The purpose of this study was to evaluate the effectiveness of TXA in reducing transfusions and hospital costs of primary TJA. The authors' hypothesis was that TXA will minimize blood loss, thereby minimizing the need for transfusion and reducing costs after TJA.

Institutional Review Board approval was granted to complete this study. All authors have participated in the research. This paper has not been submitted to any other journal. No funding was received in the production of this publication.

[a] Department of Orthopaedic Surgery, Hospital for Joint Diseases, NYU Langone Medical Centre, New York University Hospital for Joint Diseases, 301 E 17th Street, 14th Floor, New York, NY 10003, New York; [b] Department of Orthopaedic Surgery & Rehabilitation Administrative Office, Howard University Hospital Tower Building Suite 1700 Washington, DC 20064

* Corresponding author.
E-mail address: perry.evangelista@nyumc.org

METHODS

Institutional review board approval was obtained and a retrospective analysis of participants who underwent elective primary TJA at a single orthopedic specialty hospital between 2012 and 2014 was conducted. The groups were categorized into 2 distinct cohorts:

1. Those who did not receive intravenous (IV) TXA
2. Those who received IV TXA.

All data were collected retrospectively using the hospital electronic medical record system by trained research assistants.

Participants or Study Subjects

In 2012, 856 and 969 consecutive primary THA and TKA participants who did not receive TXA were identified. During 2013, 1084 and 962 primary THA and TKA participants received TXA based on a department-wide protocol, which was implemented in 2013 at the authors' institution. The medical comorbidities and demographics of these participants were not matched.

Tranexamic Acid Protocol and Venous Thromboembolic Disease Prophylaxis

Both THA and TKA participants (in year 2013) received 1 g TXA after induction of anesthesia. THA participants received an additional 1 g of TXA before wound closure, whereas TKA participants received 1 g of TXA before release of the tourniquet.[7,8] However, participants were excluded from the TXA protocol if there was a history of coronary artery disease (CAD), stroke, and/or pulmonary embolism or deep venous thrombosis (DVT), per an institutional protocol. Both the 2012 and 2013 cohorts had the same venous thromboembolic disease (VTED) prevention protocol using enoxaparin, fondaparinux, rivaroxaban, or coumadin based on surgeon preference, unless contraindicated in cases of excessive bleeding risk or elevated coagulation studies. Most participants were treated beginning postoperative day 1 with 30 mg subcutaneously twice daily of enoxaparin while hospitalized and 40 mg subcutaneously daily after discharge, for a total of 28 days postoperation.

Description of Follow-up Routine

Participants were discharged to home, or rehabilitation facility, including skilled nursing facilities, based on rehabilitation medicine discharge protocol. Postoperative antibiotics were discontinued after 24 hours.

Definition of Outcome Variables and Measures

This study assessed and reported the number of units transfused, number of participants needed to treat with TXA to prevent 1 transfusion (ie, inverse of absolute risk reduction), direct hospital costs, transfusion and TXA costs, average length of stay (ALOS) in days, percentage of participants discharged to inpatient facilities, and their relationship to transfusion, as well as incidence of VTED, myocardial infarction (MI), and stroke. Transfusion rate was defined as the number of participants transfused with packed RBCs (PRBCs) divided by the number of participants in the cohort. The cost of transfusion was estimated by the total number of units of PRBC per unit cost. Actual and projected cost estimates were calculated.

Statistical Analysis

Descriptive statistics were used to describe the cohorts and their demographics. Categorical variables were analyzed using chi-square tests, whereas continuous data were analyzed using independent t or Mann Whitney U tests (based on distribution of data). We used relative risk reduction and number needed to treat to quantify the use of TXA needed to reduce a blood transfusion compared with the comparison group. All statistical analyses were performed with SPSS version 21.0 software (SPSS, Inc, Chicago, IL, USA) or Microsoft Excel 2010 (Microsoft, Redmond, WA, USA) and significance level was set at $P<.05$.

RESULTS

The average age of the non-TXA and TXA hip cohorts was 61 and 63 years, respectively. The average age for the non-TXA and TXA knee cohorts was 69 and 65, years respectively.

Among THA participants, 427 units of blood were transfused in 194 of 856 (22.7%) participants in the non-TXA cohort, whereas 248 units of blood were transfused in 129 of 1084 (11.9%) participants in the TXA cohort ($P<.001$). Among the TKA participants, 325 units of blood were transfused in 188 of 969 (19.4%) participants in the non-TXA cohort, whereas while 121 units of blood were transfused in 67 of 962 (7%) participants in the TXA cohort ($P<.001$). The number needed to treat with TXA to prevent 1 blood transfusion was 9.3 in the THA cohort and 8.0 in the TKA cohort, a 54.2% combined relative risk reduction.

The average costs of 1 g/10 mL TXA and 1 unit (PRBC) were $25.98 and $414.43,

Table 1
Total hip arthroplasty average costs and savings for 2013 (tranexamic acid) versus 2012 (no tranexamic acid)

Year	Number Participants	Number Participants Transfused	Transfusion (Total Units PRBC)	Transfusion Rate (%)	Transfusion Cost	Cost of TXA	Actual Total Cost	Actual Cost Savings	Average Direct Hospital Costs
2012	856	194	427	22.7[a] (49.8[b])	$206,028	—	$206,028	—	$28,512
2013	1084	129	248	11.9[a] (22.9[b])	$111,198	$52,005	$163,203	$42,824	$25,428

All costs are in US dollars.
[a] Participant transfusion rate.
[b] Transfusion rate units, PRBC (packed red blood cells).

Table 2
Total hip arthroplasty projected transfusion costs for 2013 using 2012 transfusion rate (no tranexamic acid) and projected savings per case by using tranexamic acid

Participants 2013	2012 Transfusion Rate[a]	Projected Transfusion (PRBC)	Projected Cost	Projected 2013 Cost–Actual 2013 Cost	Projected Savings per Case
1084	49.8	540	$223,722.58	$64,619.30	$59.61

All costs are in US dollars.
[a] Transfusion rate units per participant.

respectively. Actual cost savings between the THA cohorts was $42,824 with a projected cost savings due to transfusion avoidance of $59.61 per case (Tables 1 and 2), whereas that for the TKA cohorts was $56,644 with a projected cost savings due to transfusion avoidance of $34.75 per case (Tables 3 and 4). The THA and TKA cohorts treated with TXA demonstrated average direct hospital cost reduction of $3083 (from $28,512 to $25,428) and $2582 (from $28,420 to $25,838), respectively, when compared with those not treated with TXA (P<.001) (see Tables 1 and 2). The incidence of VTED decreased from 1.7% in 2012 to 0.7% in 2013. The incidence of MI and stroke did not change in the cohorts.

ALOS for THA and TKA decreased in the cohort treated with TXA but did not demonstrate a statistically significant difference (P>.05). The ALOS for THA and TKA cases in 2012 was 3.7 days, whereas the 2013 ALOS for THA and TKA was 3.4 and 3.5 days, respectively. In the non-TXA THA cohort, 381 of 856 (44.5%) participants were discharged to a rehabilitation facility. Of the participants from the TXA THA cohort, 252 of 1084 (23.2%) were discharged to a rehabilitation facility (P<.05). In the 2012 TKA cohort, 489 of 969 participants (50.4%) were discharged to a rehabilitation facility. Of the TXA TKA cohort, 336 of 962 participants (34.9%) were discharged to a rehabilitation facility, (P<.05).

DISCUSSION

The results demonstrate a decrease in transfusion rates from 22.7% to 11.9% and from 19.4% to 7.0% for primary THA and TKA participants, respectively. The decrease in transfusion rates resulted in an actual cost savings of $56,644 ($34.75 per case) for TKA and $42,824 ($59.61 per case) for THA. Direct hospital costs, ALOS, and discharge to inparticipant facilities were also decreased in the TXA cohort. Fewer discharges to inpatient facilities may be related

to TXA use but a direct correlation cannot be obtained due to changes in the institutional protocol where the Bundled Payment Care Initiative through Centers for Medicare and Medicaid Services was entered to promote coordinated and efficient care by both the surgeons and the hospital system. In today's value-based health care environment, it is imperative to provide patients with cost-effective treatments that optimize care. By decreasing transfusion rates, outcomes and reduced costs are simultaneously improved. Although there are other contemporary programs aiding in these cost-effectiveness trends, TXA contributed to this trend by reducing blood loss and subsequent blood transfusions.

Various methods of TXA administration have been reported, including varying doses, direct injection, IV administration, or through drains. This study evaluated the standardization of one method of IV TXA application in large cohorts of THA and TKA participants based on an institutional protocol. The authors do not know of any other studies that report the cost-effectiveness of implementing a standardized TXA protocol in a large cohort of participants. Our study demonstrated significantly decreased transfusion rates in the TXA cohorts compared with the non-TXA cohorts with greatly reduced hospital costs. Other studies have also reported the effectiveness of TXA in reducing transfusion rates. A randomized controlled trial of 50 participants undergoing TKA treated with two doses of IV TXA versus placebo found 32% of the placebo cohort were transfused with an odds ratio of 2.32.[7] Wei and colleagues[8] conducted a randomized controlled trial of placebo versus IV TXA versus topical TXA and found similar rates of reduced blood loss in both treatment cohorts compared with placebo, and no significant difference between the two application methods.

The safety of TXA has been demonstrated in multiple studies.[4,7–12] In our study, the rates of intraoperative or postoperative MI and stroke did not increase in the TXA cohorts. However,

Table 3
Total knee arthroplasty average costs and savings for 2013 (tranexamic acid) versus 2012 (no tranexamic acid)

Year	Number Participants	Number Participants Transfused	Transfusion (Total Units PRBC)	Transfusion Rate (%)	Transfusion Cost	Cost of TXA	Actual Total Cost	Actual Cost Savings	Average Direct Hospital Costs
2012	969	188	325	19.4[a] (33.5[b])	$156,813	—	$156,813	—	$28,420
2013	962	67	121	7.0[a] (12.6[b])	$54,254	$45,915	$100,169	$56,644	$25,838

All costs are in US dollars.
[a] Participant transfusion rate.
[b] Transfusion rate units, PRBC (packed red blood cells).

Table 4
Total knee arthroplasty projected transfusion costs for 2013 using 2012 transfusion rate (no tranexamic acid) and projected savings per case by using tranexamic acid

Participants 2013	2012 Transfusion Rate[a]	Projected Transfusion (PRBC)	Projected Cost	Projected 2013 Cost–Actual 2013 Cost	Projected Savings per Case
962	33.5	325	$133,558.36	$33,426.81	$34.75

All costs are in US dollars.
[a] Transfusion rate units per participant.

we observed a decrease in the rate of VTED. These findings compare favorably with recent studies assessing the safety of TXA in TJA.[4,7–9] We did not include participants for systemic TXA treatment who had a history of DVT, stroke, or CAD, which limits the generalizability of our study to a subset of participants who may have an increased risk of developing these conditions after TJA. It provides questions that should be answered with future studies. One such study would include the use of local TXA in high-risk participants.

In our study, ALOS and associated in-hospital costs were affected by rapid rehabilitation protocols, improved pain management strategies, and increased rates of discharges from hospital to home, among other interventions aimed at maximizing patient outcomes and resource utilization. When comparing cohorts, there was a decreased ALOS, decreased discharge location to rehabilitation facilities, decreased overall average direct hospital cost, and decreased number of blood transfusions in the TXA-treated cohorts. However, these results cannot be attributed exclusively to TXA use, although TXA did contribute to the reported improved outcomes and cost savings.

Multiple limitations exist in this study. First, this study did not implement a standardized transfusion protocol. Due to the large number of surgeons participating in the study, there were several surgeon variations in regard to transfusion thresholds. However, it is important to understand that the institutional criteria for transfusions did not vary between our cohorts, the same surgeons were used in both cohorts, and their year-to-year practice did not vary in regard to transfusion trigger. For both cohorts, surgeons used a hemoglobin threshold of 8.0 or symptomatic acute blood loss anemia. Finally, participants were not randomized to different treatment arms, nor were compared groups from the same temporal period. This makes direct attribution of cost savings related to TXA alone difficult to determine because other cost saving strategies were implemented in

2013. However, we were able to calculate the cost of TXA and blood transfusions by knowing the institutional costs of these products from our pharmacy and blood banks, and to calculate the savings of transfusion avoidance. Year-to-year cost differences of these products were averaged.

SUMMARY

This retrospective analysis of TXA administration perioperatively demonstrates significantly reduced blood transfusion requirements and discharge to inpatient facilities and direct hospital costs in THA and TKA participants treated with IV TXA according to an institutional protocol compared with those not treated with TXA. Importantly, there was no increased VTED found in these treated populations. Future studies that assess the effectiveness and cost-savings of our TXA protocol while performing revision arthroplasties are needed.

REFERENCES

1. McCormack PL. Tranexamic acid: a review of its use in the treatment of hyperfibrinolysis. Drugs 2012; 72(5):585–617.
2. Huang Z, Ma J, Shen B, et al. Combination of intravenous and topical application of tranexamic acid in primary total knee arthroplasty: a prospective randomized controlled trial. J Arthroplasty 2014; 29(12):2342–6.
3. Samujh C, Falls TD, Wessel R, et al. Decreased blood transfusion following revision total knee arthroplasty using tranexamic acid. J Arthroplasty 2014;29(9):182–5.
4. Xu Q, Yang Y, Shi P, et al. Repeated doses of intravenous tranexamic acid are effective and safe at reducing perioperative blood loss in total knee arthroplasty. Biosci Trends 2014;8(3):169–75.
5. Lelubre C, Piagnerelli M, Vincent JL, et al. Association between duration of storage of transfused red blood cells and morbidity and mortality in adult patients: myth or reality? Transfusion 2009;49(7): 1384–94.

6. D'Alessandro A, Kriebardis AG, Rinalducci S, et al. An update on red blood cell storage lesions, as gleaned through biochemistry and omics technologies. Transfusion 2014;55(1):205–19.

7. Tranexamic Acid-Use in Orthopedic Surgery. Pharmacy benefits management Services, medical advisory panel and VISN pharmacist executives, veterans health administration. Washington, DC: Department of Veterans Affairs; 2014. Available at: https://vaww.cmopnational.va.gov/cmop/PBM/Clinical%20Guidance/Abbreviated%20Reviews/T RANEXAMIC%20ACID-Use%20in%20Orthopedic%20Surgery.docx.

8. Tranexamic Acid. Available at: http://www.accessdata.fda.gov/drugsatfda_docs/label/2013/019281s031lbl.pdf. Accessed February 10, 2014.

9. Bidolegui F, Arce G, Lugones A, et al. Tranexamic acid reduces blood loss and transfusion in patients undergoing total knee arthroplasty without tourniquet: a prospective randomized controlled trial. Open Orthop J 2014;8:250–4.

10. Wei W, Wei B. Comparison of topical and intravenous tranexamic acid on blood loss and transfusion rates in total hip arthroplasty. J Arthroplasty 2014;29(11):2113–6.

11. Chimento GF, Huff T, Ochsner JL Jr, et al. An evaluation of the use of topical tranexamic acid in total knee arthroplasty. J Arthroplasty 2013;28(8):74–7.

12. Shen P, Hou WL, Chen JB, et al. Effectiveness and safety of tranexamic acid for total knee arthroplasty: a prospective randomized controlled trial. Med Sci Monit 2015;22(21):576–81.

Physical Function and Physical Activity in Obese Adults After Total Knee Arthroplasty

Webb A. Smith, PhD[a],*,
Audrey Zucker-Levin, PhD, PT, MBA, GCS Emeritus[b],
William M. Mihalko, MD, PhD[c],
Michael Williams, PT, OCS[d], Mark Loftin, PhD[e],
James G. Gurney, PhD[f]

KEYWORDS

• Physical function • TKA • Obesity • Physical activity • Quality of life

---

KEY POINTS

• Obese patients are more likely to have osteoarthritis and total knee arthroplasty (TKA). This investigation sought to evaluate physical function, activity level, and quality of life (QOL) in obese TKA patients.
• Obese adults who had TKA and were near 1-year postsurgical follow-up appointment were recruited. Evaluation included QOL and activity questionnaire, medical histories, anthropometrics, strength, and aerobic capacity.
• Obese TKA patients have physical performance limitations and low physical activity levels 1 year after surgery and completion of postoperative rehabilitation.

INTRODUCTION

Obesity is associated with several health-related conditions detrimental to general health and, specifically, the musculoskeletal system.[1,2] Excess body weight directly and indirectly stresses the joints, particularly the knees, which increases the deterioration of the protective soft tissues in the joint structures.[3,4] Thus, obesity is a strong risk factor for development of osteoarthritis (OA)[5,6] and obese individuals have a substantially higher rate of total knee arthroplasty (TKA) than healthy weight individuals.[7,8]

Although the associations between obesity and OA and obesity and incidence of TKA are reasonably well described, the effects of obesity on TKA rehabilitation and long-term functional recovery are not sufficiently understood. All patients, regardless of body weight, seem to experience decreased pain and improved function following TKA.[9] However, there is some

---

Funding: This work was supported by the FedEx Institute of Technology at the University of Memphis.
Conflicts of Interest: The authors have no financial disclosures.
[a] Department of Pediatrics, University of Tennessee Health Science Center, 50 North Dunlap Street, Room 447R, Memphis, TN 38103, USA; [b] Department of Physical Therapy, College of Health Professions, University of Tennessee Health Science Center, 930 Madison Avenus, Suite 636, Memphis, TN 38163, USA; [c] Joint Graduate Program in Biomedical Engineering, Campbell Clinic Department of Orthopaedic Surgery & Biomedical Engineering, University of Tennessee Health Science Center, 956 Court Avenue, Memphis, TN 38163, USA; [d] Department of Physical Therapy, Campbell Clinic Orthopaedics, 1400 South Germantown Road, Germantown, TN 38138, USA; [e] Department of Health, Exercise Science, and Recreation Management, School of Applied Sciences, University of Mississippi, George Street House, MS 38677, USA; [f] Division of Epidemiology, Biostatistics & Environmental Health, School of Public Health, University of Memphis, 228 Robison Hall, Memphis, TN 38152, USA
* Corresponding author.
E-mail address: wsmith74@uthsc.edu

evidence indicating worse long-term outcomes among obese patients. For example, morbidly obese patients are more than 5 times more likely than healthy weight patients to experience complications and device failure within 5 years of TKA.[10,11] Obese individuals, accordingly, have higher reported need for additional surgical revision to adjust or repair the TKA and, although functional abilities improve following TKA, outcomes are significantly poorer when compared with healthy weight patients.[12] Functional abilities, such as completion of activities of daily living and exercise capacity, and factors that influence functional capacity, including persistent pain, muscle weakness, and balance impairments, are not well researched after completion of initial rehabilitation programs. Thus, the long-term benefit of the TKA intervention among obese adults requires further consideration.

The purpose of this investigation was to evaluate baseline physical function, physical activity levels, and quality of life in obese patients 1 year following TKA as part of an individually tailored exercise intervention designed to improve physical function among obese adults.

MATERIALS AND METHODS
Participants
Sixty obese (body mass index [BMI] >30 kg/m^2) patients who were 10 to 18 months post-TKA volunteered to complete surveys, a functional assessment, and 16 weeks of home-based

exercise. Patients were required to have medical clearance to participate in exercise testing and intervention. Patients were identified and recruited from surgical follow-up clinics at an orthopedic clinic based at a large health science center. Before consent, each participant was prescreened for eligibility by phone by a research nurse (**Fig. 1**). As approved by Institutional Review Boards for Human Subjects Research at the University of Tennessee Health Science Center and the University of Memphis, participants were informed of all procedures, potential risks, and benefits associated with the study, and written informed consent was obtained for each participant. Final eligibility was verified through health and medical history and a physical activity survey at the initial clinic visit.

Measurements
Anthropometrics
Height and weight were collected without shoes using a calibrated digital clinic scale and a wall-mounted stadiometer. Body composition was measured using standardized skinfold measures developed by Jackson and Pollock[13] and described in detail by the American College of Sports Medicine (ACSM).[14] Skinfolds were measured with a Lange skinfold caliper (Beta Technology, Santa Cruz, CA, USA) at the chest, abdomen, and thigh in men; and triceps, suprailiac crest, and thigh in women. Sum of skinfolds measured were used to calculate percentage

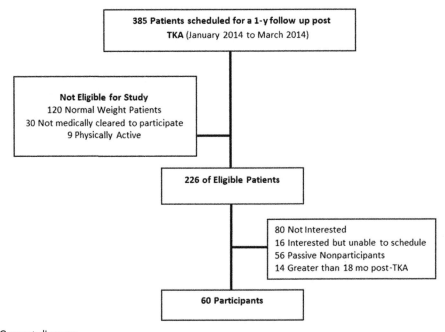

Fig. 1. Consort diagram.

body fat using 2-stage predictive equations by first calculating body density and then body fat percentage.[13,14] BMI was calculated by dividing kilograms of body weight by height in meters squared. Waist and hip circumference were measured using a (Gulick II tape, North Coast Medical Inc, Gilroy, CA) measure at the narrowest point between the umbilicus and the xiphoid process and the widest point between umbilicus and the knee, respectively.

Physical function

Heart rate, blood pressure, and respiration were measured following a 5-minute quiet, seated rest period. Walk endurance was measured using the 6-minute walk test (6-MW), which consists of continuous walking at a self-selected walk pace in accordance with the American Thoracic Society guidelines.[15] During the 6-MW, participants were encouraged to walk as quickly as possible for 6 minutes on the designated walk path. Participants could stop and rest as needed during the test; however, the test timer did not stop. The distance walked (meters) in 6 minutes was recorded for each participant. Expected normative walk distances were based on previously published predictive equations in age-matched and gender-matched healthy adults.[16]

Passive and active range of motion at the knee was measured by a licensed physical therapist using a goniometer. Participants were instructed to flex and extend the knee actively as far as possible and passive measurements made by the physical therapist were recorded at the terminal range in degrees. Knee extension strength was measured using a handheld dynamometer (Chantillion DFE, AMETEK Test & Calibration Instruments, Largo, FL). The participants were seated with the knee positioned at 60° and the dynamometer was placed 20 cm below the tibial tuberosity. The participant was instructed to extend his or her lower leg against the dynamometer as hard as possible. Three trials were performed on each leg with 1-minute rest between trials. Predicted strength values were based on previously published gender-based normative ranges in healthy adults.[17]

Self-reported knee function and health-related quality of life

The Western Ontario and McMaster University Osteoarthritis Index (WOMAC) was used to assess pain, function, and quality of life.[18] WOMAC scoring yields 1 composite (0–96) and 3 subscales: pain (0–20), stiffness (0–8), and physical function (0–68). Responses to each question range from 0, indicating none, to 4, indicating severe; thus higher scores on the composite or subscales indicate worse pain, stiffness, and/or function. The composite and subscales have reasonable validity (Spearman correlations from 0.63 to 0.67) and reliability (Cronbach's alphas from 0.86 to 0.95).[19,20]

Health-related quality of life was assessed using the Medical Outcomes Study short form 36 version 2 (SF36).[21,22] The survey is a widely applied generic health questionnaire previously used in obese and osteoarthritic populations.[23,24] Scores were calculated for 8 health domains (mental health, role physical, physical function, vitality, social function, bodily pain, role emotional, and general health) and 2 summary measures: the physical component scale and mental component scale. Survey responses were summed to generate raw scores in each subscale and health domain, and used to create general population norm-based scoring (T-scores with a population mean of 50 and a standard deviation [SD] of 10 using previously described methodology).[21,22,24] Scores were considered poor if the normalized scores (T-scores) were less than 37, which corresponds to the lowest 10th percentile of the general population.

Physical activity levels

Physical activity was assessed using the Nation Health and Nutrition Examination Survey (NHANES) Physical Activity Questionnaire (PAQ) version 2009 (available at http://www.cdc.gov/nchs/nhanes/nhanes2009-2010/PAQ_F.htm). The survey consists of questions about daily, leisure time, and sedentary activities. Weekly time spent doing vigorous or moderate physical activity was calculated from responses to daily (work) and leisure time activities. Sedentary time was collected and reported in average hours per day. Screen time was evaluated separately as television and computer time. Responses were coded as less than 1 hour, and hourly increments up to 5 hours or more per day.

All testing was completed by the same trained clinical exercise physiologist, with the exception of lower extremity range of motion and the WOMAC index, which were completed and reviewed by the same licensed physical therapist.

Data analysis

Study data was managed using REDCap electronic data capture tools.[25] REDCap (Research Electronic Data Capture, Vanderbilt University, Nashville, TN) is a secure, Web-based application designed to support data capture for research studies, providing

1. An intuitive interface for validated data entry
2. Audit trails for tracking data manipulation and export procedures
3. Automated export procedures for seamless data downloads to common statistical packages
4. Procedures for importing data from external sources.

All data reduction, processing, and analysis for this project were generated using SAS software, version 9.2 of the SAS system for Windows (SAS Institute, Cary, NC, USA). The outcomes considered in this article are primarily descriptive with statistical analysis consisting of means and SDs for each measure. Reference ranges were constructed from population-based normative equations and references when available.

RESULTS
Patient Description
This study included 39 women and 21 men with an average age of 64.7 plus or minus 8.6 years old (mean ± SD) and 14.0 plus or minus 2.6 months postsurgery (Table 1). On average, participants had a normal resting heart rate (76.5 ± 6.8 beats per minute), borderline hypertensive systolic blood pressure (131.1 ± 8.9 mm Hg), and prehypertensive diastolic blood pressure (81.1 ± 4.5 mm Hg). Three participants (5.0%) were current smokers. All had medical clearance

and none were currently receiving medical treatment of an acute medical issue.

Anthropometrics
Participants were on average 165.8 plus or minus 10.6 cm tall, weighed 103.0 plus or minus 18.3 kg, and had a BMI of 37.4 plus or minus 5.5 kg/m^2 (all patients had a BMI higher than 30 kg/m^2 indicating obesity) (see Table 1). Mean sum of skinfolds were 135.0 plus or minus 20.1 mm on average, which corresponds to an estimated body fat percentage of 41.2 plus or minus 5.6%. Men, relative to women, had lower body fat (34.8 ± 3.5% vs 44.6 ± 2.8%), BMI (36.3 ± 4.7 kg/m^2 vs 38.0 ± 5.9 kg/m^2), skinfolds (121.0 ± 17.7 mm vs 142.6 ± 17.1 mm), and higher waist to hip ratios (0.98 ± 0.09 vs 0.87 ± 0.08), respectively (see Table 1).

Knee Range of Motion
Active knee extension ranged from 8° of hyperextension to lacking 18° of full extension. The average active knee extension was lacking 2.6° plus or minus 3.9° of extension on TKA knee and lacking 2.4° plus or minus 5.4° of extension on the nonsurgery knee. Active knee extension limb difference was 3.7° plus or minus 3.3° with a range of 0° to 14°. Active knee flexion ranged from 80° to 154°. The average active knee flexion was 117.8° plus or minus 10.5° on TKA knee and 121.1 plus or minus 11.6° on

Table 1 Participant characteristics			
	Total (N = 60) N (%)	Men (n = 21) N (%)	Women (n = 39) N (%)
Smoker	3 (5.0)	0 (0)	3 (5.0)
	Mean ± SD	Mean ± SD	Mean ± SD
Age (y)	64.7 ± 8.7	63.3 ± 7.3	65.5 ± 9.3
Height (cm)	165.8 ± 10.6	175.9 ± 8.6	160.3 ± 7.0
Weight (kg)	103.0 ± 18.3	113.0 ± 18.5	97.6 ± 16.0
BMI (kg/m^2)	37.4 ± 5.5	36.4 ± 4.7	38.0 ± 5.9
Body fat (%)	—	34.8 ± 3.5	44.6 ± 2.8
Skinfolds (mm)	135.0 ± 20.1	121.0 ± 17.7	142.6 ± 17.1
Waist to hip	0.91 ± 0.10	0.98 ± 0.09	0.87 ± 0.08
WOMAC Score			
Composite (0–96)	20.5 ± 15.2	16.1 ± 12.4	23.0 ± 16.2
Function (0–68)	14.9 ± 11.6	11.3 ± 9.1	16.8 ± 12.4
Pain (0–20)	3.5 ± 3.4	2.8 ± 2.7	3.9 ± 3.6
Stiffness (0–8)	2.6 ± 1.5	2.0 ± 1.4	2.9 ± 1.5

non-TKA knee. Active knee extension limb difference was 8.2 plus or minus 6.6° with a range of 0 to 31°.

Knee Extensor Strength
Knee extension strength ranged from 8.5 kg to 45.6 kg. The average knee extension strength was 26.5 plus or minus 8.5 kg on TKA knee and 26.1 plus or minus 7.7 kg on non-TKA knee. Knee extension strength difference was 3.4 plus or minus 4.4 kg with a range of 0.2 to 11.2 kg. Percent of predicted strength based on gender-based normative data were 84.2% plus or minus 20.4%. Nineteen patients (31.7%) failed to reach 75% of their predicted knee extension strength values.

Walk Performance
Total distance walked during 6 minutes ranged from 122.0 m to 489.0 m, with a mean of 312.3 plus or minus 77.2 m. Percent of predicted walk distance, based on the gender-based prediction equation, averaged 71.7% plus or minus 16.6%. Thirty-five patients (58.3%) failed to reach 75% of their predicted walk distance during the 6-MW. Average peak heart rate during the 6-MW was 105.2 plus or minus 12.6 beats per minute. Average peak rating of perceived exertion was 10.6 plus or minus 2.9 on the Borg scale. The average rating of perceived exertion scores corresponds to very light to light exertion values on the 6 to 20 Borg scale.

Self-Reported Knee Function
WOMAC composite scores (see **Table 1**) were 20.5 plus or minus 15.2 points of a possible 96 with a minimum of 2 and maximum of 71. The function subscale scores were 14.9 plus or minus 11.6 points of a possible 68 with a minimum of 0 and maximum of 50. Pain subscale scores were 3.5 plus or minus 3.4 points of a possible 20 with a minimum of 0 and a maximum of 15. Stiffness subscale scores were 2.6 plus or minus 1.5 points of a possible 8 with a minimum of 0 and a maximum of 6.

Self-Reported Health-Related Quality of Life
Participants had a mean T-score of 40.3 plus or minus 9.3 on the SF36 Physical Component Scale (**Table 2**), including 18 participants (30.0%) who scored in the lowest 10th percentile of the general population. Only 8 participants (13.0%) scored average or better (≥40th percentile) on the physical component scale. Normative scores on the physical function subscale were 37.2 plus or minus 10.0, with 28 participants (46.6%) scoring in the lowest 10th

percentile of the general population. In addition, only 7 (11.7%) scored at or above the 40th percentile, indicating physical performance was within normal limits on the physical function subscale. Role physical subscale (42.8 ± 10.9) and bodily pain subscales (45.9 ± 9.1) were slightly below the normative values. Participants had a mean slightly above the population normal (55.5 ± 9.0) on the Mental Component Scale. Social functioning, mental health, and general health subscales were all with the normative ranges (50.5 + 8.8, 53.5 ± 9.6, and 49.6 ± 7.6, respectively).

Physical Activity Levels and Sedentary Time
No patients reported completing any vigorous physical activity during daily or leisure time activities in the past 30 days. On average, participants reported completing 14.3 plus or minus 25.9 minutes of moderate intensity physical activity per week. Forty-three participants (71.6%) reported no physical activity in the last 30 days. Participants reported 10.4 plus or minus 3.0 hours per day of sedentary time. Nineteen participants (31.7%) reported more than 5 hours per day of television watching.

DISCUSSION

The management of knee OA and its debilitating symptoms has advanced significantly in recent decades to include TKA as a viable surgical option for severe OA.[12,26] These advancements necessitate the evaluation of outcomes after TKA. Evaluation of functional limitations is particularly important because the number of obese patients receiving TKA is increasing. The authors' findings indicate that patients have substantial physical limitations and low levels of physical activity 1-year after TKA. Furthermore, patient-reported limitations are confirmed with objective assessment of physical performance.

The recovery from TKA has been reasonably well described up to about 6 months postoperation. This early period is marked by rapid recovery from surgery, restoration of independence, and significant improvements from presurgery function and quality of life.[27] After 6 months, the recovery of function, albeit based on limited data, seems to be slow.[27] Our results indicate that obese TKA patients remain well below age-predicted references on the 6-MW distance and leg extensor strength 1 year after surgery.

Although data on obese patients with 1 year of follow-up are sparse, our results seem consistent with previous studies in healthy weight patients showing about 20% deficit in knee

Table 2
Quality of life after TKA

	Mean ± SD[a]	<10th Percentile (%) n (%)	10th-29th Percentile (%) n (%)	30th-59th Percentile (%) n (%)	60th-89th Percentile (%) n (%)	>90th Percentile (%) n (%)
Summary Scores						
Physical Components Scale	40.3 ± 9.3	18 (30.0)	20 (33.3)	16 (26.7)	6 (10.0)	0 (0.0)
Mental Components Scale	55.5 ± 9.0	2 (3.3)	6 (10.0)	11 (18.3)	27 (45.0)	14 (23.4)
Component Scores						
Mental Health Scale	53.5 ± 9.6	3 (5.0)	8 (13.3)	5 (8.3)	34 (56.7)	10 (16.7)
Physical Function Scale	37.2 ± 10.0	28 (46.6)	18 (30.0)	10 (16.7)	4 (6.7)	0 (0.0)
Role Emotional Scale	48.0 ± 11.4	11 (18.3)	10 (16.7)	7 (11.7)	32 (53.3)	0 (0.0)
Role Physical Scale	42.8 ± 10.9	16 (26.7)	14 (23.3)	16 (26.7)	14 (23.3)	0 (0.0)
Social Functioning Scale	50.5 ± 8.8	6 (10.0)	6 (10.0)	17 (28.3)	31 (51.7)	0 (0.0)
Vitality Scale	51.2 ± 8.4	5 (8.3)	7 (11.7)	25 (42.7)	20 (33.3)	2 (5.0)
General Health Scale	49.6 ± 7.9	4 (6.7)	12 (20.0)	19 (31.7)	24 (40.0)	1 (1.6)
Bodily Pain Scale	45.9 ± 9.1	8 (13.3)	15 (25.0)	25 (41.7)	12 (20.0)	0 (0.0)

[a] Linear transformed T-Scores with mean of 50 and SD of 10.

extensor strength in those 6 to 33 months post-TKA compared with healthy controls.[28,29] On average, our participants achieved approximately 81% of gender-predicted strength values. However, 38% of our participants were not able to achieve 75% of their gender-based reference strength values. This represents a clinical subset of patients who are at particular risk for poor long-term satisfaction, perhaps due to excess body weight, and whose physical function may be limited by muscle weakness. These results are particularly concerning because knee extensor strength is a significant predictor of long-term satisfaction with TKA.[30]

6-MW distances were also well below age-predicted and gender-predicted values in our population. Half of the participants in our study were not able to walk at least 75% of their predicted distance based on gender and body size. Although not completely analogous, our results are in agreement with Yoshida and colleagues,[31] who noted significantly decreased walk distance in a group of normal to overweight patients at 3 months and 1 year after TKA. The 6-MW distances in our participants were notably lower than many other reported walk distances in normal to overweight but not obese patient populations.[31,32]

Additionally, our results indicate that patients report impairments in physical function on both the SF36 and WOMAC scales. This finding is similar to previously published studies in which patients self-reported physical performance limitations as long as 2 years after TKA.[12,33] Although no absolute or clinical cutoff points exist for the WOMAC scale, our participants reported mild to moderate functional limitation, pain, and stiffness in their knees, which is similar to previous reports and supports the notion of less than optimal recovery from TKA.[34] In addition, the global assessment of health-related quality of life (SF36) showed that most our participants reported poor physical function. Interestingly, despite the physical limitations that remain after TKA, participants in our study reported similar vitality, general health, and mental health compared with the general population. These findings support previous reports in which patients report physical limitation but are otherwise on par with the general population.[35]

Low level of physical activity has been a commonly reported risk factor for development and progression of knee OA. Low preoperative levels of physical activity are well-documented and commonly assumed to result from preoperative pain. Our results agree with previous reports that physical activity levels are low 1 year after TKA.[9,36] Our participants were substantially less active than healthy older adults studied by Crombie and colleagues,[37] who reported that 17% of participants completed more than 2 hours of physical activity per week and only 36% reported no physical activity at all. None of our participants reached the activity guidelines established by the ACSM and Centers for Disease Control and Prevention guidelines for older adults, which includes 120 minutes of physical activity per week.[14] Furthermore, nearly 70% of our participants reported no physical activity in the past 30 days. In addition to very low average amounts of physical activity, our participants reported high levels of sedentary behavior. The large degree of sedentary behavior and lack of physical activity likely further exacerbates the physical performance limitations and deconditioning that seems to follow TKA.

The low activity profiles reported by our participants is particularly concerning because the impact of obesity is compounded by low levels of vigorous physical activity. Physical inactivity has been reported to have negative effects similar to obesity following joint arthroplasty. Although not observed in our participants at 1-year post-TKA, inactive patients have higher surgical revision rates and loosening of the components, and lower function scores, than those who are physically active.[38] The assumption that obesity and physical inactivity were secondary to pain and physical limitations associated with OA is questionable. Obesity and physical inactivity do not seem to improve with the restored function and reduced pain following TKA, and perhaps should be thought of as separate medical issues.[9,36] This is further supported by the finding that TKA does not result in decreased body weight. In fact, it has been frequently reported that body weight often increases after TKA.[9,36,39]

Most studies indicate patients report the ability to return to regular activities, such as walking, hiking, and swimming, with some patients even returning to sports such as tennis and jogging.[12,35] Despite the ability to return to these activities, it seems that poor exercise habits that preceded surgery are likely to return following the initial recovery period, which may result in long-term functional abilities that are significantly compromised.[40] Based on the limited data available, it seems that obesity and physical inactivity, which are major contributors to the development and progression of OA, remain after TKA. Although our study did not assess presurgical weight and activity, it is clear that our participants have problematic body weight and activity profiles. Thus, functional recovery, such as general mobility, gait mechanics, walking endurance, ability to walk stairs, freedom from pain, and quality of life, may not be as thorough and lasting as could be expected.

Certain limitations should be considered when interpreting the result of this study. First, this is a cross-sectional evaluation and the authors could not evaluate the preoperative body habitus, functional abilities, or quality of life of the patient. Without such baseline data, we could not assess functional changes over time. We were not able to evaluate the surgical techniques used, complications during surgery, or postoperative therapy programs that could influence the outcomes at 1 year. Second, this was a convenience sample recruited from an orthopedic surgery follow-up clinic and, as such, may not represent the full range of obese patients who undergo TKA. In addition, our population included only obese individuals, which precludes comparisons to nonobese, postsurgical TKA patients.

Future research that involves longitudinal evaluation of obese patients, and preferably inclusion of nonobese patients for comparative purposes, is needed to determine if preoperative factors are predictive of long-term functional outcomes and the deleterious role excess body weight may play. Given that the number of obese patients receiving TKA has increased dramatically in the past decade, a careful evaluation is needed on how well postoperative rehabilitation facilitates effective functional recovery in obese patients, and how recovery of function may differ in the obese and nonobese TKA patients. Greater inclusion of lifestyle counseling and intervention, including exercise and physical activity interventions targeting the observed deficits in health-related physical fitness, offer great promise with regard to long-term function and satisfaction, and should be a priority for clinicians in patients with obesity after TKA, especially as recovery from surgery nears completion and inclusion of traditional rehabilitative services decrease.

In summary, results from this clinical evaluation of obese individuals 1-year post-TKA provides evidence that functional and physical performance limitations are problematic after patients have been released from postoperative rehabilitation. These limitations may be exacerbated by increased body weight and decreased physical activity, although we did not assess those factors explicitly. The combination of residual strength and conditioning deficits after TKA, low levels of physical activity, and increased physiologic and biomechanical pressure from excess body weight, may converge to render obese patients particularly vulnerable to poor long-term outcome following TKA.

ACKNOWLEDGMENTS

The authors would like to thank Dr Ramin Homayouni and Mr Dudley Kelso for their assistance developing and maintaining the Redcap database. Mrs Anita Kerkhof and Mr Tyler Ward for their assistance with subject recruitment and logistics on this project.

REFERENCES

1. Anandacoomarasamy A, Leibman S, Smith G, et al. Weight loss in obese people has structure-modifying effects on medial but not on lateral knee articular cartilage. Ann Rheum Dis 2012; 71(1):26–32.
2. Mihalko WM, Bergin PF, Kelly FB, et al. Obesity, orthopaedics, and outcomes. J Am Acad Orthop Surg 2014;22(11):683–90.
3. Abramson SB, Attur M, Yazici Y. Prospects for disease modification in osteoarthritis. Nat Clin Pract Rheumatol 2006;2(6):304–12.
4. Powell A, Teichtahl AJ, Wluka AE, et al. Obesity: a preventable risk factor for large joint osteoarthritis which may act through biomechanical factors. Br J Sports Med 2005;39(1):4–5.
5. Centers for Disease Control and Prevention. Prevalence of obesity among adults with arthritis — United States, 2003–2009. MMWR Morb Mortal Wkly Rep 2011;60(16):509–13.
6. Murphy L, Helmick CG. The impact of osteoarthritis in the United States: a population-health perspective. Am J Nurs 2012;112(3):13–9.
7. Bourne R, Mukhi S, Zhu N, et al. Role of obesity on the risk for total hip or knee arthroplasty. Clin Orthop Relat Res 2007;465:185–8.
8. Wright EA, Katz JN, Cisternas MG, et al. Impact of knee osteoarthritis on health care resource utilization in a US population-based national sample. Med Care 2010;48(9):785–91.
9. Unver B, Karatosun V, Bakirhan S, et al. Effects of total knee arthroplasty on body weight and functional outcome. J Phys Ther Sci 2009;21(2):201–6.
10. Dewan A, Bertolusso R, Karastinos A, et al. Implant durability and knee function after total knee arthroplasty in the morbidly obese patient. J Arthroplasty 2009;24(6):89–94.e3.
11. Ghomrawi HMK, Kane RL, Eberly LE, et al. Patterns of functional improvement after revision knee arthroplasty. J Bone Joint Surg Am 2009;91(12): 2838–45.

12. Foran JRH, Mont MA, Rajadhyaksha AD, et al. Total knee arthroplasty in obese patients. J Arthroplasty 2004;19(7):817–24.

13. Jackson AS, Pollock ML. Practical assessment of body-composition. Phys Sportsmed 1985;13(5):76.

14. Whaley MH, Brubaker PH, Otto RM, et al. ACSM's guidelines for exercise testing and prescription. Philadelphia: Lippincott Williams & Wilkins; 2006. p. 66–72.

15. American Thoracic Society. Guidelines for the six-minute walk test. Am J Respir Crit Care Med 2002;166(1):111–7.

16. Enright PL, Sherrill DL. Reference equations for the six-minute walk in healthy adults. Am J Respir Crit Care Med 1998;158(5):1384–7.

17. Andrews AW, Thomas MW, Bohannon RW. Normative values for isometric muscle force measurements obtained with hand-held dynamometers. Phys Ther 1996;76(3):248–59.

18. Quintana JM, Escobar A, Arostegui I, et al. Health-related quality of life and appropriateness of knee or hip joint replacement. Arch Intern Med 2006; 166(2):220–6.

19. Bullens PH, van Loon CJ, de Waal Malefijt MC, et al. Patient satisfaction after total knee arthroplasty: a comparison between subjective and objective outcome assessments. J Arthroplasty 2001;16(6): 740–7.

20. Dunbar MJ, Robertsson O, Ryd L, et al. Appropriate questionnaires for knee arthroplasty. Results of a survey of 3600 patients from The Swedish Knee Arthroplasty Registry. J Bone Joint Surg Br 2001; 83(3):339–44.

21. Ware JE. SF-36 Health Survey. In: Maruish M, editor. The Use of Psychological Testing for Treatment Planning and Outcome Assessment. Mahwah (NJ): Lawrence Erlbaum Associates; vol. 3. 2004. p. 693–718.

22. Ware JE, Snow KK, Kosinski M, et al. SF-36 health survey: manual and interpretation guide. Boston: New England Medical Center Hospital Health Institute; 1993. p. 238.

23. Bohannon RW, DePasquale L. Physical functioning scale of the short-form (SF) 36: internal consistency and validity with older adults. J Geriatr Phys Ther 2010;33(1):16–8.

24. Ware JE Jr. SF-36 health survey update. Spine 2000;25(24):3130–9.

25. Harris PA, Taylor R, Thielke R, et al. Research electronic data capture (REDCap)—A metadata-driven methodology and workflow process for providing translational research informatics support. J Biomed Inform 2009;42(2):377–81.

26. Van Manen MD, Nace J, Mont MA. Management of primary knee osteoarthritis and indications for total knee arthroplasty for general practitioners. J Am Osteopath Assoc 2012;112(11):709–15.

27. Mizner RL, Petterson SC, Snyder-Mackler L. Quadriceps strength and the time course of functional recovery after total knee arthroplasty. J Orthop Sports Phys Ther 2005;35(7):424–36.

28. Berman AT, Bosacco SJ, Israelite C. Evaluation of total knee arthroplasty using isokinetic testing. Clin Orthop Relat Res 1991;271:106–13.

29. Berth A, Urbach D, Awiszus F. Improvement of voluntary quadriceps muscle activation after total knee arthroplasty. Arch Phys Med Rehabil 2002; 83(10):1432–6.

30. Mizner RL, Petterson SC, Stevens JE, et al. Preoperative quadriceps strength predicts functional ability one year after total knee arthroplasty. J Rheumatol 2005;32(8):1533–9.

31. Yoshida Y, Mizner RL, Ramsey DK, et al. Examining outcomes from total knee arthroplasty and the relationship between quadriceps strength and knee function over time. Clin Biomech 2008;23(3): 320–8.

32. Kennedy DM, Stratford PW, Riddle DL, et al. Assessing recovery and establishing prognosis following total knee arthroplasty. Phys Ther 2008; 88(1):22–32.

33. Walsh M, Woodhouse LJ, Thomas SG, et al. Physical impairments and functional limitations: a comparison of individuals 1 year after total knee arthroplasty with control subjects. Phys Ther 1998; 78(3):248–58.

34. Bourne RB, Chesworth BM, Davis AM, et al. Patient satisfaction after total knee arthroplasty: who is satisfied and who is not? Clin Orthop Relat Res 2010;468(1):57–63.

35. Loughead JM, Malhan K, Mitchell SY, et al. Outcome following knee arthroplasty beyond 15 years. Knee 2008;15(2):85–90.

36. Heisel C, Silva M, Rosa MAD, et al. The effects of lower-extremity total joint replacement for arthritis on obesity. Orthopedics 2005;28(2): 157–60.

37. Crombie IK, Irvine L, Williams B, et al. Why older people do not participate in leisure time physical activity: a survey of activity levels, beliefs and deterrents. Age Ageing 2004;33(3):287–92.

38. Gschwend N, Frei T, Morscher E, et al. Alpine and cross-country skiing after total hip replacement: 2 cohorts of 50 patients each, one active, the other inactive in skiing, followed for 5-10 years. Acta Orthop Scand 2000;71(3):243–9.

39. Zeni JA, Snyder-Mackler L. Most patients gain weight in the 2 years after total knee arthroplasty: comparison to a healthy control group. Osteoarthritis Cartilage 2010;18(4):510–4.

40. Bradbury N, Borton D, Spoo G, et al. Participation in sports after total knee replacement. Am J Sports Med 1998;26(4):530–5.

Deep Vein Thrombosis and Pulmonary Embolism Considerations in Orthopedic Surgery

Jasmine Saleh, MD[a], Mouhanad M. El-Othmani, MD[b],
Khaled J. Saleh, MD, MSc, FRCS(C), MHCM, CPE[b],*

KEYWORDS

- Deep vein thrombosis • Venous thromboembolism • Pulmonary embolism • Prophylaxis
- Risk factors • Treatment • Perioperative clearance

KEY POINTS

- Deep vein thrombosis and pulmonary embolism are major complications of concern after surgical intervention.
- Older age and a history of venous thromboembolism are considered the main risk factors with strong evidence in the literature to increase the risk of venous thromboembolism.
- The current gold standard diagnostic instruments are venography for deep vein thrombosis and pulmonary angiography for pulmonary embolism. However, because these tests are invasive and expensive, alternative diagnostic tools include venous compression ultrasonography for deep vein thrombosis and ventilation-perfusion scan and computed tomographic pulmonary angiogram for pulmonary embolism.
- Multiple pharmacologic and nonpharmacologic interventions are available for the prevention and treatment of deep vein thrombosis and pulmonary embolism, and the risks associated with the use of each modality should be weighed against the benefits in its use on a case-based level.

INTRODUCTION

Both deep venous thrombosis (DVT) and pulmonary embolism (PE) are responsible for substantial patient morbidity and mortality, with PE ranking as the third most common acute cardiovascular disease.[1] Nearly 10,000 deaths were the result of PE or DVT in 2009 with PE having an estimated mortality rate of nearly 30%.[1,2] Because of the serious nature of venous thromboembolism (VTE) complications, health care providers allocate an abundance of resources to diagnose and treat this condition, resulting in an increased length of hospitalization and cost. DVT and PE account for more than 500,000 hospitalizations in the adult population and carry a large economic burden with a health care cost up to $33,200 per patient annually.[1] Orthopedic procedures, especially trauma and total joint arthroplasty, place patients at an increased risk for VTE. Complications of VTE may affect large numbers of patients, as the incidence of hospital-acquired DVT after major orthopedic surgery is 40% to 60%.[3,4] Therefore,

Funding Sources: No additional funding sources were used for this article.
Conflicts of Interest: No conflicts of interest are evident for authors of this article.
[a] Department of Research Institute, National Institute of Health, 9000 Rockville Pike Street, Bethesda, MD 20892, USA; [b] Department of Orthopaedics and Sports Medicine, Detroit Medical Center, University Health Center (UHC), 4201 Saint Antoine Street, 9B, Detroit, MI 48201-2153, USA
* Corresponding author.
E-mail address: kjsaleh@gmail.com

having a better understanding for risk factors, diagnosis, and management of DVT and PE is essential in preventing and treating patients and may achieve substantial reduction in overall perioperative morbidity, mortality, and health care cost burden.

RISK FACTORS AND DIAGNOSIS
Risk Factors
In patients undergoing total hip arthroplasty (THA), total knee arthroplasty, or hip fracture surgery, 1% to 3% will go on to have a symptomatic DVT, whereas 0.2% to 1.1% will go on to have a PE within 35 days of surgery. The first postoperative week is the period of highest risk for symptomatic PE development.[5,6] In addition to identifying the period in which patients are at risk for VTE, identifying which patients' characteristics are associated with a higher risk is essential in guiding diagnostic and management efforts.

Certain patient characteristics, such as age and a history of a previous VTE, may pose primary risk factors for unprovoked VTE in the emergent setting.[2,7] In the ninth decade of life, the incidence of emergent PE is 1 in 200 patients, whereas in the third decade of life the incidence is only 1 in 10,000 patients.[2] Risk associated with age for emergent PE development is most significant after the age of 50 and increases until the age of 80 years.[2] A history of prior VTE is also a risk factor for emergent PE, causing a 2- to 3-fold increase in risk of future unprovoked VTE in men.[2] Surgery requiring intubation, immobility, and estrogen also transiently increase the risk of provoked PE.[2] In surgical patients, the risk of VTE extends for months and even potentially for a year.[5,8] Although sex, smoking, congestive heart failure, cancer, and obesity are commonly thought to be risk factors for DVT and PE, there is not enough evidence to consider these as primary risk factors.[2] With specific regard to risk factors for VTE in orthopedic patients, the American Academy of Orthopedic Surgeons (AAOS) guidelines report that, with the exception of a history of VTE, the current evidence is inconclusive as to whether other factors increase the risk of VTE in patients undergoing elective arthroplasty and, therefore, does not recommend routinely assessing patients for these factors.[9]

Diagnosis
When suspecting DVT and PE, and before conducting any further testing, it is important to initially establish a level of pretest probability.[10] The Wells clinical prediction criteria is used to establish whether a patient has a low, intermediate, or high pretest risk for PE development.[10] It considers the presence of certain risk factors, signs of DVT, and the likelihood of an alternative diagnosis.[10] A meta-analysis of 15 studies reported that patients with the highest pretest probability had a prevalence of DVT ranging from 17% to 85%, whereas those with a moderate pretest probability had a prevalence of 0% to 38%, and patients with the lowest pretest probability had a prevalence of 0% to 13%.[11] These results suggest that Wells clinical prediction rule is not definitive and should be only used to establish probability assessment and to guide further diagnostic and screening tests.

There are several imaging modalities currently used to confirm or rule out the diagnosis of DVT and PE. The current gold standard diagnostic techniques are venography and pulmonary angiography, respectively; however, because of exorbitant cost and the invasive nature of these tests, their role in diagnosis has become limited.[10] Therefore, less-invasive tests are sought after to play a more significant role in ruling in or out DVT and PE diagnoses.[12]

Currently, one of the most common noninvasive diagnostic tests for DVT is venous compression ultrasonography (CUS).[10,12] When attempting to diagnose proximal DVT, CUS has been reported to have a sensitivity and specificity of 97% and 98%, respectively.[11] Patients with low pretest probability combined with a negative CUS can be safely withheld from anticoagulant therapy.[10] CUS is not frequently used to detect distal DVT, as the sensitivity and specificity are much lower, and controversy exists as to whether to treat isolated distal DVT.[10]

Another safe and cost-effective way of evaluation is a D-dimer assay.[13] D-dimers are products of cross-linked fibrin breakdown by plasmin produced at the site of thrombosis.[11,14] Although no biomarker exists that is both 100% sensitive and specific for VTE, D-dimer is a very sensitive laboratory test, and a negative assay in combination with a low pretest probability of VTE is useful in ruling out the presence of DVT and PE.[14] However, studies have found that an elevated D-dimer is also seen in various clinical scenarios, including sepsis, pregnancy, malignancy, and after surgery, making the test nonspecific with limited use in ruling in DVT or PE in these settings.[2,10,14] The current AAOS guidelines therefore conclude that D-dimer is not a reliable marker to screen for DVT after arthroplasty.[10] In the event of an elevated D-dimer assay in which PE may not be ruled out, imaging must be ordered. In patients with impaired renal function (glomerular filtration rate <60 mL/min), a ventilation-perfusion scan may be used.[15] In patients with a nondiagnostic ventilation-perfusion scan or adequate renal function, a computed tomographic pulmonary angiogram may be used to confirm or exclude the diagnosis of PE and to guide prospective management.[15]

MANAGEMENT IN THE ACUTE PHASE
Prophylaxis
Given the substantial morbidity and mortality and increased health care burden associated with the incidence of VTE, the most effective way to begin management is through primary prevention (**Table 1**). Because VTE is difficult to diagnose with absolute certainty, it is often misdiagnosed; therefore, treatment is not possible in every case.[5]

Pharmacologic thromboprophylaxis is commonly used in postoperative orthopedic patients to prevent VTE.[16] One of the challenges in using pharmacologic agents is balancing benefits of anticoagulation and the risk of bleeding complications.[5] To help achieve this balance, current AAOS treatment guidelines moderately recommend discontinuing antiplatelet agents before undergoing elective hip or knee arthroplasty to reduce the bleeding risk during surgery and using anticoagulation postoperatively to prevent VTE.[9]

Low-molecular-weight heparin (LMWH), fondaparinux, dabigatran, apixaban, and rivaroxaban may be used after THA or total knee arthroplasty.[5,17] Apixaban showed greater safety and similar efficacy when compared with LMWH, whereas rivaroxaban showed greater efficacy and similar safety when compared with LMWH in hip and knee arthroplasties.[17,18] LMWH and fondaparinux are preferentially used specifically in patients undergoing surgical treatment for femoral neck fracture.[17] In orthopedic patients with nonhip fractures and soft tissue injuries such as cartilage or tendon injuries or patients undergoing arthroscopy, pharmacologic thromboprophylaxis is not routinely recommended according to current guidelines.[5]

For those patients in whom warfarin is used as prophylaxis, it is recommended that it is begun the night before surgery.[19] The dose should then be adjusted postoperatively to a target international normalized ratio (INR) of 2.2.[19] When compared with a 2-step regimen in which warfarin is started 10 to 14 days preoperatively and titrated to an INR of 2.2 to 3, this regimen has an equal benefit regarding VTE prevention and may cause less perioperative bleeding.[19] Prophylaxis with warfarin has been found to decrease asymptomatic DVT by 55% and PE by 80%.[20]

When LMWH is used for prophylaxis, there are questions regarding whether it should be started preoperatively or held until the postoperative period. Enoxaparin, 30 to 40 mg twice daily, is the prophylactic dose most commonly used.[19,21] LMWH decreases the risk of DVT by 50% to 60% and the risk of PE by approximately two-thirds.[20] Some guidelines recommend starting LMWH either 12 hours or more preoperatively or 12 hours or more postoperatively in arthroplasty and hip fracture patients.[20] If LMWH is administered between 2 hours preoperatively and 4 hours postoperatively, the rate of major bleeding is 5% to 7%.[20] In comparison, starting LMWH 12 hours preoperatively or waiting until 12 to 24 hours postoperatively has a risk of major bleeding of only 1% to 3%.[20] Although LMWH has typically been given, no difference was found in the rate of PE between patients using LMWH and those using warfarin.[20] However, studies indicated that LMWH is associated with significantly less asymptomatic DVT and more major bleeding.[20] Fitzgerald and colleagues[22] reported the odds ratio in patients taking warfarin for development of DVT to be 2.52 when compared with those taking enoxaparin.[22] However, the rate of hemorrhage complications was higher in patients taking enoxaparin (7% vs 3%).

Although several pharmacologic prophylactic strategies are effective, safe, and readily available, these drugs are not without risk or drawbacks for certain patients. Some of the drawbacks to using anticoagulants for thromboprophylaxis in orthopedic patients include the need for repetitive laboratory testing, monitoring, anxiety and pain with self-injection, and the risk of postoperative bleeding complications.[23,24] Therefore, other nonpharmacologic thromboprophylactic strategies

Table 1 Venous thromboembolism prophylaxis	
Prophylactic Measure	**Recommendation**
Warfarin	Give night of surgery and allow INR to normalize to 2.2
LMWH	Start 12 h preoperatively or 12 h postoperatively
Aspirin	325 mg daily for 4–6 wk, starting the night of surgery
PCD	Use in adjunction to pharmacologic prophylaxis when patient in bed

are available as alternative options. One noninvasive, nonpharmaceutical, and inexpensive option is the use of lower extremity pneumatic compression devices (PCD). Evidence suggests that PCDs with intermittent compression are effective in preventing DVT; however, their use has been limited in the inpatient setting because of concerns with comfort and compliance.[25,26] Interestingly, one study reported that postoperative THA patients who used a mobile compression device reported an overall positive response and would choose to use this method again in the future rather than using pharmacologic thromboprophylaxis.[25] Unfortunately, there is little evidence to suggest how long patients should use PCDs postoperatively to most effectively prevent DVT occurrence. Although current AAOS guidelines moderately recommend the use of either pharmacologic or mechanical compression devices for VTE prophylaxis, they mention that current evidence is inconclusive as to which prophylactic strategy is superior.[9] Further studies comparing the relative effectiveness of different VTE prophylaxis strategies would be useful in making decisions about which methods should be used over others in various patient types.

Another method of thromboprophylaxis that may be used as a PE prevention strategy is the placement of an inferior vena cava (IVC) filter. IVC filters may be used in combination with anticoagulants for patients who are at high risk of suffering a PE.[27] When used in combination with anticoagulants or mechanical compression therapy in high-risk orthopedic patients, IVC filters are found to effectively prevent PE.[27] Additionally, IVC filters may be useful in patients who cannot tolerate anticoagulants or have a high risk of bleeding with anticoagulant use.[28] Some other indications of IVC filters include use in high-risk burn or trauma patients, patients with a free-floating iliofemoral thrombus, or in patients undergoing iliocaval thrombolysis or pulmonary thrombectomy.[28] Although there may be some benefits of using IVC filters, serious potential adverse effects include risk of recurrent DVT, IVC thrombosis, migration of the device, infection, and inability to retrieve the device.[25,28] The risk of adverse events increases with the duration of filter placement; therefore, the benefits of IVC filters are best achieved with short-term placement.[28]

Intervention

In cases of prophylaxis failure, symptomatic and potentially devastating PE may develop and must be treated aggressively. Within 1 hour of PE presentation, complications such as right ventricular (RV) strain, cardiac arrest, and heart failure may occur, resulting in mortality rates as high as 70%.[26] In the event of acute or submassive PE diagnosed by computed tomography imaging, anticoagulation with intravenous heparin and supplemental oxygen therapy is initiated.[26,29] The next step in treatment is determined by whether the patient is hemodynamically stable or unstable. In case of hemodynamic stability, echocardiography should be used to investigate the presence of RV dysfunction.[26] If RV dysfunction is not present, then conservative management with anticoagulation is indicated.[26] However, in the setting of a hemodynamically unstable patient or RV dysfunction, a surgical embolectomy is indicated.[26] If in a given setting in which a facility does not have cardiac surgical capabilities, then thrombolysis or catheter embolectomy may be indicated.[26] Evidence suggests that surgical embolectomy is a more successful treatment strategy with relatively low morbidity, mortality, and recurrence rates compared with thrombolysis.[26,29–34]

PERIOPERATIVE MANAGEMENT OF PATIENTS ON ANTICOAGULATION
Risk of Venous Thromboembolism when Anticoagulant Therapy is Discontinued Perioperatively

When determining how to treat patients on long-term anticoagulation perioperatively, one must balance the risk of thromboembolism versus major bleeding (Table 2). The risk assessment for thromboembolism in patients is based on multiple factors, including the indications for long-term anticoagulation, the presence of additional thromboembolic risk factors, and the consequences of the potential thromboembolic event.[31]

In patients taking warfarin for prior VTE, long-term anticoagulation decreases the risk of recurrence after initial VTE to 17% at 1 week, 13% at 1 month, and 3% at 3 months.[32] However, if warfarin is discontinued in the first month after VTE, the risk of recurrence increases to 40% and to 10% if discontinued in the second or third month of treatment.[32] Although the risk continues to decrease with length of treatment, the case fatality rate of 5% to 9% in patients who experience a recurrent VTE requires careful planning when discontinuing long-term warfarin treatment perioperatively at any point.[33,34]

Patients with a history of VTE are divided into high-risk, intermediate-risk, and low-risk groups based on the timing of their previous event and the presence of additional thromboembolic risk factors.[33] Patients with a high risk for VTE

Table 2 Treatment of patients on anticoagulation medication			
	Preoperatively	**Postoperatively**	**Comments**
Warfarin	Stop 5 d preoperatively to achieve a 2.0 INR	Resume at normal dose the evening of surgery	
LMWH	Last dose 24 h before surgery	Resume 12 h after surgery and full dose 24 h postoperatively	Use unfractionated heparin in patients with renal failure
Antiplatelet therapy (aspirin, clopidogrel, and ticlopidine)	Discontinue 7–10 d before surgery in patients at low risk for perioperative cardiovascular events. Aspirin therapy should be continued while clopidogrel should be held 5–10 d before surgery in patients at moderate or high risk for cardiovascular events	Resume 24 h postoperatively	Do not stop in low bleeding risk surgeries. In moderate or high bleeding risk surgeries, antiplatelet therapy decision is based on patient's risk for perioperative cardiovascular events.

include those who have had a previous event within the last 3 months; severe thrombophilia; deficiency of protein C, S, or antithrombin; antiphospholipid antibodies; or multiple thrombophilias.[35] In high-risk patients, the risk of recurrence is greater than 10% annually.[33] Intermediate-risk patients have a risk of 5% to 10% annually and include those patients whose prior VTE occurred in the last 3 to 12 months or those with recurrent VTE, nonsevere thrombophilia, recurrent VTE in association with previous discontinuation of warfarin, or active cancer.[35,36] Patients who had a VTE event more than 1 year ago are considered to be at low risk, with a less than 5% risk of recurrence annually.[31,33,36] There is evidence that anticoagulation reduces the risk of recurrent VTE by approximately 80%.[34]

Patients may also use long-term anticoagulation for mechanical heart valves (MHV) or nonvalvular atrial fibrillation (NVAF).[31–34,37,38] Patients with MHV are on long-term anticoagulants to prevent complications such as systemic embolization (ie, stroke or myocardial infarction) or occlusive valve thrombosis.[31–33] Overall, the rates of a major thromboembolic event in a patient with NVAF or an MHV who are not on anticoagulation therapy are 4.5% and 8% to 22% annually, respectively.[31,34] Although this finding correlates to a risk of 0.17% to 0.42% in 6 to 8 days perioperatively, the morbidity and mortality associated with a thromboembolic event warrants prophylaxis.[31] Studies found arterial

thromboembolism to be fatal in 15% to 40% of patients and to cause permanent disability in 20% to 40% of patients.[33,34,37] Factors that make MHV patients higher risk include mitral valve involvement, caged-ball or tilting-disc aortic valve, stroke, or transient ischemic attack (TIA) in the last 3 to 6 months.[33,38] A bileaflet aortic valve along with one or more stroke risk factors (ie, atrial fibrillation, heart failure, hypertension, age >75 years, diabetes, history of stroke or TIA) constitutes an intermediate risk, whereas a bileaflet aortic valve with no stroke risk factors is low risk.[33,38] Anticoagulation therapy has been found to reduce the risk of thromboembolism in patients with NVAF or MHV by 66% and 75%, respectively.[34]

As with VTE and MHV patients, those with NVAF are stratified into high-, intermediate-, and low-risk groups based on the CHADS$_2$ score.[33,34] The components of CHADS$_2$ score include cardiac failure, hypertension, age, diabetes, and stroke.[34,38] Patients with a CHADS$_2$ score of 5 or 6, those that have had a stroke or TIA in the last 3 months, or those with rheumatic valvular heart disease are high risk.[33,38] Those with a CHADS$_2$ score of 3 or 4 are at moderate risk, whereas those with a score of 0 to 2 and no history of prior stroke or TIA are at low risk.[33,38]

Perioperative Bleeding Risk
The risk of perioperative bleeding in patients on long-term warfarin therapy is based on several factors, including the patient's medical history

of bleeding, concurrent use of antiplatelet agents, and the type of surgery to be performed.[32,33] In orthopedic surgery, bilateral knee replacement is considered a high-bleed risk surgery, whereas unilateral hip replacement, unilateral knee replacement, shoulder surgery, foot surgery, hand surgery, and arthroscopy are all considered low risk.[33,39] The risk of a major bleeding event at postoperative day 2 is reported to be 2% to 4% in high-risk cases and 0% to 2% in low-risk cases.[33] The fatality rate of major bleeding is between 8% and 10%.[33] Given that the occurrence of thromboembolic events and major bleeding events carries a high fatality rate, every effort is made to balance these 2 risks against one another when determining periprocedural anticoagulation management.

Treatment of Patients Receiving Warfarin

As a vitamin K antagonist, warfarin exerts its effect by inhibiting the synthesis of vitamin K–dependent clotting factors, including factors II, VII, IX, and X and proteins C and S.[40,41] It takes 24 hours for warfarin to exhibit a minimal effect, and the full therapeutic effect will not be seen for 4 to 5 days.[31] Because warfarin has an elimination half-life of 36 to 42 hours, it is recommended that patients who are taking warfarin should withhold it for approximately 5 days before surgery to allow INR to normalize to 2.0 or less.[31,42]

For patients in whom warfarin is discontinued, the INR should be measured on the day it is stopped and again the day before surgery.[31,34] This action will allow surgeons to consider whether it is safe to proceed with the procedure.[43] Patients who undergo surgery with higher-than-target INR have an increased risk of postoperative bleeding complications.[31] Therefore, a low dose of oral vitamin K (1–2 mg) should be administered to these patients before surgery.[31,34,43] Warfarin should be resumed at the patient's normal dose the evening of surgery or the following morning as long as adequate hemostasis is achieved during surgery.[31,33,38,43,44] This can be done without impacting the patient's bleeding risk, as it takes 2 to 3 days for warfarin to exert a measurable effect and 5 to 7 days for the full anticoagulant effect to be achieved.[38,41,44]

Reversal of high INR is important to avoid significant delay in surgery.[45] Although vitamin K can reverse warfarin's effect, it is not sufficient to achieve immediate normalization of INR, as orally dosed vitamin K will not take effect within 24 hours.[45] Some studies reported that high doses (5–10 mg) would not further shorten the time to reverse warfarin therapy and may result in resistance to reinstating warfarin postoperatively.[31,45] Therefore, studies recommend that, for patients requiring emergent surgery, fresh-frozen plasma should be administered, as it immediately reverses anticoagulation and does not cause resistance to reinstating warfarin.[32,45]

Treatment of Patients Receiving Low-Molecular-Weight Heparin

The decision to use bridging with LMWH when interrupting warfarin therapy is based on both the thromboembolic risk and the bleeding risk.[33,39] Bridging minimizes the time of anticoagulant therapy perioperatively, thereby decreasing the thromboembolic risk.[33,39] For patients with a high perioperative bleeding risk and a low or intermediate VTE risk, warfarin can be stopped preoperatively with no bridging.[33] If the risk of VTE is high or intermediate with a low perioperative bleeding risk, bridging should be considered.[33,38]

LMWH is the preferred agent for bridging, as it does not require laboratory monitoring; is safe, effective, and inexpensive; and can be used in the outpatient setting.[32,34,39,43,46] Typically, LMWH is started 36 to 48 hours after the last warfarin dose.[33,44,46] A commonly used dosing strategy preoperatively is enoxaparin, 1 mg/kg every 12 hours.[32] Regardless of dosing regimen, the last dose of LMWH should be administered 24 hours before surgery to minimize risk of perioperative bleeding.[32,33,43] In patients with mild or moderate renal insufficiency (creatinine clearance, 30–50 mL/min), doses of LMWH should be reduced and anti-Xa levels should be monitored. However, because LMWH is predominately renally excreted and unfractionated heparin is metabolized in the liver and endothelium, unfractionated heparin should be considered for bridging in patients with significant renal impairment (creatinine clearance, <30 mL/min) who are at high risk for thromboembolism.[43,47,48]

Resumption of LMWH after surgery depends on postoperative hemostasis and the bleeding risk associated with surgery.[31] If there is active bleeding or inadequate postoperative hemostasis, resumption of LMWH should be held until the bleeding subsides or adequate hemostasis is obtained.[31,39] In patients undergoing procedures that carry a minor or moderate bleeding risk, low-dose LMWH can be resumed on the evening of surgery; however, the use of full dose should be avoided for at least 24 hours after surgery.[33,39,44,46] A previous study found that enoxaparin given within 12 to 24 hours postoperatively led to a major bleeding episode in 20% of patients undergoing major surgery and 0.7% of patients undergoing minor surgery.[38,43] These findings indicate that resumption of low-dose LMWH should be delayed for at least 24 to 48 hours and full dose up to 72 hours after surgery.[31,33,43]

Treatment of Patients Receiving Antiplatelet Therapy

Perioperative treatment of patients on antiplatelet therapy (aspirin, clopidogrel, and ticlopidine) is based on both cardiovascular and bleeding risks associated with surgery.[43,49] For surgeries associated with a low bleeding risk, antiplatelet therapy does not need to be withheld. In contrast, for surgeries associated with a moderate or high bleeding risk, the decision to continue or withhold antiplatelet therapy is based significantly on the patient's risk for perioperative cardiovascular events.[43] Furthermore, in patients at low risk for perioperative cardiovascular events, antiplatelet therapy should be discontinued 7 to 10 days before surgery.[31,37,50] However, in patients at moderate or high risk for cardiovascular events, the American College of Chest Physicians recommends continuing aspirin therapy while holding clopidogrel 5 to 10 days before surgery.[31,39,44,50,51] In patients with a coronary stent, surgery should be delayed to at least 6 weeks after bare-metal stent placement and at least 6 months after drug-eluting stent placement.[31,37,50] In contrast, the American College of Chest Physicians recommends against delaying urgent surgery (eg, hip fracture) and suggests that platelets should only be transfused if there is excessive bleeding.[52] Several studies found that patients undergoing early hip fracture surgery who are receiving antiplatelet therapy are not at increased risk for perioperative bleeding complications and mortality, whereas other studies found that they may have greater perioperative blood loss but still no significance difference in mortality.[53,54] Nevertheless, it is strongly recommended that surgical invention for hip fracture (>48 hours) or other emergent surgeries should not be delayed.[55,56]

Antiplatelet therapy should be resumed 24 hours postoperatively.[49,50,52] Resumption of aspirin would achieve the maximal antiplatelet effect within minutes.[43] Clopidogrel, however, may take up to 7 days to achieve the maximum antiplatelet effect, and a loading dose may be given initially to shorten this process.[44]

SUMMARY

DVT and PE are among the leading causes of perioperative morbidity and mortality in orthopedic patients. To reduce potentially devastating complications of DVT and PE, it is essential that orthopedic surgeons have a comprehensive understanding of risk factors, diagnosis, and medical treatment of acute DVT and PE and perioperative management of patients on anticoagulant therapy. This knowledge will lead to substantial improvement in perioperative outcomes and contribution to reducing cost and length of hospital stay, health care burden, and postoperative morbidity and mortality.

ACKNOWLEDGMENT

The authors thank Mrs Katelyn Pratt and Mr Bilal Mahmood for their assistance in writing this article.

REFERENCES

1. LaMori JC, Shoheiber O, Mody SH, et al. Inpatient resource use and cost burden of deep vein thrombosis and pulmonary embolism in the United States. Clin Ther 2015;37(1):62–70.

2. Kline JA, Kabrhel C. Emergency evaluation for pulmonary embolism, part 1: clinical factors that increase risk. J Emerg Med 2015;48(6):771–80.

3. Park SJ, Kim CK, Park YS, et al. Incidence and factors predicting venous thromboembolism following surgical treatment of fractures below the hip. J Orthop Trauma 2015;29(10):e349–54.

4. Dixon J, Ahn E, Zhou L, et al. Venous thromboembolism rates in patients undergoing major hip and knee joint surgery at Waitemata District Health Board: a retrospective audit. Intern Med J 2015; 45(4):416–22.

5. Granziera S, Cohen AT. VTE primary prevention, including hospitalised medical and orthopaedic surgical patients. Thromb Haemost 2015;113(6): 1216–23.

6. Parvizi J, Huang R, Raphael IJ, et al. Timing of symptomatic pulmonary embolism with warfarin following arthroplasty. J Arthroplasty 2015;30(6): 1050–3.

7. Saragas NP, Ferrao PN, Saragas E, et al. The impact of risk assessment on the implementation of venous thromboembolism prophylaxis in foot and ankle surgery. Foot Ankle Surg 2014;20(2):85–9.

8. Cukic V. The pulmonary thromboembolism as a risk of surgical treatments and the role of anticoagulant prophylaxiss. Mater Sociomed 2014;26(5):303–5.

9. American Academy of Orthopaedic Surgeons guideline on preventing venous thromboembolic

disease in patients undergoing elective hip and knee arthroplasty. In: American Academy of Orthopaedic Surgeons, editor. Evidence-based Guideline and Evidence Report. Rosemont (IL): American Academy of Orthopaedic Surgeons; 2011. p. 801.

10. McRae SJ, Ginsberg JS. Update in the diagnosis of deep-vein thrombosis and pulmonary embolism. Curr Opin Anaesthesiol 2006;19(1):44–51.

11. Segal JB, Eng J, Tamariz LJ, et al. Review of the evidence on diagnosis of deep venous thrombosis and pulmonary embolism. Ann Fam Med 2007; 5(1):63–73.

12. Swanson E. Ultrasound screening for deep venous thrombosis detection: a prospective evaluation of 200 plastic surgery outpatients. Plast Reconstr Surg Glob Open 2015;3(3):e332.

13. Hamidi S, Riazi M. Cutoff values of plasma d-dimer level in patients with diagnosis of the venous thromboembolism after elective spinal surgery. Asian Spine J 2015;9(2):232–8.

14. Lippi G, Cervellin G, Franchini M, et al. Biochemical markers for the diagnosis of venous thromboembolism: the past, present and future. J Thromb Thrombolysis 2010;30(4):459–71.

15. Wilbur J, Shian B. Diagnosis of deep venous thrombosis and pulmonary embolism. Am Fam Physician 2012;86(10):913–9. Available at: http://www.aafp.org/afp/2012/1115/p913.html.

16. Kester BS, Merkow RP, Ju MH, et al. Effect of postdischarge venous thromboembolism on hospital quality comparisons following hip and knee arthroplasty. J Bone Joint Surg Am 2014;96(17):1476–84.

17. Prisco D, Cenci C, Silvestri E, et al. Pharmacological prevention of venous thromboembolism in orthopaedic surgery. Clin Cases Miner Bone Metab 2014;11(3):192–5.

18. Levitan B, Yuan Z, Turpie AG, et al. Benefit-risk assessment of rivaroxaban versus enoxaparin for the prevention of venous thromboembolism after total hip or knee arthroplasty. Vasc Health Risk Manag 2014;10:157–67.

19. Unay K, Akan K, Sener N, et al. Evaluating the effectiveness of a deep-vein thrombosis prophylaxis protocol in orthopaedics and traumatology. J Eval Clin Pract 2009;15(4):668–74.

20. Falck-Ytter Y, Francis CW, Johanson NA, et al. Prevention of VTE in orthopedic surgery patients: Antithrombotic therapy and prevention of thrombosis, 9th ed: American College of Chest Physicians Evidence-Based Clinical Practice Guidelines. Chest 2012;141(2 Suppl):e278S–325S.

21. Planes A, Vochelle N, Fafola M. Venous thromboembolic prophylaxis in orthopedic surgery: Knee surgery. Semin Thromb Hemost 1999;25(Suppl 3):73–7.

22. Fitzgerald RH Jr, Spiro TE, Trowbridge AA, et al. Prevention of venous thromboembolic disease following primary total knee arthroplasty. A randomized, multicenter, open-label, parallel-group comparison of enoxaparin and warfarin. J Bone Joint Surg Am 2001;83-A(6):900–6.

23. McAsey CJ, Gargiulo JM, Parks NL, et al. Patient satisfaction with mobile compression devices following total hip arthroplasty. Orthopedics 2014; 37(8):e673–7.

24. Morris RJ, Woodcock JP. Evidence-based compression: prevention of stasis and deep vein thrombosis. Ann Surg 2004;239(2):162–71.

25. Seshadri T, Tran H, Lau KK, et al. Ins and outs of inferior vena cava filters in patients with venous thromboembolism: the experience at Monash Medical Centre and review of the published reports. Intern Med J 2008;38(1):38–43.

26. Samoukovic G, Malas T, deVarennes B. The role of pulmonary embolectomy in the treatment of acute pulmonary embolism: a literature review from 1968 to 2008. Interact Cardiovasc Thorac Surg 2010; 11(3):265–70.

27. Strauss EJ, Egol KA, Alaia M, et al. The use of retrievable inferior vena cava filters in orthopaedic patients. J Bone Joint Surg Br 2008; 90(5):662–7.

28. Berczi V, Bottomley JR, Thomas SM, et al. Long-term retrievability of IVC filters: should we abandon permanent devices? Cardiovasc Intervent Radiol 2007;30(5):820–7.

29. Aymard T, Kadner A, Widmer A, et al. Massive pulmonary embolism: surgical embolectomy versus thrombolytic therapy–should surgical indications be revisited? Eur J Cardiothorac Surg 2013;43(1): 90–4 [discussion: 94].

30. Gulba DC, Schmid C, Borst HG, et al. Medical compared with surgical treatment for massive pulmonary embolism. Lancet 1994;343(8897):576–7.

31. Douketis JD. Perioperative anticoagulation management in patients who are receiving oral anticoagulant therapy: a practical guide for clinicians. Thromb Res 2002;108(1):3–13.

32. Heit JA. Perioperative management of the chronically anti-coagulated patient. J Thromb Thrombolysis 2001;12(1):81–7.

33. Spyropoulos AC, Douketis JD. How I treat anticoagulated patients undergoing an elective procedure or surgery. Blood 2012;120(15):2954–62.

34. Kearon C, Hirsh J. Management of anticoagulation before and after elective surgery. N Engl J Med 1997;336(21):1506–11.

35. Brotman DJ, Streiff MB. Overuse of bridging anticoagulation for patients with venous thromboembolism: first, do no harm. JAMA Intern Med 2015; 175(7):1169–70.

36. Douketis JD, Spyropoulos AC, Spencer FA, et al. Perioperative management of antithrombotic therapy. Chest 2012;141(2 Suppl):e326S–50S.

37. Kearon C. Perioperative management of long-term anticoagulation. Semin Thromb Hemost 1998; 24(Suppl 1):77–83.

38. Duoketis JD. Perioperative management of patients who are receiving warfarin therapy: an evidence-based and practical approach. Blood 2011;117(19):5044–9.

39. Duoketis JD, Johnson JA, Turpie AG. Low-molecular-weight heparin as bridging anticoagulation during interruption of warfarin. Arch Intern Med 2004; 164(12):1319–26.

40. Hirsh J, Fuster V, Ansell J, et al. American Heart Association/American College of Cardiology Foundation guide to warfarin therapy. Circulation 2003; 107:1692–711.

41. Ageno W, Gallus AS, Wittkowsky A, et al. Oral anticoagulant therapy. Chest 2012;141(2 Suppl): e44S–88S.

42. Do EJ, Lenzini P, Eby CS, et al. Genetics InFormatics Trial (GIFT) of warfarin to prevent deep vein thrombosis (DVT): rationale and study design. Pharmacogenomics J 2012;12(5): 417–24.

43. McBane RD, Wysokinski WE, Daniels PR, et al. Periprocedural anticoagulation management of patients with venous thromboembolism. Arterioscler Thromb Vasc Biol 2010;30(3):442–8.

44. Ortel TL. Perioperative management of patients on chronic antithrombotic therapy. Blood 2012; 120(24):4699–705.

45. Ashouri F, Al-Jundi W, Patel A, et al. Management of warfarin anticoagulation in patients with fractured neck of femur. ISRN Hematol 2011;2011: 294628.

46. Jaffer AK, Ahmed M, Brotman DJ, et al. Low-molecular-weight heparins as peril-procedural anticoagulation for patients on long-term warfarin therapy: a standardized bridging therapy protocol. J Thromb Thrombolysis 2005;20(1):11–6.

47. Wysokinski WE, McBane RD. Clinical update: periprocedural bridging management of anticoagulation. Circulation 2012;126:486–90.

48. Capodanno D, Angiolillo DJ. Contemporary reviews in cardiovascular medicine: antithrombotic therapy in patients with chronic kidney disease. Circulation 2012;125:2649–61.

49. Chassot PG, Marcucci C, Delabays A. Perioperative antiplatelet therapy. Am Fam Physician 2010;82(12): 1484–9.

50. Hirsh J, Guyatt G, Albers GW, et al. Executive summary: american college of chest physicians evidence-based clinical practice guidelines (8th Edition). Chest 2008;133(6 Suppl):71S–109S.

51. Gleason LJ, Friedman SM. Preoperative management of anticoagulation and antiplatelet agents. Clin Geriatr Med 2014;30(2):219–27.

52. Al Khudairy A, Al-Hadeedi O, Sayana MK, et al. Withholding clopidogrel for 3 to 6 versus 7 days or more before surgery in hip fracture patients. J Orthop Surg 2013;21(2):146–50.

53. Feely MA, Mabry TM, Lohse CM, et al. Safety of clopidogrel in hip fracture surgery. Mayo Clin Proc 2013;88(2):149–56.

54. Collinge CA, Kelly KC, Little B, et al. The effects of clopidogrel (Plavix) and other oral anticoagulants on early hip fracture surgery. J Orthop Trauma 2012;26(10):568–73.

55. Chechik O, Thein R, Fichman G, et al. The effect of clopidogrel and aspirin on blood loss in hip fracture surgery. Injury 2011;42(11):1277–82.

56. Harty JA, McKenna P, Moloney D, et al. Antiplatelet agents and surgical delay in elderly patients with hip fractures. J Orthop Surg 2007;15(3): 270–2.

Trauma

Role of Systemic and Local Antibiotics in the Treatment of Open Fractures

David C. Carver, MD, Sean B. Kuehn, MD,
John C. Weinlein, MD*

KEYWORDS

- Open fractures • Systemic antibiotics • Infection • Local antibiotics • PMMA • Chitosan sponge
- Calcium sulfate

KEY POINTS

- Systemic antibiotics have been shown to decrease infection rates after open fracture.
- Controversy continues to exist over the ideal systemic antibiotic prophylaxis, particularly for type III open fractures.
- Local antibiotic delivery, although not new, is an area of renewed interest.
- Local antibiotics allow delivery of high concentrations of antibiotic without systemic toxicity.
- Many modes of local antibiotic delivery currently exist.

INTRODUCTION

Open fractures can be problematic for the patient, orthopedic surgeon, and society in general. An open fracture occurs when communication exists between fracture or fracture hematoma and the outside environment. This communication potentially allows bacteria from the environment to colonize the fracture site. Colonization of the fracture site with pathogenic bacteria may result in infection, which is known to be one of the more common causes of fracture nonunion.[1] Infection and nonunion result in significant cost to the patient and society.[2,3]

Antibiotics work in many different ways to disrupt the life cycle of bacteria. Antibiotics can be administered systemically or locally to a fracture site. Both methods of administration have been used in attempts to reduce infection after open fracture. This article reviews the data supporting both systemic and local antibiotics.

SYSTEMIC ANTIBIOTICS

History, Incidence of Infection, and Infecting Organisms

Patzakis and colleagues[4] in 1974 were the first to demonstrate in a prospective randomized trial the efficacy of systemic antibiotics in decreasing infection rates after open fractures. Patients (310 open fractures) were randomized to 3 groups: no antibiotics, penicillin/streptomycin, or cephalothin. Patients receiving cephalothin had a lower incidence of infection (2.4%) than those receiving penicillin/streptomycin (9.8%) and patients not receiving antibiotics at all (13.9%).

Gustilo and Anderson[5] in 1976 reported antibiotic sensitivity data as part of analysis of more than 1000 open fractures; 50.7% of open fractures were colonized on admission and an additional 20.0% of patients had a positive culture at wound closure. Sensitivity analysis of cultured organisms led to the investigators' recommendation that a first-generation cephalosporin was the antibiotic of choice for open fractures. All *Staphylococcus* species, both coagulation

---

Disclosures: Senior author, J.C. Weinlein, receives royalties from Mosby-Elsevier for contributions to Campbell's Operative Orthopaedics.

Department of Orthopaedic Surgery, University of Tennessee-Campbell Clinic, Memphis, TN, USA

* Corresponding author. 1211 Union Avenue, Suite 500, Memphis, TN 38104.

E-mail address: jweinlein@campbellclinic.com

positive and negative, were sensitive to cephalothin. Fifty-seven of 143 isolates reported were gram negative. Of these 57 gram-negative isolates, 23 were either *Pseudomonas* or *Enterobacter* and were not sensitive to cephalothin. Interestingly, the investigators cautioned about the nephrotoxic effects of adding aminoglycosides and advocated doing so only when "the anticipated beneficial effects are deemed essential after careful weighing of the potential benefits and dangers."[5]

Gustilo and colleagues[6] in 1984 further classified type III open fractures (Table 1).[6] Subclassifications of type III open fractures were found to be predictive of infection and need for amputation. The infection rate was found to be 4%, 52%, and 42% for type IIIA, type IIIB (Fig. 1), and type IIIC open fractures, respectively. Of the infections reported after type III open fractures, 77% (24/31) were caused by gram-negative bacteria. Ten of 24 gram-negative infections were secondary to *Enterobacter* or *Pseudomonas* species, 2 organisms previously shown not to be sensitive to cephalothin.[5] The investigators did recommend a change in antibiotic prophylaxis for type III open fractures. They recommended adding an aminoglycoside to a first-generation cephalosporin or using a

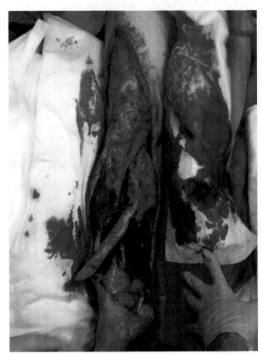

Fig. 1. Clinical photo of patient with type IIIB open tibia fracture.

third-generation cephalosporin with the goal of "avoiding potential aminoglycoside toxicity."[6]

Templeman and colleagues[7] retrospectively evaluated infection rate based on the Gustilo and Anderson[5] classification; 11.3% of open tibia shaft fractures were complicated by infection with infection rates of 0%, 3%, and 21% for type I, II, and III open tibial shaft fractures, respectively. Patzakis and Wilkins[8] reported similar infection rates based on the Gustilo and Anderson[5] classification. They reported infections rates of 1.4%, 3.6%, and 22.7% for type I, II, and III open fractures, respectively, with an overall incidence of 10.5%. They also reported that the rate of infection is dependent on anatomic site, with the tibia having a 10% infection rate versus a 5.3% infection rate for other sites combined.

In a more contemporary study, Chen and colleagues[9] reported the most common infecting organisms after open fracture. Overall, the investigators reported a 10% infection rate after 202 open fractures. *Staphylococcus* was the most common organism cultured (55% of infections), with coagulase-negative *Staphylococcus* and methicillin-resistant *Staphylococcus aureus* (MRSA) representing 30% and 25% of infections, respectively. Interestingly, 67% (4/6) of coagulase-negative *Staphylococcus* infections

Table 1 Gustilo and Anderson classification of open fractures	
Type	**Description**
I	Wound <1 cm; clean; simple fracture pattern; minimal comminution; minimal soft tissue injury.
II	Wound 1–10 cm; simple fracture pattern; moderate soft tissue injury.
IIIA	Extensive soft tissue injury but with adequate soft tissue coverage over bone; high-energy, comminuted, or segmental injuries.
IIIB	Extensive soft tissue injury with soft tissue loss and periosteal stripping; inadequate soft tissue coverage over bone.
IIIC	Open fracture with associated vascular injury requiring repair.

From Gustilo RB, Anderson JT. Prevention of infection in the treatment of one thousand and twenty-five open fractures of long bones: retrospective and prospective analyses. J Bone Joint Surg Am 1976;58A:453–8; and Gustilo RB, Mendoza RM, Williams DN. Problems in the management of type III (severe) open fractures: a new classification of type III open fractures. J Trauma 1984;24:742–6.

included a second organism. Overall, 55% of infections included at least 1 gram-negative organism. Thirty-two percent of type IIIB open fractures were complicated by infection. Overall, 2.5% of open fractures were complicated by infection with MRSA.

Another contemporary study reported the most common infecting organisms after treatment of both open and closed fractures. A total of 214 infections were analyzed, of which 103 involved the tibia. S aureus was responsible for 56% of infections, with MRSA being responsible for 32% of infections. In type III open fractures, S aureus was responsible 21% of the time with gram-negative rods (GNR) and anaerobes being responsible 14% and 7%, respectively. Of the GNR infections found after open fracture, 35% were found in type III open fractures compared with 18% in type II open fractures and 0% in type I open fractures. However, there was no statistically significant difference in comparing rates of GNR infection between type III open fractures and types I and II combined. Interestingly, 32% of open fractures and 33% of closed fracture infections involved GNR. Although "barnyard-type" injuries did receive penicillin, type III open fractures did not routinely receive aminoglycosides for prophylaxis.[10]

Timing of Antibiotic Administration

Time to antibiotic administration was first shown to be predictive of infection by Patzakis and Wilkins[8] in 1989. These investigators reported a 4.7% infection rate when antibiotics were administered within 3 hours of injury and a 7.4% infection rate when antibiotics were administered after 3 hours. This series included all types of open fractures and only 35.5% of open fractures received antibiotics within 3 hours. Several different antibiotic regimens were used during the course of the study. The investigators concluded that "the single most important factor in reducing the infection rate was the early administration of antibiotics that provide antibacterial activity against both gram-positive and gram-negative microorganisms." This conclusion appears at least partly based on the fact that patients who received cefamandole and tobramycin did have the lowest infection rates after open fractures and more specifically open tibia fractures (4.5%).[11] A confounding variable is that wound care differed throughout the study among groups.

Lack and colleagues[12] also reported that time to antibiotic administration is predictive of infection. The investigators reported on 137 type III open tibia fractures, of which 94.9% received antibiotics within 3 hours of injury. Cefazolin was the only agent given in 93.4% of cases. The overall deep infection rate was 17.5%. Patients who received antibiotics within 1 hour of injury had a 6.8% infection rate compared with 27.9% in those receiving antibiotics after 90 minutes. The organisms responsible for deep infection were not reported.

One of the shortcomings of the Gustilo and Anderson[5] classification includes lack of interobserver reliability. Brumback and Jones[13] recommended delaying fracture classification until the first operative debridement. With fractures not classified until the first debridement, appropriate antibiotic treatment could be delayed. As more and more data suggest that time to debridement is not predictive of infection,[14–18] the average time to debridement is likely to increase. If time to debridement increases, then time to classification and appropriate antibiotic treatment could be delayed. An example would be an open tibia fracture that was thought on initial physical examination to be a type II open fracture. Based on many protocols, this patient would prophylactically receive a first-generation cephalosporin. If at surgery, the patient's fracture was classified as a type IIIB open fracture, he or she would have had a delay in administration of an antibiotic with effective gram-negative coverage. The importance of the time to administration of an antibiotic with effective gram-negative coverage is not well established in the literature.

Established Guidelines (Agent and Duration)

Eastern Association for the Surgery of Trauma (EAST) Practice Management Guidelines strongly advocate for gram-positive coverage in type I and II open fracture wounds with the addition of gram-negative coverage for type III open wounds. Guidelines also advocate for the addition of penicillin with open fracture wounds at risk for fecal or clostridial contamination, discontinuation of antibiotics by 24 hours after wound closure in type I and II open fractures, and discontinuation of antibiotics in type III wounds by 72 hours after injury or by 24 hours after closure or coverage, whichever occurs first.[19,20]

The Surgical Infection Society Guidelines differed from the EAST Practice Management Guidelines concluding that insufficient evidence existed to advocate using gram-negative antibiotics and antibiotics with clostridial coverage. These guidelines advocated using a first-generation cephalosporin in conjunction with modern wound care techniques.[21]

Additional guidelines published in 2011 regarding combat-related injuries, endorsed by both the Surgical Infection Society and the Infectious Diseases Society of America, recommended cefazolin (clindamycin in patients with allergy to β lactams) for extremity wounds. The guidelines did not advocate for addition of gram-negative coverage nor did they advocate for addition of penicillin. These guidelines call for duration of antibiotic therapy of 1 to 3 days.[22]

Dellinger and colleagues[23] in a randomized trial reported no differences in infection rates comparing 1 day of antibiotic coverage with 5 days of antibiotic coverage. Patients were randomized to 1 of 3 groups: cefonicid × 1 day, cefonicid × 5 days, cefamandole × 5 days. There also was no significant difference in infection rates for type III open fractures treated with 1 day versus 5 days. Although S aureus was the most common infecting organism identified (58%), GNRs were identified in 33% of infections. Patzakis and colleagues[11] also concluded that antibiotic duration is not a significant predictor of infection and have not advocated routinely extending duration beyond 3 days.

Clindamycin has been supported as an alternative to first-generation cephalosporin in patients with β lactam allergy. Benson and colleagues[24] reported no difference in infections rates in a prospective study of open fractures comparing clindamycin with cefazolin. In a separate prospective study of open fractures, patients treated with prophylactic clindamycin had a lower incidence of infection than those treated with cloxacillin (9.3% infection in clindamycin group; 20.0% infection in cloxacillin group). All infections in type I and II open fractures were secondary to gram-positive organisms. Both antibiotics were associated with high infection rates in type III open fractures, with the investigators recommending additional gram-negative coverage for type III open fractures.[25]

Nephrotoxicity with Aminoglycosides?

Although Gustilo and colleagues, in 1976[5] and 1984,[6] warned about the potential systemic toxicity associated with gentamicin, the EAST Practice Management Guidelines have given some support for the safety of once-daily aminoglycoside administration.[19,20] This guideline was based on data published by Sorger and colleagues[26] in 1999 and Russell and colleagues[27] in 2001. Sorger and colleagues[26] compared once-daily dosing of gentamicin with twice-a-

day dosing of gentamicin in 71 patients with type II and III open fractures. In addition to gentamicin, patients received cefazolin. Antibiotics were continued for 48 hours after each operation and until wound closure or coverage. Incidence of infection was 6.4% in the once-daily dosing of gentamicin compared with 13.6% in the twice-a-day dosing; however, this difference was not statistically significant. No patients in either group treated with prophylactic gentamicin experienced renal complications. Two patients receiving extended therapeutic treatment with gentamicin for diagnosis of infection did have an increase in serum blood urea nitrogen (BUN)/creatinine ratio and both patients were receiving twice-daily therapeutic treatment with gentamicin. Of note is that patients with renal insufficiency were excluded from the trial.[26] Russell and colleagues[27] reported a very small series of patients (n = 16) treated with cefazolin and once-daily dosing of gentamicin for types II and III open tibia fractures. BUN and creatinine were followed and no patients in this series showed evidence of nephrotoxicity.

Recently, Bell and colleagues[28] reported an increased rate of acute kidney injury (AKI) in orthopedic patients in Scotland after surgical prophylaxis was changed from cefuroxime to flucloxacillin and gentamicin. Gentamicin was administered as a single dose, 4 mg/kg. This study included 12,482 patients; of those patients, 7666 underwent orthopedic procedures. The mean age of orthopedic patients was 71. Patients undergoing surgery for femoral neck fracture were excluded because of concern of administering gentamicin to this patient population. The incidence of AKI in orthopedic patients increased from 6.2% to 10.8% after protocol change.

Risk factors associated with nephrotoxicity after once-daily dosing of aminoglycoside usage have recently been reported. Oliveira and colleagues[29] reported an increased rate of AKI with aminoglycoside usage in the intensive care unit in patients with a history of diabetes mellitus, hypotension, iodinated contrast, and administration of other nephrotoxins. Unfortunately, the mortality rate of patients who experienced AKI was 44.5% (vs 29.1% in the group without AKI). The average duration of usage of aminoglycoside between patients who developed AKI (9.4 days) was similar to patients not developing AKI (9.9 days).

Usage of aminoglycosides among orthopedic trauma surgeons remains high, with 76.3% of respondents in a recent survey using aminoglycosides in contaminated type IIIB open fractures.

Interestingly, aminoglycosides also are being used in lower-grade open fractures, with 29.8% of respondents using aminoglycosides in contaminated type I open wounds and 15% of respondents using aminoglycosides in nonconta-minated type II open wounds.[30] Patient and fracture characteristics and AKI have to be considered in the care of patients with open fracture, as AKI has been shown to be an inde-pendent risk factor for mortality[31] and even un-complicated AKI is associated with a 10% risk of mortality.[32,33]

Contemporary Antibiotic Options

Recently, studies have challenged the traditional antibiotic regimen for type III open fractures and fractures with potential fecal or clostridial contamination. Rodriguez and colleagues[34] re-ported no statistically significant difference in infection rates for type III open fractures primar-ily treated with ceftriaxone compared with a traditional antibiotic regimen including a first-generation cephalosporin and aminoglycoside. Gram-negative organisms comprised 33.3% of cultured organisms with the traditional antibiotic regimen and 40.0% of cultured organisms with the ceftriaxone regimen. The investigators effec-tively reduced the use aminoglycosides, vanco-mycin, and penicillin (53.5% usage in the traditional antibiotic group vs 16.4% usage in the ceftriaxone group).

Similarly, Redfern and colleagues[35] reported on 72 type III open fractures treated with piper-acillin/tazobactam versus cefazolin/gentamicin. Patients treated with piperacillin/tazobactam did have a lower infection rate at 30 days compared with cefazolin/gentamicin (11.4% vs 21.6); however, this difference was not statisti-cally significant. There was no statistically signif-icant difference in infection at 1 year.

Johnson and colleagues[36] in an earlier study also provided some support for usage of a third-generation cephalosporin in higher-grade open tibia fractures. The investigators compared cefazolin with cefotaxime in a prospective ran-domized trial. Forty-six open tibia fractures (type II, IIIA, IIIB) were randomized to treatment with either cefazolin or cefotaxime. Patients treated with cefotaxime had a lower infection rate (19% vs 25%); however, this difference was not statistically significant. Interestingly, only 1 of 4 infections in the cefotaxime group involved a gram-negative organism compared with 4 of 6 in the cefazolin group.

Recently, the results of a large retrospective study of 1539 open fractures comparing

traditional antibiotic prophylaxis of cefazolin and a gentamicin (CG) with a new regimen of vancomycin and cefepime (VC) were presented. No differences were found in overall infection. However, the vancomycin/cefepime group demonstrated a significantly lower infection rate (3.1% vs 6.8%) in the type III open fractures; 22% of infections were secondary to MRSA with 8 infections in each group. Overall, 1% of open fractures were complicated by infection with MRSA. Significantly fewer infections secondary to Enterococcus (0 VC, 6 CG) and Pseudomonas (2 VC, 9 CG) occurred in the VC group. The in-vestigators reported a zero incidence of AKI in patients presenting with normal renal function.[37] Saveli and colleagues[38] reported the results of a randomized trial comparing cefazolin with cefa-zolin plus vancomycin for the treatment of open fractures. Overall, the investigators re-ported a 16.8% infection rate with no difference between treatment groups. The rate of infection in type III open fractures was 29%. MRSA was responsible for 1 infection in each group (overall, 18% of infections); 27% of infections involved gram-negative bacilli. Enterococcus was involved in 18% of infections (1 vancomycin-susceptible Enterococcus; 1 vancomycin-resis-tant Enterococcus). Although appearing safe, neither study appears to show a significant benefit of vancomycin in the prophylaxis of open fractures. Cefepime and potentially other fourth-generation cephalosporins show promise and deserve further investigation.

Importance of Body Weight on Dosing?

Previous recommendations and doses of cefa-zolin frequently appearing in the literature include 1 g in patients weighing 80 kg or less and 2 g in patients weighing more than 80 kg. Recent guidelines for routine surgical antibiotic prophylaxis developed jointly by the American Society of Health-System Pharmacists, the Infectious Diseases Society of America, the Sur-gical Infection Society, and the Society for Healthcare Epidemiology of America recom-mend 2 g of cefazolin in adult patients weighing less than 120 kg and 3 g of cefazolin in adult patients weighing 120 kg or more.[39] Underdos-ing of antibiotics has been found to be rela-tively common, as 21% of patients in a study by Collinge and colleagues[40] did not receive appropriate weight-based dosing of antibiotic before implementation of a performance-improvement initiative. The clinical implications of underdosing weight-based antibiotics are not yet clear.

Potential Implications of Changing Wound Care on Infecting Organisms

Most early studies from which our antibiotic recommendations have largely been derived treated open fractures by initially leaving wounds open or partially open.[11,24] At the very least, most type III wounds were left open after initial debridement.[6,7] Early studies supported the concept that infections were most likely due to nosocomial organisms. Of 21 infections associated with type IIIB open tibia fractures, 57% were due to organisms not cultured within the first 2 weeks.[41] Similarly, Lee[42] reported that the organism responsible for infection after open fracture was not present in 78% of predebridement and 58% of postdebridement cultures. Current treatment of open fractures is more aggressive with regard to early wound closure and negative pressure wound therapy (NPWT) is more frequently used in wounds that are not closed. These 2 changes in wound management may lead to decreased nosocomial infection. Jenkinson and colleagues[43] recently reported a lower incidence of infection when open fractures (types I, II, and IIIA) were closed primarily (4.1%) versus delayed (17.8%). Although 3 of 73 patients closed primarily developed infection, none of the 3 was infected by a clostridial or gram-negative organism.

Unfortunately, a prospective randomized trial illustrating the benefit of NPWT in high-energy open fractures failed to describe any differences in identity of infecting organisms between groups. Nine infections occurred overall in this series with an infection rate of 28% in the gauze-dressing group and 5.4% in the NPWT group. Ten organisms were identified, including 7 gram-positive and 3 gram-negative organisms. Clostridium was not cultured in this study.[44] Blum and colleagues[45] reported similar findings in a retrospective study of open tibia fractures. The investigators reported an 8.4% infection rate with NPWT versus 28% with conventional dressings. The incidence of polymicrobial infection was decreased with NPWT (17% vs 47%). Dedmond and colleagues[46] reported results of using NPWT in the treatment of 50 type III open tibia fractures; 29.2% of type III open tibia fractures required debridement for deep infection. Ten deep infections occurred, with at least 6 involving MRSA (3 MRSA alone; 3 polymicrobial including MRSA). The identity of the other organisms identified in the polymicrobial infections was not reported.

Moues and colleagues[47] investigated bacterial counts after treatment with NPWT versus gauze dressings. Although the total bacterial load did not differ between groups, gram-negative bacilli load was decreased with NPWT. The basic science indicates that NPWT does reduce levels of *Pseudomonas* compared with wet to dry dressing changes in a goat wound model. This same reduction was not observed with NPWT and *Staphylococcus aureus*.[48] Whether NPWT decreases the level of contamination of gram-negative organisms in open fracture wound or serves as a barrier to colonization with nosocomial gram-negative organisms is not completely clear in clinical practice.

Systemic Antibiotic Recommendations in 2017

Choice of antibiotic is guided by the Gustilo and Anderson classification.[5,6] Patients with type I and II open fractures should be given a first-generation cephalosporin (cefazolin). In patients with serious β lactam allergy, clindamycin is an appropriate alternative.[24,25] Patients with type III open fractures also should be given an agent with gram-positive coverage but consideration should be given to adding an agent with effective gram-negative coverage or using an agent with both effective gram-positive and gram-negative coverage (**Table 2**). Traditionally,

Table 2
Recommended systemic antibiotic prophylaxis (2017)

Open Fracture Type	Recommended Systemic Antibiotic Prophylaxis
Gustilo and Anderson Type I	First-generation cephalosporin (cefazolin) Alternative: clindamycin with β lactam allergy
Gustilo and Anderson Type II	First-generation cephalosporin (cefazolin) Alternative: clindamycin with β lactam allergy
Gustilo and Anderson Type III	First-generation cephalosporin (or clindamycin with β lactam allergy) *plus* aminoglycoside (gentamicin) Alternatives: Third-generation cephalosporin (ceftriaxone or piperacillin/tazobactam)
Fecal or potential clostridial contamination	Consider addition of penicillin to above regimen (cefazolin/gentamicin)

patients with type III open fractures have been given cefazolin and gentamicin. Penicillin or an agent with anaerobic coverage should be considered for fractures associated with fecal or clostridial contamination.[19,20] If gentamicin is administered, patient and injury characteristics need to be considered. Duration and dosing schedule should be monitored, as a short course of once-daily dosing of gentamicin in a patient without risk factors for AKI appears relatively safe. Other agents with potential promise for treatment of type III open fractures include ceftriaxone,[34] piperacillin/tazobactam,[35] and cefepime.[37] All 3 agents deserve further study.

LOCAL ANTIBIOTICS
History and Potential Advantages
The use of locally applied antibiotics is not a novel concept. Locally applied antiseptics date back to the mid-1800s when Joseph Lister began using carbolic acid as an antiseptic on surgical wounds.[49] In 1939, Jenson and colleagues[50] were able to reduce their infection rate for open fractures from 30% to 5% by placing sulfanilamide powder directly into wounds before wound closure. The modern use of local antibiotics in orthopedics began in Europe with the use of polymethylmethacrylate (PMMA) cement impregnated with antibiotics to treat infected joint prostheses.[51,52] The use of locally applied antibiotics allows delivery of high concentrations of antibiotics without significant risk of systemic toxicity. High concentrations of antibiotics have been shown be effective against biofilms[53] and therefore local antibiotics may have a significant role in reducing infections from biofilm-producing bacteria.

Various methods and techniques have been developed that allow for the direct placement of antibiotics into open wounds. Although PMMA cement is the "gold standard," it is not the ideal delivery system. PMMA beads and cement spacers can be bulky, which can prove difficult in open fractures without significant bone loss. Additionally, PMMA cement requires a second procedure for removal. The optimal antibiotic delivery system provides high concentrations of antibiotics over an extended period, without causing systemic toxicity or adverse effects to the local host environment, and does not require subsequent surgical removal. Avoidance of surgical removal has motivated the development of several different bioabsorbable delivery systems that are reviewed in the following sections.

Polymethylmethacrylate
PMMA has been used for antibiotic delivery for more than 40 years and is still considered the gold standard of local delivery.[54] PMMA is a synthetic polymer that is nonbiodegradable by nature with favorable biocompatibility and high mechanical strength.[55] In orthopedics, it has been used extensively as an anchoring platform in arthroplasty components and as a local antibiotic delivery agent in orthopedic trauma and osteomyelitis treatment.

In the trauma literature, PMMA has been used in many applications. Broadly, it is used as a treatment for soft tissue infection or osteomyelitis and in infection prevention of open fractures (**Fig. 2**). PMMA antibiotic administration has many different forms. Specifically, it is used in the form of beads,[56] spacers, and antibiotic nails or antibiotic-coated nails.[57] The membranes formed in reaction to PMMA spacers have been found to be biologically active and usage of spacers with the goal of membrane formation is called the Masquelet technique.[58,59]

Advantages of PMMA include its structural properties and space-filling capacity. These advantages are lacking in other forms of local antibiotic administration, such as antibiotic powder, aqueous solutions, gels, and collagen or chitosan sponges. Like many other forms of local

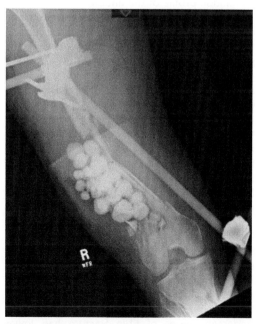

Fig. 2. Radiograph of patient with type IIIA open femur fracture treated initially with debridement and irrigation, placement of vancomycin/tobramycin-impregnated PMMA beads, and placement of external fixator.

antibiotic delivery, PMMA beads provide a method of delivery of high local antibiotic concentrations without associated high systemic levels.[60,61] Disadvantages include its nonbiodegradable nature and need for subsequent surgical removal. PMMA beads, spacers, or nails, if left in place, may act as a foreign body actually harboring biofilm and antibiotic-resistant bacteria.[62]

Antibiotics mixed with the PMMA must have certain qualities. They must be available in powder form, have broad antibiotic coverage with little resistance, and be thermally stable due to the exothermic polymerization process of PMMA formation. Commonly used antibiotics include vancomycin, tobramycin, gentamycin, erythromycin, and cefuroxime.[63]

The elution profile of antibiotic PMMA has been well delineated in multiple studies. There appears to be a rapid release of a high concentration of antibiotic during the first several days after implantation, the amount of which is quite variable among different subjects.[61] This rapid release is followed by a sustained release of antibiotic below a therapeutic concentration allowing biofilm formation in in vitro studies.[64] Additionally, this low-level release may also contribute to antibiotic resistance.[63] The type and combination of antibiotics used along with the type of PMMA used also has an effect on the elution profile of the antibiotic.[65]

Recent literature has focused on improving the consistency and duration of antibiotic elution from PMMA. In one study, addition of a hydrophilic additive, Pluronic F68, showed sustained release of vancomycin for approximately 11 weeks and allowed almost 100% release of the antibiotic without affecting the mechanical properties of the cement.[63] In another study, low-frequency ultrasound was used to increase both short-term and long-term antibiotic elution without compromising mechanical strength.[66] These newer additions to PMMA and mixing techniques may make PMMA antibiotic delivery more efficacious and possibly expand indications.

Literature supports the efficacy of PMMA delivery of local antibiotic in the treatment of open fractures. The adjunctive use of local antibiotics in addition to systemic antibiotics for open tibia fractures undergoing intramedullary nailing was recently analyzed with a systematic review and meta-analysis. In that study, all Gustilo and Anderson[5] types of tibia fracture had lower infection rates when local antibiotics were used in addition to systemic antibiotics. For type III open fractures, patients receiving only systemic antibiotics had an infection rate of 14.4%, compared with an infection rate of 2.4% when local antibiotics were used. For type IIIB and IIIC fractures, the risk of infection was 31.2% for those receiving only systemic antibiotics, but was lowered to 8.8% with the addition of local antibiotics. The studies that used local antibiotics, almost exclusively used PMMA beads impregnated with vancomycin or tobramycin. A gentamicin-coated intramedullary nail was used in a very small number of patients.[67]

Ostermann and colleagues[68] reported the results of 1085 open fractures treated with an antibiotic bead pouch and systemic antibiotics versus systemic antibiotics alone. The investigators reported a 3.7% incidence of acute infection and/or chronic osteomyelitis in the group treated with the addition of the bead pouch versus a 12% incidence in the group treated without the bead pouch. Higher-grade open fractures (type IIIB) obtained the greatest benefit from the addition of the tobramycin-impregnated beads.[68]

Polymethylmethacrylate will likely continue to have a role in the management of high-grade open fractures, infections, bone defects, and arthroplasty. Its unique advantages include its ability to fill dead space and confer certain mechanical properties not available in other antibiotic delivery methods. The recent additions and modifications to the PMMA mixing process may improve its antibiotic elution profile and increase its effectiveness and potential uses.

Antibiotics Without Carrier

In the simplest form, antibiotics can be directly placed into wounds without the use of a carrier substrate. The use of topical vancomycin in powder form is well described in the orthopedic literature, with most applications describing its use in spinal surgery for the prevention of surgical site infection, but with mixed results.[69–71] However, little has been described for the use of open fractures. Recent animal studies have evaluated the use of vancomycin powder in a contaminated fracture model in rats. Tennent and colleagues[72] found that vancomycin powder was effective at reducing bacterial counts when applied within 6 hours of contamination; however, when the powder was applied 24 hours after contamination, there was no significant reduction in the bacterial counts. Similar results were found when vancomycin-impregnated PMMA beads were placed into the wounds. However, vancomycin was detectable in the blood of all animals at 6 and 24 hours postapplication when vancomycin powder was used. These levels declined over time, with fewer than 30%

of the animals having detectable quantities of vancomycin in their serum by day 14. In contrast, those animals that received vancomycin-impregnated PMMA beads had negligible levels of serum vancomycin at 6 and 24 hours postapplication.

Other investigators have evaluated the use of injected aqueous antibiotic solutions for infection prophylaxis. Lawing and colleagues[73] in a retrospective review studied 351 open fractures that were treated with systemic antibiotics alone (183 fractures) or a combination of systemic antibiotics plus locally injected aminoglycosides at the time of index surgical procedure (168 fractures). For the local antibiotic group, an aqueous solution of either gentamicin or tobramycin was injected into the wound cavity after wound closure. For select high-grade fractures, a catheter was placed into the wound and irrigated with the antibiotic aqueous solution every 6 hours for 3 to 5 days postoperatively. The aqueous aminoglycoside group had a significantly lower infection rate (9.5%) compared with the control group (19.7%). After adjusting for potential confounding variables, the administration of aqueous aminoglycoside was found to be an independent predictor of lower infection rates in both deep and superficial infections. There was no impact, however, on the rate of nonunion between the 2 groups. Interestingly, there was no apparent benefit in the group of select high-grade fractures that received postoperative irrigations of the antibiotic solution.

Aqueous antibiotic solutions have been used in other orthopedic specialties. Lovallo and colleagues[74] studied the use of aqueous gentamicin in shoulder arthroplasty. They compared 164 patients treated with systemic antibiotics alone with 343 patients treated with systemic antibiotics plus an intra-articular injection of gentamicin at the conclusion of the procedure. The patients with systemic antibiotics alone had a 3.0% infection rate, compared with an infection rate of 0.29% in those who received intra-articular gentamicin.

Similar results have been reported in animal studies. Cavanaugh and colleagues[75] evaluated the use of injected antibiotics in a contaminated surgical site infection model. They found that the use of systemic cefazolin plus locally injected gentamicin lowered the rate of postoperative infection approximately sevenfold. The use of systemic cefazolin alone lowered the rate of postoperative infection only approximately twofold. Another animal model of contaminated surgical sites previously showed that aqueous gentamicin injected after wound closure was

significantly better at reducing bacterial counts than systemic gentamicin alone.[76] Similar results have been found using animal models for total knee arthroplasty in which local cefazolin and local vancomycin were more effective at lowering bacterial counts than the same dose of antibiotic given systemically.[77] More studies are needed to evaluate the possible systemic effects of locally applied antibiotics, but it appears as though antibiotics applied to contaminated wounds can lower bacterial counts more than systemic antibiotics alone.

Gels

A novel approach to local antibiotic delivery is the recent development of bioabsorbable gels. Few studies have been published, but a recent animal study suggests that further clinical investigations are warranted. Penn-Barwell and colleagues[78] investigated the use of a bioabsorbable phospholipid gel (DFA-02; Dr Reddy's Laboratories Inc, Bridgewater, NJ) that delivers vancomycin and gentamicin and compared this gel with the traditional use of PMMA cement beads. This study used a segmental defect rat model contaminated with *S aureus*. In the gel group, 1 mL of gel containing vancomycin and gentamicin was spread throughout the wound. In the bead group, four 3-mm beads containing vancomycin and tobramycin were placed within the wound. After 2 weeks, 19 of the 20 specimens that used only antibiotic-laden PMMA beads had detectable bacteria. In the gel group, only 8 of the 20 specimens had detectable bacteria. All 20 of the control specimen (no local antibiotics placed) had detectable bacteria. Additionally, quantitative cultures demonstrated significantly less bacteria in the wounds treated with the gel than in the control or bead group.[78] However, in a separate study by the same group using fewer subjects per study group, they found that there was no difference in bacterial eradication when using PMMA beads or bioabsorbable gel.[79] Regardless, the combination of systemic antibiotics plus either antibiotic-impregnated PMMA beads or gel was superior to the use of systemic antibiotics alone at eradicating infection. Although not yet approved by the Food and Drug Administration for use, bioabsorbable gels do provide certain advantages to traditional PMMA beads and do warrant additional research.

Collagen Sponge

Collagen sponges have been used in clinical practice for more than 3 decades,[80] having first been used for wound dressings and hemostasis.[81] The collagen sponge is unique when compared with PMMA in that it is characterized by complete dissolution by phagocytosis and enzymatic degradation,[82] thus eliminating the need for a second procedure for PMMA removal. This process takes, on average, approximately 8 weeks for full absorption of the sponge.[83] The collagen sponge also is characterized by rapid release of antibiotic from the sponge. In vitro studies have compared the release of gentamicin from collagen sheets with PMMA beads. With the collagen sheet, 95% of the gentamicin was released within 1.5 hours, whereas only 8% had been released from the PMMA beads.[84] However, in vivo studies suggest that the release appears to be dependent on the fluid supply of the surrounding tissues. Effective local concentrations of antibiotics can be maintained in bony sites for approximately 1 week, but for less than 24 hours in well-perfused areas.[85]

Studies evaluating the use of gentamicin-collagen sponges in orthopedic trauma are encouraging.[86,87] Chaudhary and colleagues[88] recently reviewed a series of 35 patients presenting acutely with open fractures. These patients underwent irrigation and debridement, immediate open reduction and plate fixation, along with placement of an antibiotic-eluting collagen sponge around the plate just before wound closure. Deep infection subsequently developed in 6.5% of patients (2 of 31 available for follow-up). No patient required implant removal and no patient developed nonunion.

Gentamicin-collagen sponges have been used extensively for the treatment of osteomyelitis. Leung and colleagues[89] report on a cohort of 50 patients treated for chronic osteomyelitis. All patients underwent surgical debridement, intravenous (IV) antibiotics, and placement of a collagen sponge infused with gentamicin. They reported a 12% recurrence rate of infection, compared with a recurrence rate of 20% to 30% often reported in the literature. A prospective randomized study of 20 patients with long-bone osteomyelitis directly compared collagen sponges with PMMA beads, both infused with gentamicin. Complete resolution of the infection was noted in 80% of the patients with collagen sponge and in 90% of the patients with PMMA. As expected, gentamicin was rapidly released from the collagen sponge, leading to high levels of antibiotic in the wound exudate and in the urine within the first 48 hours, whereas gentamicin was more slowly released from the PMMA beads.[90] Ipsen and colleagues[91] previously reported on a series of 10 patients

treated with gentamicin-collagen sponge, in which no recurrence of infection was observed in any of the patients. Similar studies have previously been reported, in which gentamicin-collagen sponges show good results in eradicating osteomyelitis.[92]

Studies evaluating the use of gentamicin-collagen sponges in clean surgical wounds are mixed. In a multicenter randomized controlled trial of nearly 700 patients receiving hemiarthroplasty for femoral neck fracture, the addition of gentamicin-eluting collagen sponge had no impact on deep or superficial infection rates.[93] However, in a meta-analysis of randomized trials evaluating the nonorthopedic use of gentamicin-containing collagen sponges, there was a significant decrease in surgical site infection in both clean and clean-contaminated surgeries.[94]

Adverse effects also have been reported with the use of gentamicin-collagen sponges. In a series of 12 patients being treated for infected total hip arthroplasty with gentamicin-impregnated collagen sponges, 7 of the 12 patients were found to have toxic serum levels of gentamicin (>2 mg/L). In 3 cases, there was a significant drop in renal clearance that persisted, and in 3 other patients there was a temporary decrease in renal clearance that resolved. Each patient in that study received between 4 and 6 sponges implanted, with each sponge containing 130 mg gentamicin.[95]

Other studies have shown a possible increased risk of infection with collagen sponges. In a large prospective trial evaluating the use of gentamicin-collagen sponge for infection prophylaxis in colorectal surgery, investigators found that patients treated with the collagen sponge actually had a higher infection rate, presumably because the antibiotics eluted quicker than the sponge degraded, leaving foreign material within the wound.[96]

Additionally, collagen sponges have been available commercially only as sponges infused with gentamicin. Gentamicin has previously been shown to have detrimental effects on fracture healing,[97–100] making them less desirable for use in open fractures.

Chitosan Sponge

Another type of sponge that has recently come into use is the chitosan sponge (Fig. 3). Similar to the collagen sponge, it is an antibiotic-impregnated sponge that is absorbed by the host tissue if left in place. Chitosan is the second-most abundant polysaccharide after cellulose and is made from shellfish sources, such as shrimp and crab.[101] Chitosan is a deacetylated

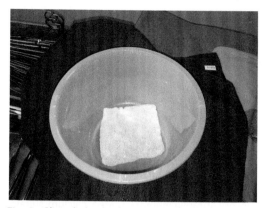

Fig. 3. Clinical photo of chitosan sponge.

derivative of chitin,[102] both of which are well known to have positive effects on wound healing.[103–105] Animal studies have shown that chitosan accelerates infiltration of polymorphonuclear cells into wounds at the early stages of wound healing, followed by the increased production of collagen by fibroblasts within granulation tissue as compared with control materials.[106]

Studies evaluating the elution of antibiotic from chitosan sponges show quick delivery of antibiotic. In one study, in vitro elution of amikacin was 85% complete after 1 hour and 96% complete after 72 hours. For daptomycin, 31% was released by 1 hour and 88% was released at 72 hours. For both agents tested, the eluted antibiotic was able to inhibit the growth of S aureus, indicating that the eluted antibiotic retained its antimicrobial activity.[107] A follow-up in vitro study from the same group showed similar results. In that study, the release of vancomycin from the chitosan sponge remained above the minimum inhibitory concentration (MIC) for S aureus for 72 hours and the release of amikacin remained above the MIC for Pseudomonas aeruginosa for 48 hours.[108]

Few clinical studies are available to demonstrate the in vivo effectiveness of antibiotic-eluting chitosan sponges for orthopedic applications. In a recent animal study, chitosan sponges eluting either vancomycin or amikacin were effective in decreasing bacterial counts in contaminated wounds. Serum antibiotic concentrations remained less than 15% of the target serum level for systemic treatment. Additionally, by 42 hours, the sponges were, on average, 85% dissolved.[101] Additional studies are needed to evaluate the chitosan sponge as a potential alternative to traditional PMMA beads. Furthermore, the chitosan sponge is available without antibiotics already infused. The surgeon can thus select which antibiotics they want to

incorporate, unlike the gentamicin-collagen sponge. The surgeon also has more antibiotic options available than with PMMA beads, as antibiotic thermal stability is not a concern.

Calcium Sulfate

Another potential drug-delivery device is calcium sulfate. Calcium sulfate impregnated with antibiotics (**Fig. 4**) has been used for decades in the treatment and prevention of orthopedic infections.[109,110] Calcium sulfate is an osteoconductive material that is resorbed at a rate similar to that of bone formation.[111]

Animal studies have evaluated the local and systemic levels of tobramycin after impregnated calcium sulfate beads are implanted into tissues. Local tobramycin levels have been found to rapidly rise over the first 24 hours, and then rapidly decline. Levels of tobramycin were found to still be therapeutic at 14 days after implantation. Some animal subjects, however, had elevated local tobramycin levels for at least 28 days. Serum levels, however, rose quickly and peaked during the first hour after implantation. Serum levels became undetectable after 24 hours.[112] In vitro testing has compared the elution of daptomycin and tobramycin from calcium sulfate beads. Similar to other studies, both antibiotics are rapidly released from the beads over the first 24 hours, followed by a rapid decline in the following days. However, after a 28-day period, the daptomycin-containing beads released only 35% of the total antibiotic incorporated into the beads, whereas 68% of the total tobramycin had been released.[113] Other in vitro studies have shown that the peak local concentration of vancomycin when eluted from calcium sulfate beads occurs 48 hours after implantation.[114] Other variations of calcium sulfate beads have been developed that elute

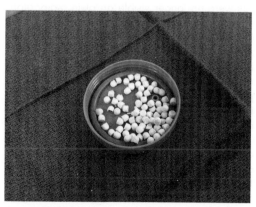

Fig. 4. Clinical photo of vancomycin/tobramycin-impregnated calcium sulfate beads.

antibiotics quicker and dissolve over only a few days,[115] which may pose a clinical advantage in certain situations.

Few clinical studies are available to document the effectiveness of calcium sulfate in preventing and treating infection. One study evaluated the use of calcium sulfate beads in open long-bone fractures treated with internal fixation. That study of 28 patients had 15 type II open fractures, 11 type IIIA open fractures, and 2 type IIIC open fractures as classified by Gustilo and Anderson.[5] All fractures were treated with vancomycin-impregnated calcium sulfate beads and internal fixation. At an average follow-up of 10.5 months, no infection was present in the 26 patients available for follow-up. Two patients were found to have exudation from the wound or drain incision, but both were treated with local wound care only. The calcium sulfate beads were no longer visible on plain radiographs at 1 month (15 cases) and 2 months (11 cases).[116] Other case series have documented the beneficial use of antibiotic-impregnated calcium sulfate in combat-related fractures.[117]

Several studies have evaluated the use of tobramycin-impregnated calcium sulfate beads in osteomyelitis. A prospective randomized clinic trial evaluated the effectiveness of traditional PMMA beads with tobramycin-impregnated calcium sulfate beads in patients with chronic osteomyelitis and/or infected nonunions. At 24 months, both groups had eradiation of infection in 86% of patients (12 of 14 patients in each group). As expected, the PMMA group required more repeat surgical procedures for removal of the PMMA beads.[118] One study evaluated the addition of tobramycin-impregnated calcium sulfate to the standard treatment of surgical debridement and IV antibiotics. In that study, infection was eradicated in 23 (92%) of the 25 study participants. The calcium sulfate pellets were no longer visible on plain radiographs at 1 month (1 case), 2 months (12 cases), 3 months (10 cases), and 6 months (2 cases), with the average time to resorption being 2.7 months. Eight patients developed a sterile draining sinus, which closed on average at 2 to 3 months postoperatively, around the same time that the calcium sulfate was no longer visible on plain radiographs.[119]

One retrospective review evaluated the use of commercially available tobramycin-impregnated calcium sulfate beads as adjunctive treatment for chronic osteomyelitis. The addition of local antibiotics to the standard treatment of surgical debridement plus IV antibiotics resulted in eradication of infection in 20 of 21 patients at an average follow-up of 16 months. Seven of the 21 cases were complicated by wound drainage. Three-quarters of these cases went on to have wound-healing problems as compared with one-third of the cases without wound drainage. Accordingly, serous drainage appears to double the relative risk of wound-healing problems ($P = .06$). Additionally, 1 patient developed transient AKI.[120] A similar study evaluated 65 patients also receiving surgical debridement, IV antibiotics, and implantation of tobramycin-impregnated calcium sulfate beads for chronic osteomyelitis. That study showed that the addition of tobramycin-impregnated calcium sulfate pellets did not have a significant impact on infection eradication, except in a small subset of patients who had normal immune systems.[121]

Several animal studies are available evaluating the use of calcium sulfate. Animal studies show that tobramycin-impregnated calcium sulfate beads are equally as effective as traditional tobramycin-impregnated PMMA beads in preventing infections in a contaminated open fracture model.[122] Similar efficacy also was shown when the tobramycin-impregnated calcium sulfate was combined with demineralized bone matrix, resulting in similar reduced bacterial counts compared with tobramycin PMMA beads.[123] Additionally, there appears to be equal effectiveness between "hand-made" tobramycin PMMA beads, commercially available tobramycin PMMA beads, and commercially available tobramycin calcium sulfate beads.[124]

The most common complication associated with the use of calcium sulfate is serous drainage from the wound, which occurs in from 4% to 51% of cases[125,126]; however, as shown previously, this tends to resolve as the calcium sulfate is resorbed. Regardless, calcium sulfate has been shown effective for use in acute open fractures as well as for the treatment of established osteomyelitis.

SUMMARY

The orthopedic community has learned much about the treatment of open fractures from the tremendous work of Ramon Gustilo, Michael Patzakis, and others. However, open fractures continue to be very difficult challenges. Type III open fractures continue to be associated with high infection rates. Some combination of systemic and local antibiotics may be most appropriate in these high-grade open fractures. Further research is still necessary in determining optimal systemic antibiotic regimens, as well as the role of local antibiotics. Any new discoveries related to novel systemic antibiotics or local antibiotic carriers also will need to be evaluated related to cost.

REFERENCES

1. Harley BJ, Beaupre LA, Jones CA, et al. The effect of time to definitive treatment on the rate of nonunion and infection in open fractures. J Orthop Trauma 2002;16:484–90.
2. Antonova E, Le TK, Burge R, et al. Tibial shaft fractures: costly burden of nonunions. BMC Musculoskelet Disord 2013;14:42.
3. Brinker MR, Hanus BD, Sen M, et al. The devastating effects of tibial nonunion on health-related quality of life. J Bone Joint Surg Am 2013;95(24):2170–6.
4. Patzakis MJ, Harvey JP, Ivier D. The role of antibiotics in the management of open fractures. J Bone Joint Surg Am 1974;56:532–41.
5. Gustilo RB, Anderson JT. Prevention of infection in the treatment of one thousand and twenty-five open fractures of long bones: retrospective and prospective analyses. J Bone Joint Surg Am 1976;58A:453–8.
6. Gustilo RB, Mendoza RM, Williams DN. Problems in the management of type III (severe) open fractures: a new classification of type III open fractures. J Trauma 1984;24:742–6.
7. Templeman DC, Gulli B, Tsukayama DT, et al. Update on the management of open fractures of the tibial shaft. Clin Orthop Relat Res 1998;(350):18–25.
8. Patzakis MJ, Wilkins J. Factors influencing infection rate in open fracture wounds. Clin Orthop Relat Res 1989;(243):36–40.
9. Chen AF, Schreiber VM, Washington W, et al. What is the rate of methicillin-resistant *Staphylococcus aureus* and gram-negative infections in open fractures. Clin Orthop Relat Res 2013;471:3135–40.
10. Torbert JT, Joshi M, Moraff A, et al. Current bacterial speciation and antibiotic resistance in deep infections after operative fixation of fractures. J Orthop Trauma 2015;29:7–17.
11. Patzakis MJ, Wilkins J, Moore TM. Use of antibiotics in open tibial fractures. Clin Orthop Relat Res 1983;(178):31–5.
12. Lack WD, Karunakar MA, Angerame MR, et al. Type III open tibia fractures: immediate antibiotic prophylaxis minimizes infection. J Orthop Trauma 2015;29:1–6.
13. Brumback RJ, Jones AL. Interobserver agreement in the classification of open fractures of the tibia: the results of a survey of two hundred and forty-five orthopaedic surgeons. J Bone Joint Surg Am 1994;76:1162–6.
14. Khatod M, Botte MJ, Hoyt DB, et al. Outcomes in open tibia fractures: relationship between delay in treatment and infection. J Trauma 2003;55:949–54.
15. Srour M, Inaba K, Okoye O, et al. Prospective evaluation of treatment of open fractures: effect of time to irrigation and debridement. JAMA Surg 2015;150:332–6.
16. Tripuraneni K, Ganga S, Quinn R, et al. The effect of time delay to surgical debridement of open tibia shaft fractures on infection rate. Orthopaedics 2008;31(12).
17. Al-Arabi YB, Nader M, Hamidian-Jahromi AR, et al. The effect of the timing of antibiotics and surgical treatment on infection rates in open long-bone fractures: a 9-year prospective study from a district general hospital. Injury 2007;38:900–5.
18. Weber D, Dulai SK, Bergman J, et al. Time to initial operative treatment following open fracture does not impact development of deep infection: a prospective cohort study of 736 subjects. J Orthop Trauma 2014;28:613–9.
19. Luchette FA, Bone LB, Born CT, et al. EAST Practice Management Guidelines work group: practice management guidelines for prophylactic antibiotic use in open fractures. Eastern Association for the Surgery of Trauma; 2000. Available at: http://www.east.org/tgp/openfrac.pdf. Accessed July 31, 2016.
20. Hoff WS, Bonadies JA, Cachecho R, et al. EAST Practice Management Guidelines work group: update to practice management guidelines for prophylactic antibiotic use in open fractures. J Trauma 2011;70:751–4.
21. Hauser CJ, Adams CA, Eachempati SR, et al. Surgical Infection Society guideline: prophylactic antibiotic use in open fractures: an evidence-based guideline. Surg Infect (Larchmt) 2006;7:379–405.
22. Hospenthal DR, Murray CK, Andersen RC, et al. Guidelines for the prevention of infections associated with combat-related injuries: 2011 update. J Trauma 2011;71:s210–34.
23. Dellinger EP, Caplan ES, Weaver LD, et al. Duration of preventive antibiotic administration for open extremity fractures. Arch Surg 1988;123:333–8.
24. Benson DR, Riggins RS, Lawrence RM, et al. Treatment of open fractures: a prospective study. J Trauma 1983;23:25–30.
25. Vasenius J, Tulikoura I, Vainionpaa S, et al. Clindamycin versus cloxacillin in the treatment of 240 open fractures. A randomized prospective study. Ann Chir Gynaecol 1998;87:224–8.
26. Sorger JI, Kirk PG, Ruhnke CJ, et al. Once daily, high dose versus divided low dose gentamicin

for open fractures. Clin Orthop Relat Res 1999;(366):197–204.

27. Russell GV, King C, May CG, et al. Once daily high-dose gentamicin to prevent infection in open fractures of the tibial shaft: a preliminary study. South Med J 2001;94:1185–91.

28. Bell S, Davey P, Nathwani D, et al. Risk of AKI with gentamicin as surgical prophylaxis. J Am Soc Nephrol 2014;25:2625–32.

29. Oliveira JF, Silva CA, Barbieri CD, et al. Prevalence and risk factors for aminoglycoside nephrotoxicity in intensive care units. Antimicrob Agents Chemother 2009;53:2887–91.

30. Obremskey W, Molina C, Collinge C, et al. Current practice in the management of open fractures among orthopaedic trauma surgeons. Part A: initial management. A survey of orthopaedic trauma surgeons. J Orthop Trauma 2014;28: e198–202.

31. Levy EM, Viscoli CM, Horwitz RI. The effect of acute renal failure on mortality. A cohort analysis. JAMA 1996;275:1489–94.

32. Liano F, Pascual J, Madero R, et al. The Madrid Acute Renal Failure Study Group: the spectrum of acute renal failure in the intensive care unit compared with that seen in other settings. Kidney Int Suppl 1998;66:s16–24.

33. Uchino S, Bellamo R, Goldsmith D, et al. As assessment of the RIFLE criteria for acute renal failure in hospitalized patients. Crit Care Med 2006;34:1913–7.

34. Rodriguez L, Jung HS, Goulet JA, et al. Evidence-based protocol for prophylactic antibiotics in open fractures: improved antibiotic stewardship with no increase in infection rates. J Trauma Acute Care Surg 2014;77:400–8.

35. Redfern J, Wasilko SM, Groth ME, et al. Surgical site infections in patients with type-III open fractures: comparing antibiotic prophylaxis with cefazolin plus gentamicin versus pipercillin/tazobactam. J Orthop Trauma 2016;30:415–9.

36. Johnson KD, Bone LB, Scheinberg R. Severe open tibia fractures: a study protocol. J Orthop Trauma 1988;2:175–8.

37. Maxson B, Serrano-Riera R, Bender M, et al. Vancomycin and cefepime antibiotic prophylaxis for open fractures reduces infection rates in grade III open fractures compared to cefazolin and gentamicin, avoids potential nephrotoxicity, and does not result in antibiotic resistance with MRSA. Read at the annual meeting of the Orthopaedic Trauma Association. San Diego (CA), October 10, 2015.

38. Saveli CC, Morgan SJ, Belkap RW, et al. Prophylactic antibiotics in open fractures: a pilot randomized clinical safety study. J Orthop Trauma 2013; 27:552–7.

39. ASHP Therapeutic Guidelines. Clinical practice guidelines for antimicrobial prophylaxis in surgery. Available at: http://www.ashp.org/surgical-guidelines. Accessed July 31, 2016.

40. Collinge CA, McWilliam-Ross K, Kelly KC, et al. Substantial improvement in prophylactic antibiotic administration for open fracture patients: results of a performance improvement program. J Orthop Trauma 2014;28:620–5.

41. Fischer MD, Gustilo RB, Varecka TF. The timing of flap coverage, bone-grafting, and intramedullary nailing in patients who have a fracture of the tibial shaft with extensive soft-tissue injury. J Bone Joint Surg Am 1991;73:1316–22.

42. Lee J. Efficacy of cultures in the management of open fractures. Clin Orthop Relat Res 1997;(339): 71–5.

43. Jenkinson RJ, Kiss A, Johnson S, et al. Delayed wound closure increases deep-infection rate associated with lower-grade open fractures: a propensity-matched cohort study. J Bone Joint Surg Am 2014;96:380–6.

44. Stannard JP, Volgas DA, Stewart R, et al. Negative pressure wound therapy after severe high open fractures: a prospective randomized study. J Orthop Trauma 2009;23:552–7.

45. Blum ML, Esser M, Richardson M, et al. Negative pressure wound therapy reduces deep infection rate in open tibial fractures. J Orthop Trauma 2012;26:499–505.

46. Dedmond BT, Korteis B, Punger K, et al. The use of negative-pressure wound therapy (NPWT) in the temporary treatment of soft-tissue injuries associated with high-energy open tibial shaft fractures. J Orthop Trauma 2007;21:11–7.

47. Moues CM, Vos MC, van den Bemd GJ, et al. Bacterial load in relation to vacuum-assisted closure wound therapy: a prospective randomized trial. Wound Repair Regen 2004;12:11–7.

48. Lalliss SJ, Stinner DJ, Waterman SM, et al. Negative pressure wound therapy reduces *Pseudomonas* wound contamination more than *Staphylococcus aureus*. J Orthop Trauma 2010;24: 598–602.

49. Pitt D, Aubin JM. Joseph Lister: the father of modern surgery. Can J Surg 2012;55(5):E8–9.

50. Jenson NK, Johnsrud LW, Nelson MN. The local implantation of sulfanilamide in compound fractures. Surgery 1939;6:1–12.

51. Buchholz HW, Elson RA, Engelbrecht E, et al. Management of deep infection of total hip replacement. J Bone Joint Surg Br 1981;63-B: 342–53.

52. Hedstrom SA, Lidgren L, Torholm C, et al. Antibiotic containing bone cement beads in the treatment of deep muscle and skeletal infections. Acta Orthop Scand 1980;51:863–9.

53. Castaneda P, McLaren A, Tavaziva G, et al. Biofilm antimicrobial susceptibility increases with antimicrobial exposure time. Clin Orthop Relat Res 2016;474:1659–64.
54. Nelson CL. The current status of material used for depot delivery of drugs. Clin Orthop Relat Res 2004;(427):72–8.
55. Xinlong M, Yang Y, Jianxiong M, et al. Comparison of mechanical properties of polymethylmethacrylate of different mixing ratios. J Med Eng Technol 2011;35(1):54–8.
56. Decoster TA, Bozorgnia S. Antibiotic beads. J Am Acad Orthop Surg 2008;16(11):674–8.
57. Thonse R, Conway J. Antibiotic cement-coated interlocking nail for the treatment of infected nonunions and segmental bone defects. J Orthop Trauma 2007;21(4):258–68.
58. Masquelet AC, Begue T. The concept of induced membrane for reconstruction of long bone defects. Orthop Clin North Am 2010;41(1):27–37.
59. Mauffrey C, Hake ME, Chadayammuri V, et al. Reconstruction of long bone infections using the induced membrane technique: tips and tricks. J Orthop Trauma 2016;30(6):e188–93.
60. Wahlig H, Dingeldein E, Bergmann R, et al. The release of gentamicin from polymethylmethacrylate beads. An experimental and pharmacokinetic study. J Bone Joint Surg Br 1978;60-B(2):270–5.
61. Anagnostakos K, Wilmes P, Schmitt E, et al. Elution of gentamicin and vancomycin from polymethylmethacrylate beads and hip spacers in vivo. Acta Orthop 2009;80(2):193–7.
62. Nuet D, van de Belt H, van Horn JR, et al. Residual gentamicin-release from antibiotic-loaded polymethylmethacrylate beads after 5 years of implantation. Biomaterials 2003;24(10):1829–31.
63. Oh EJ, Oh SH, Lee IS, et al. Antibiotic-eluting hydrophilized PMMA bone cement with prolonged bactericidal effect for the treatment of osteomyelitis. J Biomater Appl 2016;30(10):1534–44.
64. van de Belt H, Neut D, Schenk W, et al. Gentamicin release from polymethylmethacrylate bone cements and Staphylococcus aureus biofilm formation. Acta Orthop Scand 2000;71(6):625–9.
65. Penner MJ, Duncan CP, Masri BA. The in vitro elution characteristics of antibiotic-loaded CMW and palacos-r bone cements. J Arthroplasty 1999;14(2):209–14.
66. Wendling A, Mar D, Wischmeier N, et al. Combination of modified mixing technique and low frequency ultrasound to control the elution profile of vancomycin-loaded acrylic bone cement. Bone Joint Res 2016;5(2):26–32.
67. Craig J, Fuchs T, Jenks M, et al. Systematic review and meta-analysis of the additional benefit of local prophylactic antibiotic therapy for infection rates in open tibia fractures treated with intramedullary nailing. Int Orthop 2014;38(5):1025–30.
68. Ostermann PA, Seligson D, Henry SL. Local antibiotic therapy for severe open fractures. A review of 1085 consecutive cases. J Bone Joint Surg Br 1995;77(1):93–7.
69. Tubaki VR, Rajasekaran S, Shetty AP. Effects of using intravenous antibiotic only versus local intrawound vancomycin antibiotic powder application in addition to intravenous antibiotics on postoperative infection in spine surgery in 907 patients. Spine 2013;38(25):2149–55.
70. Molinari RW, Khera OA, Molinari WJ. Prophylactic intraoperative powdered vancomycin and postoperative deep spinal wound infection: 1,512 consecutive surgical cases over a 6-year period. Eur Spine J 2012;21(Suppl 4):S476–82.
71. Kanj WW, Flynn JM, Spiegel DA, et al. Vancomycin prophylaxis of surgical site infection in clean orthopedic surgery. Orthopedics 2013;36(2):138–46.
72. Tennent DJ, Shiels SM, Sanchez CJ, et al. Time dependent effectiveness of locally applied vancomycin powder in a contaminated traumatic orthopaedic wound model. J Orthop Trauma 2016;30(10):531–7.
73. Lawing CR, Lin FC, Dahners LE. Local injection of aminoglycosides for prophylaxis against infection in open fractures. J Bone Joint Surg Am 2015;97(22):1844–51.
74. Lovallo J, Helming J, Jafari SM, et al. Intraoperative intra-articular injection of gentamicin: will it decrease the risk of infection in total shoulder arthroplasty? J Shoulder Elbow Surg 2014;23(9):1272–6.
75. Cavanaugh DL, Berry J, Yarboro SR, et al. Better prophylaxis against surgical site infection with local as well as systemic antibiotics. J Bone Joint Surg Am 2009;91(8):1907–12.
76. Yarboro SR, Baum EJ, Dahners LE. Locally administered antibiotics for prophylaxis against surgical wound infection: an in vivo study. J Bone Joint Surg Am 2007;89(5):929–33.
77. Young SW, Roberts R, Johnson S, et al. Regional intraosseous administration of prophylactic antibiotics is more effective than systemic administration in a mouse model of TKA. Clin Orthop Relat Res 2015;473(11):3573–84.
78. Penn-Barwell JG, Murray CK, Wenke JC. Local antibiotic delivery by a bioabsorbable gel is superior to PMMA bead depot in reducing infection in an open fracture model. J Orthop Trauma 2014;28(6):370–5.
79. Rand BC, Penn-Barwell JG, Wenke JC. Combined local and systemic antibiotic delivery improves eradication of wound contamination: an animal

experimental model of contaminated fracture. Bone Joint J 2015;97-B(10):1423–7.

80. Ascherl R, Stemberger A, Lechner F, et al. Treatment of chronic osteomyelitis with a collagen-antibiotic compound – preliminary report. Unfallchirurg 1986;12(3):125–7 [in German].

81. Chvapil M. Collagen sponge: theory and practice of medical applications. J Biomed Mater Res 1977;11(5):721–41.

82. Diefenbeck M, Mückley T, Hofmann GO. Prophylaxis and treatment of implant-related infections by local application of antibiotics. Injury 2006; 37(Suppl 2):S95–104.

83. El-Husseiny M, Patel S, MacFarlane RJ, et al. Biodegradable antibiotic delivery systems. J Bone Joint Surg Br 2011;93(2):151–7.

84. Sørensen TS, Sørensen AI, Merser S. Rapid release of gentamicin from collagen sponge. In vitro comparison with plastic beads. Acta Orthop Scand 1990;61(4):353–6.

85. Schlapp M, Friess W. Collagen/PLGA microparticle composites for local controlled delivery of gentamicin. J Pharm Sci 2003;92(11):2145–51.

86. Feil J, Bohnet S, Neugebauer R, et al. Bioresorbable collage-gentamicin compound as local antibiotic therapy. Aktuelle Probl Chir Orthop 1990;34:94–103 [in German].

87. Ascherl R, Stemberg A, Lechner F, et al. Local treatment of infection with collagen gentamicin. Aktuelle Probl Chir Orthop 1990;34:85–93 [in German].

88. Chaudhary S, Sen RK, Saini UC, et al. Use of gentamicin-loaded collagen sponge in internal fixation of open fractures. Chin J Traumatol 2011;14(4):209–14.

89. Leung AH, Hawthorn BR, Simpson AH. The effectiveness of local antibiotics in treating chronic osteomyelitis in a cohort of 50 patients with an average of 4 years follow-up. Open Orthop J 2015;9:372–8.

90. Letsch R, Rosenthal E, Joka T. Local antibiotic administration in osteomyelitis treatment – a comparative study with two different carrier substances. Aktuelle Traumatol 1993;23(7):324–9 [in German].

91. Ipsen T, Jørgensen PS, Damholt V, et al. Gentamicin-collagen sponge for local applications. 10 cases of chronic osteomyelitis followed for 1 year. Acta Orthop Scand 1991;62(6):592–4.

92. Wernet E, Ekkernkamp A, Jellestad H, et al. Antibiotic-containing collagen sponge in therapy of osteitis. Unfallchirurg 1992;95(5):259–64 [in German].

93. Westberg M, Frihagen F, Brun OC, et al. Effectiveness of gentamicin-containing collagen sponges for prevention of surgical site infection after hip arthroplasty: a multicenter randomized trial. Clin Infect Dis 2015;60(12):1752–9.

94. Chang WK, Srinivasa S, MacCormick AD, et al. Gentamicin-collagen implants to reduce surgical site infection: systematic review and meta-analysis of randomized trials. Ann Surg 2013;258(1):59–65.

95. Swieringa AJ, Tulp NJ. Toxic serum gentamicin levels after the use of gentamicin-loaded sponges in infected total hip arthroplasty. Acta Orthop 2005;76(1):75–7.

96. Bennett-Guerrero E, Pappas TN, Koltun WA, et al. Gentamicin-collagen sponge for infection prophylaxis in colorectal surgery. N Engl J Med 2010; 363(11):1038–49.

97. Rathbone CR, Cross JD, Brown KV, et al. Effect of various concentrations of antibiotics on osteogenic cell viability and activity. J Orthop Trauma 2011;29(7):1070–4.

98. Isefuku S, Joyner CJ, Simpson AH. Gentamicin may have an adverse effect on osteogenesis. J Orthop Trauma 2003;17(3):212–6.

99. Ince A, Schütze N, Karl N, et al. Gentamicin negatively influenced osteogenic function in vitro. Int Orthop 2007;31(2):223–8.

100. Chang Y, Goldberg VM, Caplan AI. Toxic effects of gentamicin on marrow-derived human mesenchymal stem cells. Clin Orthop Relat Res 2006; 452:242–9.

101. Stinner DJ, Noel SP, Haggard WO, et al. Local antibiotic delivery using tailorable chitosan sponges: the future of infection control? J Orthop Trauma 2010;24(9):592–7.

102. Di Martino A, Sittinger M, Risbud MV. Chitosan: a versatile biopolymer for orthopaedic tissue-engineering. Biomaterials 2005;26(30):5983–90.

103. Cho YW, Cho YN, Chung SH, et al. Water-soluble chitin as a wound healing accelerator. Biomaterials 1999;20(22):2139–45.

104. Azuma K, Izumi R, Osaki T, et al. Chitin, chitosan, and its derivatives for wound healing: old and new materials. J Funct Biomater 2015;6(1):104–42.

105. Burkatovskaya M, Tegos GP, Swietlik E, et al. Use of chitosan bandage to prevent fatal infections developing from highly contaminated wounds in mice. Biomaterials 2006;27(22):4157–64.

106. Ueno H, Yamada H, Tanaka I, et al. Accelerating effects of chitosan for healing at early phase of experimental open wound in dogs. Biomaterials 1999;20(15):1407–14.

107. Noel SP, Courtney H, Bumgardner JD, et al. Chitosan films: a potential local drug delivery system for antibiotics. Clin Orthop Relat Res 2008;466(6): 1377–82.

108. Noel SP, Courtney HS, Bumgardner JD, et al. Chitosan sponges to locally deliver amikacin and vancomycin: a pilot in vitro evaluation. Clin Orthop Relat Res 2010;468(8):2074–80.

109. Mackey D, Varlet A, Debeaumont D. Antibiotic loaded plaster of Paris pellets: an in vitro study

of a possible method of local antibiotic therapy in bone infection. Clin Orthop Relat Res 1982;(167): 263–8.

110. Dacquet V, Varlet A, Tandogan RN, et al. Antibiotic-impregnated plaster of Paris beads. Trials with teicoplanin. Clin Orthop Relat Res 1992;(282):241–9.

111. Tay BK, Patel VV, Bradford DS. Calcium sulfate- and calcium phosphate-base bone substitutes. Mimicry of the mineral phase of bone. Orthop Clin North Am 1999;30(4):615–23.

112. Turner TM, Urban RM, Hall DJ, et al. Local and systemic levels of tobramycin delivered from calcium sulfate bone graft substitute pellets. Clin Orthop Relat Res 2005;(437):97–104.

113. Richelsoph KC, Webb ND, Haggard WO. Elution behavior of daptomycin-loaded calcium sulfate pellets: a preliminary study. Clin Orthop Relat Res 2007;461:68–73.

114. Aiken SS, Cooper JJ, Florance H, et al. Local release of antibiotics for surgical site infection management using high-purity calcium sulfate: an in vitro elution study. Surg Infect 2015;16(1): 54–61.

115. Jackson SR, Richelsoph KC, Courtney HS, et al. Preliminary in vitro evaluation of an adjunctive therapy for extremity wound infection reduction: rapidly resorbing local antibiotic delivery. J Orthop Res 2009;27(7):903–8.

116. Cai X, Han K, Cong X, et al. The use of calcium sulfate impregnated with vancomycin in the treatment of open fracture of long bones: a preliminary study. Orthopedics 2010;33(3).

117. Helgeson MD, Potter BK, Tucker CJ, et al. Antibiotic-impregnated calcium sulfate use in combat-related open fractures. Orthopedics 2009;32(5):323.

118. McKee MD, Li-Bland EA, Wild LM, et al. A prospective, randomized clinical trial comparing an antibiotic-impregnated bioabsorbable bone substitute with standard antibiotic-impregnated cement beads in the treatment of chronic osteomyelitis and infected nonunion. J Orthop Trauma 2010;24(8):483–90.

119. McKee MD, Wild LM, Schemitsch EH, et al. The use of an antibiotic-impregnated, osteoconductive, bioabsorbable bone substitute in the treatment of infected long bone defects: early results of a prospective trial. J Orthop Trauma 2002; 16(9):622–7.

120. Humm G, Noor S, Bridgeman P, et al. Adjuvant treatment of chronic osteomyelitis of the tibia following exogenous trauma using OSTEOSET-T: a review of 21 patients in a regional trauma centre. Strategies Trauma Limb Reconstr 2014;9(3): 157–61.

121. Chang W, Colangeli M, Colangeli S, et al. Adult osteomyelitis: debridement versus debridement plus Osteoset T pellets. Acta Orthop Belg 2007; 73(2):238–43.

122. Thomas DB, Brooks DE, Bice TG, et al. Tobramycin-impregnated calcium sulfate prevents infection in contaminated wounds. Clin Orthop Relat Res 2005;441:366–71.

123. Beardmore AA, Brooks DE, Wenke JC, et al. Effectiveness of local antibiotic delivery with an osteoinductive and osteoconductive bone-graft substitute. J Bone Joint Surg Am 2005;87(1): 107–12.

124. Wenke JC, Owens BD, Svoboda SJ, et al. Effectiveness of commercially-available antibiotic-impregnated implants. J Bone Joint Surg Br 2006;88(8):1102–4.

125. Kelly CM, Wilkins RM, Gitelis S, et al. The use of a surgical grade calcium sulfate as a bone graft substitute. Results of a multicenter trial. Clin Orthop Relat Res 2001;(382):42–50.

126. Ziran BH, Smith WR, Morgan SJ. Use of calcium-based demineralized bone matrix/allograft for nonunions and posttraumatic reconstruction of the appendicular skeleton. J Trauma 2006;63: 1324–8.

The Antibiotic Nail in the Treatment of Long Bone Infection: Technique and Results

Kenneth L. Koury, MD, John S. Hwang, MD, Michael Sirkin, MD*

KEYWORDS

- Antibiotic nail - Local antibiotic delivery - Infection - Long bone infection

KEY POINTS

- Antibiotic nails are made primarily of polymethyl methacrylate and local antibiotics.
- Antibiotic nails can provide fracture stability, manage intramedullary dead space, and allow delivery of local antibiotics.
- Antibiotic nails have proven very successful in the treatment of intramedullary bone infection.

INTRODUCTION

Antibiotic cement nails are implants created to provide an intramedullary antibiotic delivery device that also provides fracture stability. Although techniques vary by individual surgeons, these antibiotic nails are typically fashioned from metal coated with antibiotic-impregnated polymethyl methacrylate in the shape of an intramedullary nail or antibiotic cement coating an existing intramedullary nail.[1–14] Paley and Herzenberg[6] were the first to describe the utility of this device for the treatment of intramedullary osteomyelitis.

Since then, the technique has become widely described in the literature with reported indications ranging from the treatment of diagnosed intramedullary osteomyelitis to prophylactic use in damage control situations whereby there is a high risk of intramedullary osteomyelitis.[1] There are several relatively small case series documenting the utility of this device as a component of intramedullary osteomyelitis treatment in addition to adequate boney debridement and systemic antibiotics.[2,5–8,10,15] Additionally, there are several articles describing modifications to the fabrication technique of these devices.[3,4,13] The purpose of this article is to review the rationale, indications, techniques, and outcomes of antibiotic nail use in the treatment of long bone infections.

RATIONALE

The rationale for intramedullary antibiotic cement rods is an extension of the known utility of antibiotic-impregnated bone cement in the treatment of osteomyelitis. There are several studies describing the effective use of bone cement as a delivery device of antibiotics directly to an area of musculoskeletal infection.[16–23] The importance of local antibiotics in the treatment of bone infection has been well accepted and become a standard component of current osteomyelitis management.[16,23–26]

Cierny and colleagues[25,27–29] described 4 key principles in the treatment of osteomyelitis:

1. Debridement and dead space management
2. Stabilization
3. Soft tissue coverage
4. Adequate antibiotic administration

Disclosure: The techniques in this article of using intramedullary antibiotic rods and antibiotic beads to treat osteomyelitis are off-label usage of a Food and Drug Administration–approved product or device.
Department of Orthopaedics, Complex Fractures, Nonunions and Osteomyelitis, University Physician Associates, North Jersey Orthopaedic Institute, New Jersey Medical School, Rutgers, The State University of New Jersey, 140 Bergen Street, Suite D1610, Newark, NJ 07103, USA
* Corresponding author.
E-mail address: sirkinms@njms.rutgers.edu

0030-5898/17/© 2016 Elsevier Inc. All rights reserved.

The implementation of an antibiotic nail as part of long bone osteomyelitis management directly addresses 3 of these 4 principles. Clearly an antibiotic nail satisfies the need for local antibiotic administration to the intramedullary canal; however, the cement nail infused with antibiotics uniquely provides a method of filling the canal dead space as well as providing stability to the bone.[6]

The antibiotic nail's stability will vary depending on the amount of antibiotics placed in the cement, as this alters the integrity of the cement after curing, as well as the metal device on which the surgeon molds the cement.[9,11,30] Although the strength of these different nail techniques has not been compared scientifically, it makes sense to hypothesize that a larger metal device at the center of the nail would provide greater stability. Coating an intramedullary nail in cement would likely create an antibiotic nail most resistant to deformity, which Thonse and Conway[9] described; but an antibiotic implant with such stability is unnecessary in most chronic osteomyelitis cases.

In addition to the stability that antibiotic nails offer, there are several advantages provided by the nail. Antibiotic beads are a proven method of treating osteomyelitis.[16,17,21] Problems cited with bead use within the intramedullary canal include lack of dead space filling as well as potential extraction difficulty if left in place for a long duration.[6] In contrast, the antibiotic nail can be sized in a custom fashion to fill the patients' canal, filling the dead space as well as maximizing the amount of antibiotic cement introduced into the canal. The duration of which the antibiotic nail can be left in place as well as the relative ease of extraction are further unique advantages of the nail over beads. Paley and Herzenberg[6] described removal of a nail after 753 days with relative ease.

INDICATIONS AND CONTRAINDICATIONS

Given the numerous advantages of the antibiotic cement nail and relative ease of implementation as well as extraction, there is expanding use of this technique. The original description of its use entailed treatment of intramedullary osteomyelitis. Most of these patients required a long duration of external fixation for deformity correction with subsequent infection of the intramedullary canal.[6] Since that time, additional case series have documented utilization of the antibiotic nail in other circumstances, which include treatment of chronic osteomyelitis and infected nonunions of the diaphysis.[4–10,14,15] Moreover, other surgeons advocate the use of

an antibiotic nail as a prophylactic modality in the setting of prolonged external fixation either in the face of severe trauma requiring staged fixation or in lengthy deformity correction.[1]

There are no absolute contraindications to the use of an antibiotic nail in the treatment of long bone infection. Open physes in children may limit the use of antibiotic nails because of the potential harm caused to the growth plate by insertion of the nail. Nonetheless, Bar-On and colleagues[12] were able to use antibiotic rods in the intramedullary canal without disrupting the physes in children as young as 4.5 years of age. Shyam and colleagues[8] reported concern with bone defects greater than 6 cm because of a lack of stability provided by antibiotic nails in their study. It is unclear that this is valid for all antibiotic nail constructs, and it does not seem to be reason for not using the antibiotic nail as much as it is reason to augment the nail with another form of stabilization.

TREATMENT METHODOLOGY

Effective utilization of antibiotic nails for the treatment of long bone infection consists of several important treatment steps. These steps are consistently described throughout the literature reporting antibiotic-infused cement nail use. The sequence of appropriate infection treatment with antibiotic nails includes infection diagnosis, debridement, antibiotic nail placement, and antibiotic nail removal with or without definitive hardware placement.

Diagnosis
To begin, patients must have an accurate diagnosis, which includes culture identification of the infectious agent as well as sensitivities and susceptibilities. Thorough patient history is important to identify any factors that will affect treatment, such as immune-compromise, or aid in treatment, such as surgical and infection history. In particular, the history of an intramedullary device is an important factor in diagnosing long bone infection. Laboratory evaluation should include white blood cell count, erythrocyte sedimentation rate, C- reactive protein, and blood cultures. These studies will potentially aid in diagnosing infection and will certainly help with monitoring the effectiveness of treatment.

Imaging is an important part of diagnosing intramedullary osteomyelitis. Radiographic signs are not present in an acute infection but in chronic osteomyelitis include diffuse demineralization, soft tissue swelling, periosteal reaction, involucrum formation, and trabecular destruction with a change in bony architecture. Of note, these findings may be minimal if an intramedullary device is in place from previous surgery. Advanced imaging, such as MRI, computed tomography (CT), and bone scans, are useful to identify areas affected by infection.

Signs of osteomyelitis on CT scan include cortical bone destruction, new bone formation, and soft tissue swelling or abscess formation. In addition, signs of increased bone marrow density and gas in the medullary canal are highly specific for osteomyelitis.[31–33] An additional finding that can be seen with CT in the chronic setting is sequestrum. The CT results will also provide important information about the suspected stability of the bone, which may require the intramedullary stability of a cement Intramedullary Nail (IMN).

MRI will show the soft tissue extent of the infection and importantly the spread of infection within the intramedullary canal. The presence of an intramedullary device obviates this step, as intramedullary infection is present along the length of the implant and the metal will obstruct the image quality. Studies have demonstrated up to 95% sensitivity and 91% specificity in the diagnosis of osteomyelitis with MRI.[31,34] Because MRI delineates the proximal and distal bone marrow involvement, it provides the best overall impression of the extent of the infection.

Because treatment to eradicate the infection can occur only after knowing the offending bacteria, biopsy and culture are part of the diagnostic process. Culturing should consist of sampling from multiple areas within the location of concern in a sterile, operating room setting.[35] Aerobic and anaerobic tissue culture bottles with an agar medium are ideal as they increase the culture yield. With an IMN in place, the interlocking screw sites are important locations to culture, as they provide information about the extent of infection spread along the nail.

Debridement

Debridement is performed at the same operating room trip as biopsy and culture. The goal of debridement is to remove infected tissue as well as dead tissue, which is a nidus for further bacterial colonization. The debridement must decrease the bacterial load to less than 10^5 colonies so that antibiotic therapy and host defenses can complete the eradication of infection.[36] Once the area of infected bone is identified, debridement of the bone should continue until healthy bleeding bone is encountered. Instruments such as burrs, rongeurs, and curettes are useful tools to achieve a sufficient debridement. Often 1 debridement is inadequate, as Patzakis and colleagues[37]

demonstrated that 26% of patients with chronic osteomyelitis of the tibia had positive intraoperative cultures during their second debridement. When there is gross purulence or a significant amount of necrotic tissue present, additional debridement should be performed.

When considering long bone infection, there is often extensive intramedullary canal involvement. Intramedullary reaming provides an effective option to debride the canal without creating extensive incisions.[25] Standard reaming may be performed; but a vent hole must be used to avoid increasing intramedullary canal pressures, which can drive infectious material into the circulatory system. Intramedullary reaming and irrigation device allows for simultaneous reaming, irrigation, and aspiration of the medullary canal that can be sent for culture.[38] The use of irrigation and suction while reaming decreases the amount of heat generation, which in turn decreases the risk of endosteal thermal necrosis. A study by Goplen and colleagues[39] demonstrated that RIA produced pressures less than atmospheric pressure, making the RIA less likely to force bacteria into the blood stream than standard reaming.

Antibiotic Nail Placement

As discussed previously, the antibiotic rod provides both stability and local antibiotics to the canal. Stabilization of the bone is a vital component in eradicating infection, as it stabilizes bone and soft tissue for healing, which decreases the likelihood of persistent infection.[25,27–29] Many studies support the use of local antibiotics to decrease infection when used in conjunction with systemic antibiotics.[40,41]

There are several techniques for antibiotic nail formation, but the basic principles are the same for all nails described in the literature.[1–10,12–14] The nail typically consists of antibiotic-impregnated cement coating a rigid object with a method for extraction built into the design. The greatest variation seems to be in the object used for the core of the nail, with investigators reporting use of ender nails, Ilizarov threaded rods, intramedullary nails, carbon fiber nails, as well as cut guidewires.[1–10,12–15]

Antibiotic Nail Removal and Definitive Hardware Placement

Nail removal occurs after a period of adequate treatment with the local antibiotics as well as systemic antibiotics based on culture results. During this time, erythrocyte sedimentation rate (ESR) and C-reactive protein (CRP) are monitored to ensure downward to normal values

Table 1
Summary of case reports and case series for using antibiotic nails in the treatment of intramedullary bone infection

Article, Year	N	Resolved	Mean Age (y)	Location	F/U (mo)	Equipment	Antibiotics in Cement (per Bag of Cement)	Length of Antibiotic Nail Treatment	Length of Systemic Antibiotics (wk)	Complications
Kanakaris et al,[2] 2014	24	23	45 (17–75)	14 Femurs 10 Tibias	21 (8–36)	Not specified	0.5 g Gentamicin in cement 2 g Vancomycin Antifungal as needed	2.6 (1–5) mo	3–18	4% Recurrence leading to amputation
Wasko & Borens,[10] 2013	10	10	42 (20–59)	10 Tibias	72 (60–84)	K wire Chest tube	2 g Gentamicin	6 wk	6–8	None
Selhi et al,[42] 2011	16	14	39 (18–54)	8 Femurs 7 Tibias 1 Humerus	39 (18–54)	Kuntscher nail Steel wire Interlocking nail	0.5 g Gentamicin in cement 4 g Vancomycin	—	12–18	12% Infected nonunion
Bar-On et al,[12] 2010	4	4	9 (5.5–14.6)	2 Tibias 2 Femurs	41 (36–46)	1.2-mm K wire 28-G Chest tube	Gentamicin (amount not specified)	16–62 d	16	50% Wound complication
Bhadra & Roberts,[1] 2009	30	—	47 (20–79)	24 Tibias 6 Femurs	26 (4–40)	Ender nail Chest tube	1.2 g Tobramycin 1 g Vancomycin	42 d Average	5–8	Unknown
Shyam et al,[8] 2009	25	20	33 (21–58)	23 Femurs 2 Tibias	29 (18–40)	6 or 7 mm Nail	2 g Vancomycin 2 g Gentamicin	8 (6–12) wk	—	20% Recurrence

Study			Age	Bones	F/U	Technique	Antibiotic	Duration		Complications
Sancineto & Barla,[14] 2008	19	17	37 (18–52)	4 Femurs 14 Tibias	37 (10–54)	Chest tube Ender nail	4 g Vancomycin, +/– Gentamicin, tobramycin, imipenem	6–76 wk	Unknown	5% Septic knee 5% abx vancomycin hypersensitivity
Qiang et al,[7] 2007	19	18	38 (22–78)	6 Femurs 13 Tibias	16 (6–28)	Chest tube 3-mm Guidewire	2 g Vancomycin	35–123 d	6–8	32% Partial union 5% Nonunion 5% Rod fracture 5% Septic knee
Thonse & Conway,[9] 2007	20	18	47 (15–79)	7 Femur 3 Tibia 5 Knee arthrodesis 5 Ankle arthrodesis	16 (7–40)	Custom molds coating nail	1 g Vancomycin 3.6 g Tobramycin	Unknown	Unknown	5% Nonunion 10% Nails debonded 5% Amputation
Paley & Herzenberg,[6] 2002	9	9	30 (8–70)	6 Femur 2 Tibia 1 Humerus	41 (32–48)	Chest tube 3-mm Beaded guidewire	2.4 g Tobramycin 2 g Vancomycin	29–753 d	Unknown	33% Nonunions 11% Rod fracture

Abbreviations: abx, antibiotics; F/U, follow-up; K, Kirschner.

indicating sufficient treatment of the infection. If the initial treatment is found to be inadequate based on these values, then the authors repeat debridement and insert a new antibiotic nail. Once the treatment is adequate and ESR and CRP values remain normal off of systemic antibiotics, then nail removal and definitive bone fixation can occur as needed. In the review of case series, there is minimal difficulty reported when attempting to remove these antibiotic implants (Table 1).

SENIOR AUTHOR'S PREFERRED NAIL TECHNIQUE

The senior author's (M.S.) preferred technique consists of fashioning a cement nail from the following: 40-g bag of medium viscosity cement, 1.2 g powder tobramycin and/or 1.0 g powder vancomycin, 400-mm Ilizarov threaded rod, and a female hinge from the Ilizarov set (Fig. 1A). The authors also routinely use a 40-F chest tube, which corresponds with a 10.0-mm diameter nail, as well as a cement injection gun equipped with a narrow nozzle (see Fig. 1B).

To begin, vancomycin and/or tobramycin are added to the prepackaged dry cement powder based on culture results, if available. After performing a dry mix, the prepackaged polymer is then added and mixing is performed again until achieving a thick liquid consistency. The surgeon cuts the chest tube to a desired length based on the canal depth gauge measurement or prior nail length and then fills the tube using the cement gun (Fig. 2). The threaded Ilizarov rod, with female hinge attached to one side, is cut to the same length as the chest tube.

With the cement still soft, the surgeon inserts the Ilizarov rod into the chest tube with the female hinge left just outside the chest tube and not covered by cement. An appropriate bend should be placed to match the bow of the femur or Herzog curve needed to insert into the tibia (Fig. 3). The cement cures, and the chest tube is cut away from the cement rod (Fig. 4). Insertion of the nail is done primarily with manual force and gentle mallet taps on the female hinge to finalize the positioning (Fig. 5). The final position of the nail should allow access to the female hinge such that the surgeon can insert and remove a bone hook.

PEARLS AND PITFALLS

Pearls

1. A 40-F chest tube will form a 10.0-mm diameter cement nail. If the surgeon prefers a larger nail, then use of dilation and

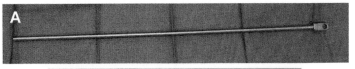
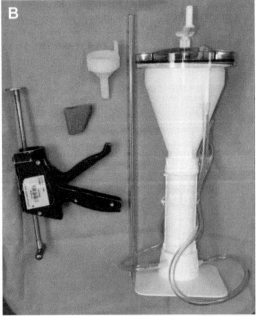

Fig. 1. (A) A 400-mm Ilizarov threaded rod with female hinge. (B) A 40-F chest tube and a cement injection gun equipped with a narrow nozzle.

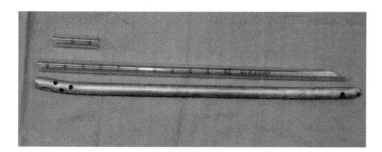

Fig. 2. The chest tube cut to the desired length by using the prior nail length as a reference.

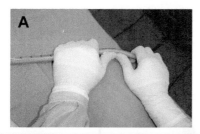

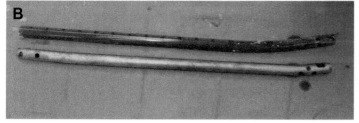

Fig. 3. (A) The surgeon manually bending the antibiotic rod to match the Herzog curve of a tibial nail. (B) The Herzog curve of the antibiotic rod compared with that of the previous implanted tibialnail.

Fig. 4. Once the cement is cured, the surgeon cuts the chest tube away from the antibiotic rod.

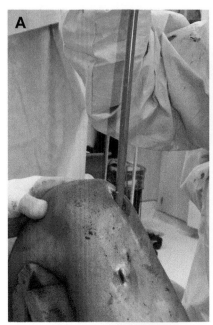
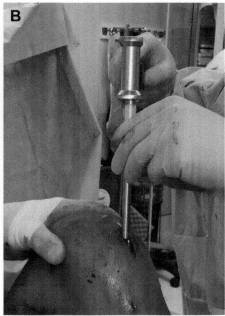
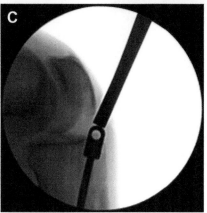

Fig. 5. The nail is inserted (*A*), and gentle mallet taps are used to finalize the position of the nail (*B*). This position is confirmed on fluoroscopy (*C*).

curettage tubing will yield a 12.5-mm diameter nail.

2. Using a threaded Ilizarov rod prevents delamination of the cement from the metal when removal from an intramedullary location.

3. The female hinge attached to the Ilizarov rod allows for reliable and easy nail removal with a bone hook.

4. A 40-g bag of cement is adequate for most nails; the cement will fill the chest tube halfway with cement, but on insertion of the threaded rod there will be enough cement to fill the entire chest tube.

5. When filling the chest tube with cement use a cement gun with a narrow nozzle to pressurize the cement. Maintain a thumb over the far end of the tube to ensure pressurization of the cement while the threaded rod is inserted into the tube (**Fig. 6**). This pressurization will prevent the creation of cement voids.

6. Target antibiotics in the cement to the culture and sensitivities identified on cultures from the initial debridement. When cultures are not available, empirical antibiotics should consist of vancomycin and tobramycin.

7. RIA is a useful tool to debride the canal, obtain specimen for culture (**Fig. 7**A), and irrigate the canal after debridement (see **Fig. 7**B).

8. The cement IMN may provide enough stability to allow fracture healing, eliminating the need for a secondary fixation procedure.

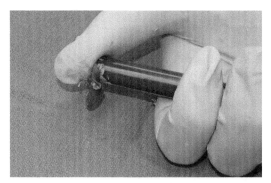

Fig. 6. A thumb over the far end of the tube is used to ensure pressurization of the cement during filling.

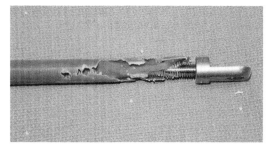

Fig. 8. Improper pressurization of the cement, leading to voids in the cement and incomplete rod coverage.

Pitfalls

1. Using a smooth metal core risks cement delamination and weakness of the cement nail risking breakage as well as leaving cement from the nail in the canal. Delamination of the cement away from the nail can occur during insertion or extraction.
2. Using a nail without a means of easy extraction will risk extraction difficulty and possible nail breakage.
3. Failure to properly pressurize the cement can lead to poor cement coverage of the nail leading to voids in the cement or incomplete threaded rod coverage (**Fig. 8**).
4. Standard reaming can lead to increased pressure within the canal, which can force infectious material into the blood stream. Instead ventilate the canal with a distal hole and suction or use the RIA system.
5. Failure to target the antibiotics based on culture results can lead to treatment failure or promote bacterial antibiotic resistance.
6. Opening the knee joint should be avoided when gaining access to the tibial canal for hardware removal, debridement, and cement nail placement. Entering the joint risks septic arthritis.

OUTCOMES

The success rates of antibiotic nails for intramedullary bone infection range from 80% to 100%.[1–10,12–14] The antibiotics incorporated into the cement are normally vancomycin, tobramycin, gentamicin, or a mixture of these antibiotics. Typically, the antibiotic nail remains in place for 1.5 to 4.0 months. In addition to treating the infection itself, the antibiotic rods may also promote healing of previous nonunions. **Table 1** summarizes several case reports and case series.

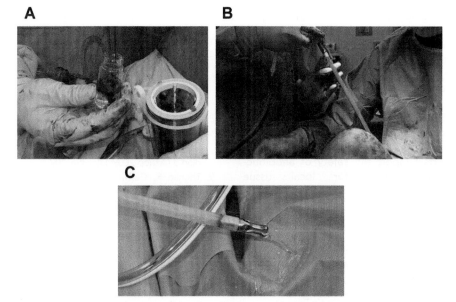

Fig. 7. The RIA can be used to obtain specimen for culture (A) as well as irrigate the canal (B, C).

Although the antibiotic nail is an effective means of treating intramedullary infection and infected nonunion, it is not without complications. There is a risk of contaminating the knee joint during the reaming and nail insertion process. Because of this risk of septic arthritis, surgeons should reserve antibiotic rod use for confirmed intramedullary osteomyelitis. Thorough irrigation of the joint following the removal of an infected nail is absolutely critical, though this does not completely eliminate the risk of a septic joint.[7,14]

Other complications can arise from the intramedullary rod itself. There are multiple reports of the antibiotic rod breaking within the canal.[7] Because infections frequently cause nonunions, antibiotic rods may not be strong enough to resist the forces of full weight bearing like a standard intramedullary nail. Surgeons should supplement grossly unstable limbs with an external fixator to avoid nail failure, prevent deformity, and increase stability of the limb for healing. Limbs with more stability but with unhealed fractures benefit from casting or use of fracture braces in the authors' experience.

Cement may debond from a smooth metal material. Thonse and Conway[9] reported debonding of the cement from the nail in 20% of their cases. This debonding typically occurred during nail insertion. The investigators recommend over-reaming by 2 mm in order to prevent this. In the authors' experience, debonding also occurs during nail removal and may leave cement in the bone making further instrumentation of the intramedullary canal difficult. One benefit from using a threaded rod, compared with using a smooth nail, is that the threads provide an irregular surface for cement bonding, which prevents the cement mantle from sliding off of the nail.

Finally, hypersensitivity reactions and nephrotoxicity to antibiotics are still theoretic possibilities, though very uncommon. There is one report of a hypersensitivity reaction to a vancomycin-impregnated rod.[14] The authors have not seen this in their experience, and multiple reports support the safety of antibiotic-impregnated cement for local tissue administration.

SUMMARY

Antibiotic cement nails provide a useful and relatively simple technique to treat intramedullary osteomyelitis of the long bones. These devices provide stability as well as local, targeted antibiotics, which are both critical aspects of osteomyelitis management. In the authors' experience, the RIA system is an effective method for debriding, culturing, and irrigating the canal. Additionally, the use of a threaded core, an Ilizarov rod in the authors' practice, is a critical component of successful cement nail assembly. The threaded core prevents cement debonding and allows for easy attachment of a female hinge from the Ilizarov set for simple rod extraction. With adherence to the simple principles outlined in this review, surgeons can expect reliably good results using these drug-delivery implants.

REFERENCES

1. Bhadra AK, Roberts CS. Indications for antibiotic cement nails. J Orthop Trauma 2009;23(5 Suppl): S26–30.
2. Kanakaris N, Gudipati S, Tosounidis T, et al. The treatment of intramedullary osteomyelitis of the femur and tibia using the Reamer-Irrigator-Aspirator system and antibiotic cement rods. Bone Joint J 2014;96-B(6):783–8.
3. Kim JW, Cuellar DO, Hao J, et al. Custom-made antibiotic cement nails: a comparative study of different fabrication techniques. Injury 2014;45(8): 1179–84.
4. Madanagopal SG, Seligson D, Roberts CS. The antibiotic cement nail for infection after tibial nailing. Orthopedics 2004;27(7):709–12.
5. Ohtsuka H, Yokoyama K, Higashi K, et al. Use of antibiotic-impregnated bone cement nail to treat septic nonunion after open tibial fracture. J Trauma 2002;52(2):364–6.
6. Paley D, Herzenberg JE. Intramedullary infections treated with antibiotic cement rods: preliminary results in nine cases. J Orthop Trauma 2002; 16(10):723–9.
7. Qiang Z, Jun PZ, Jie XJ, et al. Use of antibiotic cement rod to treat intramedullary infection after nailing: preliminary study in 19 patients. Arch Orthop Trauma Surg 2007;127(10):945–51.
8. Shyam AK, Sancheti PK, Patel SK, et al. Use of antibiotic cement-impregnated intramedullary nail in treatment of infected non-union of long bones. Indian J Orthop 2009;43(4):396–402.
9. Thonse R, Conway J. Antibiotic cement-coated interlocking nail for the treatment of infected nonunions and segmental bone defects. J Orthop Trauma 2007;21(4):258–68.
10. Wasko MK, Borens O. Antibiotic cement nail for the treatment of posttraumatic intramedullary infections of the tibia: midterm results in 10 cases. Injury 2013;44(8):1057–60.
11. Wasko MK, Kaminski R. Custom-made antibiotic cement nails in orthopaedic trauma: review of

outcomes, new approaches, and perspectives. Biomed Res Int 2015;2015:387186.

12. Bar-On E, Weigl DM, Bor N, et al. Chronic osteomyelitis in children: treatment by intramedullary reaming and antibiotic-impregnated cement rods. J Pediatr Orthop 2010;30(5):508–13.

13. Mauffrey C, Chaus GW, Butler N, et al. MR-compatible antibiotic interlocked nail fabrication for the management of long bone infections: first case report of a new technique. Patient Saf Surg 2014; 8(1):14.

14. Sancineto CF, Barla JD. Treatment of long bone osteomyelitis with a mechanically stable intramedullar antibiotic dispenser: nineteen consecutive cases with a minimum of 12 months follow-up. J Trauma 2008;65(6):1416–20.

15. Makridis KG, Tosounidis T, Giannoudis PV. Management of infection after intramedullary nailing of long bone fractures: treatment protocols and outcomes. Open Orthop J 2013;7:219–26.

16. Hake ME, Young H, Hak DJ, et al. Local antibiotic therapy strategies in orthopaedic trauma: practical tips and tricks and review of the literature. Injury 2015;46(8):1447–56.

17. Hanssen AD. Local antibiotic delivery vehicles in the treatment of musculoskeletal infection. Clin Orthop Relat Res 2005;(437):91–6.

18. Hanssen AD, Osmon DR, Patel R. Local antibiotic delivery systems: where are we and where are we going? Clin Orthop Relat Res 2005;(437):111–4.

19. Klemm K. Gentamicin-PMMA-beads in treating bone and soft tissue infections (author's transl). Zentralbl Chir 1979;104(14):934–42 [in German].

20. Klemm K. The use of antibiotic-containing bead chains in the treatment of chronic bone infections. Clin Microbiol Infect 2001;7(1):28–31.

21. Nelson CL. The current status of material used for depot delivery of drugs. Clin Orthop Relat Res 2004;(427):72–8.

22. Seligson D, Popham GJ, Voos K, et al. Antibiotic-leaching from polymethyl methacrylate beads. J Bone Joint Surg Am 1993;75(5):714–20.

23. Zalavras CG, Patzakis MJ, Holtom P. Local antibiotic therapy in the treatment of open fractures and osteomyelitis. Clin Orthop Relat Res 2004;(427):86–93.

24. Calhoun JH, Cierny G 3rd, Holtom P, et al. Symposium: current concepts in the management of osteomyelitis. Contemp Orthop 1994;28(2):157–85.

25. Cierny G 3rd. Surgical treatment of osteomyelitis. Plast Reconstr Surg 2011;127(Suppl 1):190S–204S.

26. Mouzopoulos G, Kanakaris NK, Kontakis G, et al. Management of bone infections in adults: the surgeon's and microbiologist's perspectives. Injury 2011;42(Suppl 5):S18–23.

27. Cierny G, Mader JT. Adult chronic osteomyelitis. Orthopedics 1984;7(10):1557–64.

28. Cierny G 3rd, Mader JT. Approach to adult osteomyelitis. Orthop Rev 1987;16(4):259–70.

29. Cierny G 3rd, Mader JT, Penninck JJ. A clinical staging system for adult osteomyelitis. Clin Orthop Relat Res 2003;(414):7–24.

30. Anagnostakos K, Kelm J. Enhancement of antibiotic elution from acrylic bone cement. J Biomed Mater Res B Appl Biomater 2009;90(1):467–75.

31. Lazzarini L, Mader JT, Calhoun JH. Osteomyelitis in long bones. J Bone Joint Surg Am 2004;86-A(10): 2305–18.

32. Kuhn JP, Berger PE. Computed tomographic diagnosis of osteomyelitis. Radiology 1979;130(2): 503–6.

33. Ma LD, Frassica FJ, Bluemke DA, et al. CT and MRI evaluation of musculoskeletal infection. Crit Rev Diagn Imaging 1997;38(6):535–68.

34. Johnson PW, Collins MS, Wenger DE. Diagnostic utility of T1-weighted MRI characteristics in evaluation of osteomyelitis of the foot. AJR Am J Roentgenol 2009;192(1):96–100.

35. Patzakis MJ, Wilkins J, Kumar J, et al. Comparison of the results of bacterial cultures from multiple sites in chronic osteomyelitis of long bones. A prospective study. J Bone Joint Surg Am 1994;76(5): 664–6.

36. Marshall KA, Edgerton MT, Rodeheaver GT, et al. Quantitative microbiology: its application to hand injuries. Am J Surg 1976;131(6):730–3.

37. Patzakis MJ, Greene N, Holtom P, et al. Culture results in open wound treatment with muscle transfer for tibial osteomyelitis. Clin Orthop Relat Res 1999;(360):66–70.

38. Kanakaris NK, Morell D, Gudipati S, et al. Reaming Irrigator Aspirator system: early experience of its multipurpose use. Injury 2011;42(Suppl 4): S28–34.

39. Goplen G, Wilson JA, McAffrey M, et al. A cadaver model evaluating femoral intramedullary reaming: a comparison between new reamer design (Pressure Sentinel) and a novel suction/irrigation reamer (RIA). Injury 2010;41(Suppl 2):S38–42.

40. Henry SL, Ostermann PA, Seligson D. The prophylactic use of antibiotic impregnated beads in open fractures. J Trauma 1990;30(10):1231–8.

41. Ostermann PA, Seligson D, Henry SL. Local antibiotic therapy for severe open fractures. A review of 1085 consecutive cases. J Bone Joint Surg Br 1995;77(1):93–7.

42. Selhi HS, Mahindra P, Yamin M, et al. Outcome in patients with an infected nonunion of the long bones treated with a reinforced antibiotic bone cement rod. J Orthop Trauma 2012;26(3):184–8.

The Impact of Negative Pressure Wound Therapy on Orthopaedic Infection

Lawrence X. Webb, MD[a,b,c,]*

KEYWORDS

- Negative pressure wound therapy • Topical negative pressure • Surgical site infection
- Quorum sensing • Tissue demarcation • Integra • Antibiotic beads • Wound coverage

---

KEY POINTS

- Topical negative pressure wound therapy (TNP) is used as a dynamic dressing for high-energy wounds following surgical debridement. The author provides support for its utility in this setting as a means of minimizing tissue demarcation (tissue death), the "fuel" of infection.
- TNP is helpful in effecting early wound coverage by eliminating edema and by acting as a dynamic bolster for an applied split skin graft or "artificial skin."
- TNP has been shown to enhance the survival of random pattern flaps—not infrequently a consequence of the surgical extensions placed on a limb's transversely directed traumatic wound.
- The use of TNP in the setting of closed surgical wounds has emerged as a safeguard to surgical site infection in certain problematic wound types such as those occurring in the obese patient or those occurring in periarticular fractures of the ankle and tibial plateau.

INTRODUCTION

The author's personal experience dates from the early 1990s when negative pressure was first introduced by 2 of his colleagues at Wake Forest Medical Center, Lou Argenta, MD and Michael Morykwas, PhD, as a strategy for potentially shortening the hospital stay of patients with decubitus ulcers. The author was one of a small group of clinicians at Wake Forest who gained an early experience with "the VAC" (vacuum-assisted closure, or formerly, the "DecubiVAC"). Given his subspecialty in orthopedic trauma, his proximity to Drs Argenta and Morykwas, and the ready availability of the product, his use of topical negative pressure in wound management quickly became a commonality. He has been a strong proponent of its use in different clinical settings. Those settings, which are relevant to infection, are elaborated upon in this article.

DEBRIDEMENT

> *Bernard a raison. La peste est rien. C'est la terrain qui est tout.*
> *(Bernard is right. The germ is nothing. It is the environment which is everything.)*
> —*Louis Pasteur*

Ramon Gustilo, MD, teacher, author, and mentor to virtually all orthopedic traumatologists, cited the above in his book entitled, *Orthopaedic Infection* and wrote, "*It behooves every surgeon to understand fully the implications of Pasteur's statement.*"[1] Wounded nonviable tissue is the

---

Disclosure Statement: The author is a consultant to Biocomposites, Inc, Wilmington, NC, USA.
[a] Department of Orthopaedic Trauma, Medical Center Navicent Health, 840 Pine Street, Macon, GA 31201, USA;
[b] Department of Surgery, Mercer University School of Medicine, 1400 Coleman Avenue, Macon, GA 31217, USA;
[c] Department of Orthopaedic Surgery, Medical Center, Wake Forest University, Medical Center Boulevard, Winston-Salem, NC 27157, USA
* Department of Orthopaedic Trauma, Medical Center Navicent Health, 840 Pine Street, Suite 500, Macon, GA 31201, USA.
E-mail address: Webb.Lawrence@navicenthealth.org

Orthop Clin N Am 48 (2017) 167–179
http://dx.doi.org/10.1016/j.ocl.2016.12.004
0030-5898/17/© 2017 Elsevier Inc. All rights reserved.

fuel of infection and needs to be excised by surgical debridement. For high-energy wounds, the policy of following the initial debridement with a return to the operating room for a "second look" at 36 to 72 hours has become a protocol at many centers, knowing that the tissues in or adjacent to the zone of injury commonly "demarcate" during that span of time.[2] Tissue "demarcation" is an ill-defined but widely acknowledged concept.

An interesting feature noted in the author's early experience with topical negative pressure wound therapy (TNP) was the fact that when it was used for high-energy wounds following an initial debridement (the author's preference was to set the transmitted negative pressure at −50 mm Hg or −75 mm Hg continuous), there was no or minimal secondary necrosis seen at 36 to 72 hours.[3–5] In other words, there appeared to be something about TNP that prevented the cascade of cellular events that would otherwise proceed to tissue necrosis (or "demarcation") in those patients.

Relevant to these observations was the study by Morykwas and colleagues[6] on the histology of porcine skin burn wounds, half (on one side of the midline) were managed with saline dressing changes and half (on the other side of the midline) were managed with TNP. Punch biopsies of the burn wounds were obtained on postburn days 1, 3, 5, and 9 (Fig. 1). The basis for the demise of the tissues managed with saline dressing changes is the lack of dynamic microcirculatory flow through the capillary bed probably due to an engorged interstitium in the tissues. Additional support for this statement is provided by the study of Langfitt and colleagues.[7] It is now understood that the reason high-energy wounds "demarcate" by the time of the "second look" is the same as was exhibited in the above described porcine burn study of Morykwas.[6] Given this, one might logically predict that the same phenomenon should apply not only to the tissues at risk in a high-energy extremity wound, a skin burn in a porcine model, but also to any tissue whose initial insult is followed by a second wave of necrosis, such as any infarct with a "reperfusion injury." This line of thought foreshadowed the results of recent studies by Lindstedt and colleagues,[8] Argenta and colleagues,[9] and Jordan and colleagues[10] on preservation of blood flow effected by TNP in an ischemic porcine heart

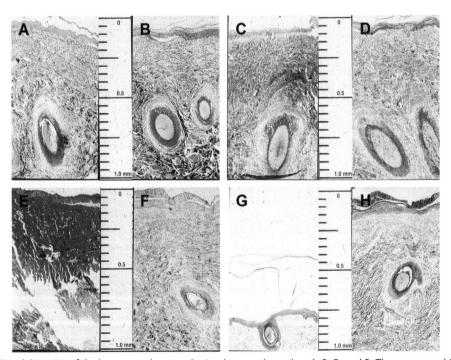

Fig. 1. Punch biopsies of the burn wounds were obtained on postburn days 1, 3, 5, and 9. There were no histologic changes seen on either the saline dressing side (A) or the TNP side (B) at day 1. On day 3, the notable finding on the saline dressing side was a significant zone of coagulation necrosis (C). There were no changes on the TNP side (D). On day 5, there is a clear zone of cleavage between the necrotic zone and the underlying living tissue on the saline dressing side (E). There were no changes on the TNP side (F). On day 9, there was significant sloughing of necrotic tissue with loss of specialized skin elements (G). There were no significant changes on the TNP side (H). From Morykwas MJ, David LR, Schneider AM, et al. Use of subatmospheric pressure to prevent progression of partial-thickness burns in a swine model. J Burn Care Rehabil 1999;20(1):15–21; with permission.

model as well as Argenta and colleagues[11] in preservation of tissue in a traumatic rat brain model evidenced by water content, histologic sectioning, MRI spectroscopy, injury cavity area, and cortical volume. Zheng and colleagues[12,13] later obtained similar findings for ameliorating spinal cord injury and traumatic brain injury. A subatmospheric pressure of 100 mm Hg was found to be more efficacious in this porcine model of traumatic brain injury.[13]

Morykwas, in his original study of the effects on the porcine animal model,[14] showed that the setting of −125 mm Hg on intermittent mode maximized the granulation tissue response. Thus, there may be several ideal pressures: one for maximizing blood flow in the setting of porcine myoischemia[15] (−50 mm Hg, continuous); one for minimizing the immediate and shortly thereafter effects following a porcine traumatic brain injury (−100 mm Hg)[13]; and one for maximizing porcine growth of healthy granulation tissue (−125 mm Hg, intermittent).[14]

Given the success at avoidance or minimization of secondary necrosis in high-energy wounds, the author has continued to use and recommend[3–5] the use of continuous TNP at the −50 mm Hg level applied at the time of completion of the initial debridement. An intermediary layer of xeroform or "artificial skin" (eg, Integra; Integra Lifesciences, Plainsboro, NJ, USA) for desiccation-prone tissue is commonly used. At the time of the "second look" at 48 to 72 hours, the wound is excisionally debrided if any dead ("demarcated") tissue is present and closed with incisional TNP application. The ideal pressure for sparing tissue demarcation following high-velocity trauma has yet to be completely derived. The concept of a "dose response curve" may apply depending on the nature of the tissue and the nature of the inciting event, which resulted in the demarcation. Supportive of a −50 mm Hg negative pressure level is the author's experience as well as the work of Lindstedt and colleagues[15] demonstrating a dose response curve where topical negative pressure levels were correlated with maximum myocardial microvascular blood flow as well as the work of Langfitt and colleagues[7] on skeletal muscle.

In the clinical arena, one wound that generates significant soft tissue trauma is the war wound inflicted by shrapnel. Peterson and colleagues[16] start their recent paper on the topic with a 1914 quote from William Osler while attending to British casualties of WWI: "This is an artillery war in which shrapnel do the damage, tearing flesh, breaking bones and always causing jagged irregular wounds. And here comes in the great tragedy—sepsis everywhere, unavoidable sepsis!... The surgeons are back in the pre-Listerian days and have wards filled with septic wounds. The wound of shrapnel and shell is a terrible affair, and infection is well nigh inevitable."[17] Dr Peterson's commentary is: "Ninety years later, his (Osler's) quote remains pertinent. War wounds are distinct from peacetime traumatic injuries because these higher velocity projectiles and/or blast devices cause a more severe injury and accompanying wounds are frequently contaminated by clothing, soil, and environmental debris."[16] Peterson and colleagues[16] were stationed on the USNS Comfort, an echelon 3 facility during the Iraq war. They reported that "surgical management of wounds was similar for all patients—WIA (wounded in action), as well as Iraqi civilians. Aggressive debridement of all necrotic tissue was performed in the operating room upon arrival to the USNS Comfort. Further wound care included daily wet-to-dry dressing changes and wound VAC therapy (TNP) depending on the availability of suction on board USNS Comfort. Additional wound debridements were performed as necessary and dressing changes on large wounds were performed in the operating room to assist in patient comfort." Therefore, in essence, these investigators reported on 211 patients, 56 of whom had shrapnel wounds, managed with initial debridement in the operating room and with subsequent daily wet-to-dry dressing changes in the "follow-on" (postoperative) period and sporadically applied TNP "depending on availability of suction on board Comfort." The reported infection rate among the shrapnel-wounded patients in their series was 32.7%.

In November 2006, Leininger and colleagues[18] reported their series of 88 high-energy shrapnel wounds in 77 patients also managed in Iraq at an echelon 3 US Air Force field hospital facility in Balad, with a similar patient demographic consisting of American WIA, prisoners of war, and Iraqi civilians. All were high-energy shrapnel wounds treated with aggressive debridement and irrigation. However, unlike the Peterson report, negative pressure (TNP) dressings were placed at the time of the initial procedure.

To quote the investigators, We believe the most significant benefit was the protection of the wound from the ward environment.

The VAC system isolated the tissue injury, yet still kept it clean and free of exudate. Dressing changes could be accomplished every 2 or 3 days, rather than 3 times per day, allowing us to do them in the cleaner environment of the operating room. The physiologic benefits of such a dressing include the clearance of wound exudate, enhanced granulation from local vasodilatation, and mechanical wound contraction because of pressure differential. . . ." Their wound infection rate was 0%. The overall wound complication rate was 0%. The investigators conclude with the statement, "experience with these patients suggests that conventional wound management doctrine may be improved with the wound VAC (TNP), resulting in earlier more reliable primary closure of wartime injuries."[18]

Of interest is that these 2 studies were contemporaneous, and the patient demographic for each study was similar, a combination of high-velocity shrapnel-wounded soldiers and civilians. Both facilities were echelon 3 centers, which is a rough measure of injury severity according to the Department of Defense triage system. Acknowledged is the fact that both studies were retrospective and without control groups (level 4 evidence). In any case, the question arises, was the difference in infection rate attributable to differences in the timing and fidelity of the application of TNP, and if so, was there more secondary necrosis in the Peterson and colleagues series to account for their higher infection rate?

COVERAGE

Topical negative pressure can be used for staging the coverage of an open fracture wound following debridement and stabilization of the fracture. The use of TNP in this setting helps to accelerate the resolution of edema as well as coverage of small areas of exposed bone, implant, or tendon.[19] The same can be said about fasciotomy wounds after debridement, where topical negative pressure can act as a bridge between the initial (often edema-laden) fasciotomy wound and later closure or skin grafting. If skin grafting is elected, then TNP can act as a dynamic bolster for the applied graft.[20] The author typically uses a 3:1 split graft in this setting to enable continued evacuation of edema and promotion of epithelialization from the graft.

One of the properties demonstrated in the initial series of basic studies done by Morykwas was that survival of random pattern pedicle flaps was higher (by 20%) with TNP. When surgical extensions are put on transversely directed traumatic wounds or when an extension of the original open wound is needed to better expose a fracture for appropriate debridement or osteosynthesis, the application of a topical negative pressure dressing may for that reason help to thwart the development of a partial wound necrosis (and secondary infection) in this setting (**Fig. 2**).[6,14,21]

ARTIFICIAL SKIN

John Burke, MD and Ionnas Yannas, PhD and their team of researchers at Harvard/MIT developed an artificial skin in the late 1970s primarily as a means of providing coverage for burn patients following an escharotomy.[22] It consisted of 2 layers: the superficial one was a thin layer of silicone serving as a bacterial moisture barrier and the second was a composite of bovine collagen within a glycosaminoglycan matrix. The latter was to serve as a matrix for ingrowing host cells derived from the underlying tissue bed over which it was applied. Once this layer "took," a very thin skin graft was applied. This overall process took about a month, and although wound-healing time in the setting of the burn patient was reported to be better than autograft, allograft, or xenograft, wound infection and "percentage of graft take" were problematic.[23]

These latter issues were "surmounted" by Drs Anthony DeFranzo and Joseph Molnar, who were both early users of "the VAC" (TNP) at Wake Forest.[24] Each were fully aware of the properties of enhancing the "take" of skin grafts both in their own practice and as reported earlier by their colleagues, Schneider and colleagues.[20] Molnar and colleagues[24] reported the results of Integra grafting with a VAC for their first 8 consecutive cases. The treated wounds included exposed bone in 62.5%, tendon in 37.5%, joint in 50%, and bowel in 25%. The mean time for clinically assessed vascularization of the Integra was 7.25 days (range 4–11 days), with an average incorporation of 96%. The split-thickness skin graft adhered to the bed by 4 days, with a success rate of 93%.[24]

Currently, the incorporation of a dermal substitute (Integra or ACell [ACell Inc, Columbia, MD, USA] and similar) is greatly enhanced by the use of TNP as a dynamic bolster. The reliability of the technique has enabled it to assume the last "rung" on the "reconstructive ladder"[4] for treating soft tissue defects before resorting to a soft tissue flap. Thus, the use of TNP either alone or as a bolster for a skin graft or an "artificial skin" graft is an option for providing early, stable coverage over desiccation-prone tissue such as bone devoid of periosteum, tendon without paratenon, joint capsule, and fascia.[4,19,20] One should

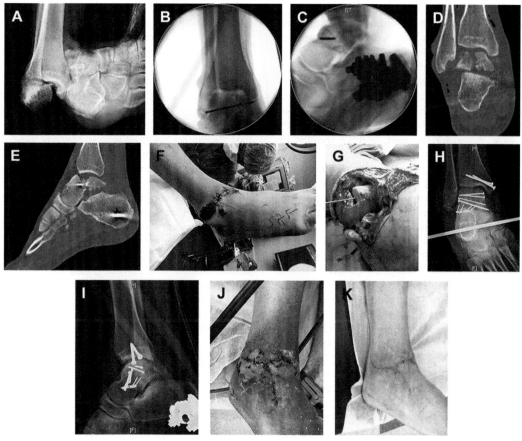

Fig. 2. Radiograph of an open, right talus fracture dislocation in a 66-year-old male bicyclist struck by a car (A). Initially managed by referring surgeon with debridement, reduction of the subtalar joint, pin fixation, and bridging external fixation (B, C). A postoperative computed tomographic scan revealed a persisting significant intra-articular displacement (D, E). The original wound had a surgical extension (done at the time of initial debride-ment) from the anterior-most point of the traumatic wound directed medially (roughly from edge of sponge) (F). To expose the talus adequately, a surgical extension was needed from roughly the mid portion of the existing wound taken 2 or 3 inches toward the base of the fourth metatarsal (G). The reflected flaps warrant careful scrutiny in the postoperative period for viability and healing. The use of TNP in this setting is supported by improvement in the survival of at-risk flaps by 20% in the porcine model reported by Morykwas and colleagues.[14] The postoperative x-rays and wound are seen in figures (H–J). There was a healthy granulation at their apex (J), which went on to heal uneventfully (K).

keep in mind the provision of early stable wound coverage is one of the essential tenets of open fracture management and is a key to the avoidance of infection.[25,26] High-energy wounds are not infrequently devoid of coverage of bone, tendon, and/or implants.

TOPICAL NEGATIVE PRESSURE WOUND THERAPY: ROLE IN MANAGEMENT OF THE IIIB FRACTURE

The author recently reviewed his own experience with the use of combined TNP and Integra for type IIIB open fractures. This work was submitted and accepted for presentation at the 2016 Georgia Orthopedic Society Annual Meeting. This study was a retrospective study of 18 consecutive type IIIB open fractures in 17 patients needing soft tissue coverage. Two patients died during their hospital stay, leaving 16 fractures in 15 patients for analysis. There were 7 tibial shaft fractures, 6 fractures of the ankle, 2 fractures of the foot, and 1 fracture of the humerus. Wound dimensions averaged 52 cm^2. All had exposed bone at the base of the wounds.

Fixation constructs were intramedullary nail (6), plate and screws (5), bridging external fixation with supplemental screws/pins/plate (4), or screws alone (1). Follow-up averaged

14.8 months (6–37). All wounds healed, although 2 of the 16 required a reapplication of the Integra and one patient required 2 (a small fraction of the total) reapplications. Total time to bone healing (inclusive of a patient with bone loss who successfully underwent the Masquelet technique and consolidated their fracture and bone graft) was 5.5 months (range: 3–11) for the tibia, 3.4 months (range: 3–6) for the ankle, 6.2 months (range: 3.3–9) for the foot, and 3.5 months for the humerus.

The author's experience with this coverage technique includes the fact that the wounds can take on a worrisome appearance, and it is understandable why many surgeons "throw in the towel" on the technique (**Fig. 3**). The author is reminded of the observation of Ioannis Yannas, the MIT materials scientist, who, along with Harvard surgeon Dr John Burke, developed Integra in the 1970s.[27] The last molecule category he tested was collagen, and the experiments on animals "didn't look so good." Rather than accept defeat in this decade-long research effort, Dr Yannas had the courage to look carefully at their "failures." The "ah-ha" moment was when he realized that the prolongation of the time for incorporation of the graft was due to the fact that the collagen was actually impairing formation of scar tissue, and by so doing, was allowing precursor cells from the underlying muscle tissue to be drawn unencumbered to the surface and grow as primordial skin (without hair follicles and sweat glands).

A literature review reveals an earlier report by Barnett and Shilt[28] of 7 consecutively managed pediatric patients with type IIIB open lower extremity injuries. All 7 healed without the need for flap coverage, and one patient required bone grafting for a nonunion.

The topic of the role of TNP in the management of the IIIB fracture is the subject of a very recent and comprehensive literature review of 6 large databases for studies reporting the use of TNP in type IIIB open tibial fractures by Schlatterer and colleagues.[29] The investigators identified one randomized controlled trial and 12 retrospective studies (not inclusive of the paper presented at the 2016 Georgia Orthopedic Society Meeting) that they considered relevant to the topic. They conclude the following: "There is an increasing body of data supporting negative pressure wound therapy as an adjunctive modality at all stages of treatment of Grade IIIB tibia fractures." The investigators point out an association between decreased infection rates with negative pressure wound therapy

versus gauze dressings in surgical wounds. Schlatterer and colleagues[29] further state "…There is evidence to support negative pressure wound therapy beyond 72 hours without increased infection rates and to support a reduction in flap rates with negative pressure wound therapy." The investigators summarize their discussion of this topic with the observation that there is limited evidence to date. They conclude that, "negative pressure wound therapy use for Grade IIIB tibia fractures requires extensive additional study." The lone randomized controlled trial included in the systematic review compared TNP with gauze dressings (control group). Debridement and irrigation were followed by TNP (or gauze dressing) application with a repeat debridement and TNP (or gauze dressing) application every 48 to 72 hours until wound closure. The control group had 2 acute infections (8%) and 5 delayed infections (20%) for a total of 8 deep infections (28%). TNP patients had 0 acute infections, 2 delayed infections (5.4%), for a total of 2 deep infections (5.4%). This difference was significant ($P = .024$).[30]

CLOSED SURGICAL INCISIONS

The use of TNP on closed surgical incisions had its origins in the early 1990s, when the author and his residents were rounding on an obese patient in the intensive care unit (ICU). On the prior day, the patient had undergone a reduction and fixation of his acetabulum. Given his multiple system injuries, the patient was edematous and "third spacing" fluid from his surgical wound. The saturation of the patient's wound dressings required frequent changes, and given his body morphotype, the imploring request from the nurses who were tasked with pushing the patient up on his side several times each shift to perform this arduous duty was, "…. is there anything you can do?" After some consideration, the author's early TNP experience prompted his response, and thus, instead of gauze dressings, it was "the VAC" set at −50 mm Hg, which continuously and effectively enabled a real-time collection of the fluid from the above referenced patient's weeping wound. Over the days following, when the collection of the fluid in the canister dropped to zero and remained at zero, the wound was inspected. To the delight of the author, the wound was perfectly healthy in appearance, dry, and pristine. Given this "remedy," topical negative pressure set at −50 mm Hg was then applied to other patients with weeping wounds

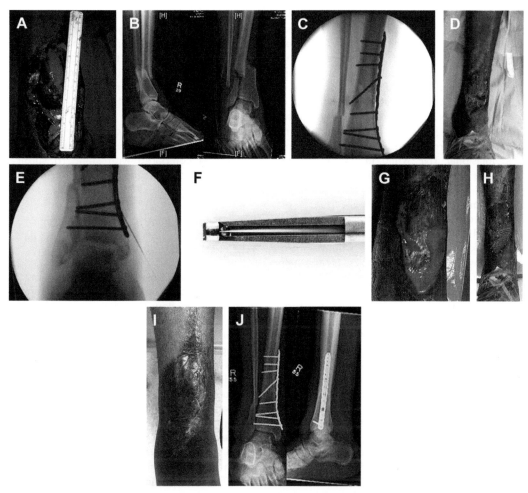

Fig. 3. Patient is a 20-year-old man whose injury was incurred by a crush from a forklift. (A) Surgical extensions were applied to the traumatic wound as depicted. Following a meticulous surgical debridement with saline irrigation, an open reduction and internal fixation of the tibial fracture (B) was performed (C), and a sterile dressing with TNP was applied with a negative pressure of −50 mm Hg. On day 2, the wound was reinspected and an Integra graft was applied and TNP re-established at −50 mm Hg. On postoperative day 14, a split-thickness skin graft was applied (meshed 3:1) and TNP was re-established at −50 mm Hg. The graft incompletely "took" on the lower portion of the recipient bed, and despite continued TNP and subsequent serial dressing changes, the area took on an escharlike appearance, worrisome for an underlying infection (D), An aspirate of the plate/bone was performed (E), which was negative on Gram stain and culture. An excisional debridement of the worrisome tissue was performed with a trauma jet tangential excision device (Courtesy of [F] Smith & Nephew, Soft Tissue Division, Tampa, FL, USA, with permission.) (F), which revealed an underlying stable vascular bed of tissue (G). A split-thickness skin graft incorporated well, and the underlying fracture healed uneventfully (H–J).

with similar results. The practice quickly morphed its way into being applied in the sterile environment of the operating room for acetabular fracture cases, morbidly obese patients, and those with other operative procedures whose surgical wounds were thought to present a potential for infection with continued serous weeping or compromised healing. (Technical point: "The width of the negative pressure strip used is about an inch with an intermediary strip of Xeroform [Medline, Mundelein, IL, USA] or Adaptic [Acelity, San Antonio, TX, USA] [of the same width] sandwiched between the underlying closed wound and the TNP sponge.")

The experience with 235 operated acetabulum fracture patients whose wound closure was supplemented with the application of an incisional TNP (August 1996 through April 2005) versus 66 consecutive antecedent patients serving as historical controls was published in 2010.[31] The infection rate was 1.27% in the group with incisional TNP (set at −50 to −75 mm Hg continuous) versus 6.06% in the historical control group (P = .04014). A subgroup of 19 of these acetabular fracture patients was the subject of a separate report. All were morbidly obese (body mass index [BMI] >40 kg/m^2), and all surgical closures were accompanied by placement of an incisional TNP while in the operating room. The wound complication rate in this group was 0%.[32] This rate stands in contrast to the report by Porter and colleagues[33] of 435 consecutive acetabular fracture surgery patients, 41 of whom were morbidly obese (BMI >40 kg/m^2). Their surgical wounds were managed with standard dressings. Nearly half of these patients (19 or 46%) had wound complications.

Stannard and colleagues[34] conducted a prospective multicenter trial of patients undergoing surgery of the tibial plateau, tibial plafond, or calcaneus randomized to either routine closure versus closure supplemented with TNP. The pressure setting used in this study was −125 mm Hg continuous. There were a total of 23 (18.8%) infections in the group without supplemental TNP and 14 (9.9%) in the group with TNP. These findings were consistent with a significant lowering of the infection rate in patients whose treatment included incisional TNP (P = .049).

A recent systematic literature review of negative pressure wound therapy in preventing complications of closed surgical incisions by TNP was authored by Scalise and colleagues.[35] In the words of the investigators, they "… reviewed published articles in databases including PubMed, Google Scholar and Scopus Database from 2006 to March 2014. Supplemental searches were included using reference lists and conference proceedings. Study selection was based on predetermined inclusion and exclusion criteria and data extraction regarding study quality, model investigated, epidemiologic and clinical characteristics and type of surgery, and the outcomes were applied to all the articles included: 1 bioengineering study, 2 animal studies, 15 human studies for a total of 6 randomized controlled trials, 5 prospective cohort studies, 7 retrospective analyses were included. Human studies investigated the outcomes of 1042 incisions on 1003 patients. The literature shows a decrease in the incidence of infection, sero-haematoma formation and on the

re-operation rates when using TNP.…" Semsarzadeh and colleagues[36] reported on a meta-analysis of the literature in September 2015 and concluded "the results suggest that closed incision negative pressure therapy is a potentially effective method for reducing surgical-site infections." A meta-analysis by Sandy-Hodgetts and Watts[37] revealed a statistically significant difference in favor of the use of negative pressure wound therapy as compared with standard surgical dressings for a lower incidence of surgical site infections.

HOW DOES THE TOPICAL NEGATIVE PRESSURE WOUND THERAPY WORK IN THE SETTING OF A CLOSED WOUND?

In the original porcine wound model work by Morykwas and colleagues,[14] a 4-fold increase in local blood flow was demonstrated with a continuous −125 mm Hg pressure exerted via an open cell polyurethane foam. Timmers and colleagues[38] demonstrated a heightened cutaneous blood flow by means of noninvasive laser Doppler probes within the foam. A range of pressures up to −300 mm Hg continuous were applied to the forearm skin in human volunteers via the 2 types of foams tested and resulted in up to a 5-fold increase in the skin blood flow. Kilpadi and Cunningham[39] used a porcine model and introduced 2 types (30 and 50 nm) of radiolabeled nanospheres into the subcutaneous tissue of each of the wounds with closure by suture. On one side of the ventral midline, wounds were dressed with continuous negative 125 mm Hg topical pressure via foam sponges and on the other side with a semipermeable film dressing (control). At 4 days, there was 63% less hematoma/seroma on the wounds managed with negative pressure. In dissected (preidentified for harvesting) regional lymph nodes, there was 50% more 30- and 50-μm nanospheres than from control sites. Lymphatic clearance was significantly greater on the side dressed with TNP, and this was true for both 30-μm and 50-μm neutron-activated nanospheres cleared to the lymph nodes (P<.04 and P<.05, respectively). The conclusion was that the use of topical negative pressure on surgically closed wounds is associated with less hematoma/seroma formation and that this is either attributable to or accompanied by a heightened dynamic in the lymphatic system.[39] This conclusion is also supported by the earlier cited work of Langfitt and colleagues.[7]

TREATMENT

The author has used topical negative pressure as an adjunct in the treatment of established infection. This use is exemplified by 2 recent cases.

Case 1

A 50-year-old woman presented as a consultation in the hospital (**Fig. 4**). Before presentation, she had been diagnosed with an infected neuropathic diabetic foot ulcer and had undergone a biopsy by her podiatrist to determine the staging of the lesion. Unfortunately, the patient broke her calcaneus while walking after the biopsy, and after being seen in the emergency department, was admitted to the hospital. Her wound was purulent and foul smelling. A clinical picture (see **Fig. 4**A) and radiograph (see **Fig. 4**B) are shown. The patient underwent a deep culture of the wound, which grew *Streptococcus* group D, *Escherichia coli*, and *Enterococcus* and was started on culture and sensitivity-directed intravenous (IV) antibiotics determined and managed by the infectious disease consultant. While cultures were growing, the patient underwent an excisional surgical debridement and a thorough irrigation of the wound along with reduction and stabilization of her calcaneus using two 7.3-mm cannulated lag screws percutaneously placed from the posterior aspect of the calcaneal tuberosity (see **Fig. 4**D). Resorbable antibiotic (vancomycin and tobramycin) beads [Biocomposites Inc., Wilmington, NC, USA] were used to fill the dead space and TNP was applied at −50 mm with the resorbable beads. The beads were fully absorbed by 8 weeks. By 12 weeks, the patient's wound was healed, but

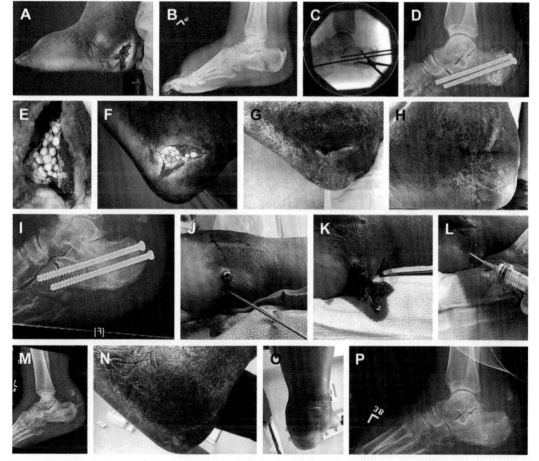

Fig. 4. (A) Clinical picture of the patient's ulcer. (B) Radiograph of the newly acquired fracture. (C) Debrided, reduced, and fixed. (D) Radiograph at 4 weeks. (E) Clinical picture of ulcer at 4 weeks. (F) At 5 weeks. (G) At 10 weeks. (H) At 22 weeks, healed. (I) X-ray at 24 weeks showing lucency about the screws. (J) Cannulated screws are removed. (K) Tracts are debrided and curetted. Lavaged and suctioned. (L) Vancomycin-impregnated CaSO₄ placed as a bone void filler [Biocomposites, Inc, Wilmington, NC, USA] (M, N). Lateral (N) and (O) posterior view of the hindfoot clinically healed; (P) radiograph with the former screw tracts faintly visible. Patient was actively mobile and weight bearing at this time.

there was a resorption line around the retained screws, indicating a possible implant-related low-grade infection; this was evidenced also by a small blister at the site of screw insertion. These findings prompted the removal of the retained screws, clearance of each tract with a curette, and filling of the dead space with more antibiotic-impregnated $CaSO_4$ while still in the "preset" (thickening liquid) state. Two weeks later, the patient's wounds were completely healed, and she was ambulatory and without pain.

Case 2

A 73-year-old woman was involved in a motor vehicle accident and injured her right wrist and femur with a minimally displaced distal radius fracture and a displaced, open, segmental distal femoral fracture with a pre-existing and now fully healed fracture of the ipsilateral hip with a retained sliding hip screw and side plate in place cephalad on the femur (Fig. 5). Notables on her medical history were chronic bronchitis, diet-controlled diabetes mellitus, and new onset atrial fibrillation. She underwent a debridement and internal fixation of her distal femoral fracture on the day of presentation. Her distal radius was splinted on that day as well. Her course was complicated by a prolonged stay in the ICU due to pneumonia and ventilator dependence. At the beginning of week 3, she developed some redness about the surgical wound, which prompted an aspiration that was sent for culture and grew Clostridium hostolyticum and Entero-bacter cloacae. Culture and sensitivity studies were ordered and IV antibiotics were initiated and managed by the infectious disease consul-tant. The patient was taken back to surgery, and the surgical wound as well as the original open fracture wound (anterior thigh) were opened, debrided, and thoroughly irrigated with 9 L of saline by gravity flow. Resorbable antibiotic beads were placed to bone level in each wound, and the wounds were closed after placement of suction drains (sewn in at their point of exit some distance from the incisions). Incisional TNP was established over each wound and set at −50 mm Hg. The drains and incisional VAC were left in place until the drainage drop-ped to 0 both for the suction drains and for the VAC canister and remained dry for 2 days. In addition, the character of the drainage was monitored: it remained clear and transudative. The patient's erythrocyte sedimentation rate (ESR) and C-reactive protein (CRP) were also followed and were also dropping as the beads slowly resorbed, as evidenced by serial radiographs. Both of these patients had a full

clinical resolution of their infection despite the depth of infection with contiguity of bone and implant.

COMMONALITIES AND RATIONALE

The above-described cases were managed early in the course of their infection with surgical debridement, fracture stabilization, appropriate dead space management, arrangement for high local concentration antibiotic levels sustainable for several weeks, with provision for drainage (dy-namic dead space management) and medical management supervised by an infectious disease consultant. These principles were the tenets taught by George Cierny and Jon Mader.[40,41] The infection milieu is influenced by many factors, including quorum sensing, which simply stated is the regulation of bacterial virulence by the con-centration of bacterial signal molecules (reflective of the population density of the bacteria).[42] As the concepts and corollaries of quorum-sensing emerge, the use of competitive inhibitors of acti-vator signal molecules is thought to theoretically provide a strategy for the development of a whole new class of antibiotics.[43] Proof of concept has shown the strategy to be effective in a mouse model.[44] To the author's knowledge, however, no such drugs are close to approval for human use. As that process wends its way forward, the use of high-concentration conventional anti-biotic/antibiotics locally to effect the lowering of the bacterial population will continue to be the major pharmacologic approach to the problem (fewer bacteria = fewer activator signal molecules = avoidance of activation of virulent bacterial gene cassettes). Given these facts, it would make sense that one way to keep the con-centration of bacterial signal molecules down is to keep the number of bacteria producing them down with a high concentration of conventional antibiotic and a continued dilution of bacterial signal molecules as well as resident bacteria with appropriate drainage of the wound seroma in which they reside (to analogize, the swamp needs to be converted into a river). Theoretically, if the virulent genes that enable glycocalyx- mediated adhesion can be kept from expression, perhaps the advantages conveyed to bacterial pathogens in the setting of bone and implant can be minimized.[44–46]

LONGSTANDING BONE AND IMPLANT-RELATED INFECTION

The management of longstanding deep infec-tions, particularly when involving dead bone

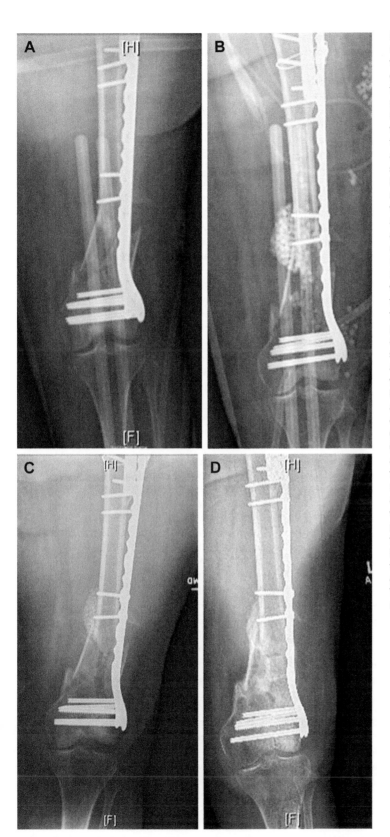

Fig. 5. A 73-year-old woman with multiple injuries from a motor vehicle accident, including an open periprosthetic (healed hip fracture with retained fixation plate proximally) distal supraintercondylar femoral fracture is managed with debridement of the open fracture and open reduction and periarticular plate fixation (A). She spent 2 weeks in the ICU with ventilator assistance, and at the beginning of week 3, was off the ventilator and in a step-down unit and developed some redness about the open fracture wound, now healed. An aspirate grew Clostridium histolyticum and Enterobacter cloacae and the patient was started on culture sensitive antibiotics supervised by the infectious disease consultant. The patient was returned to surgery and debrided to the bone and the surgical wound was thoroughly lavaged as was the original traumatic wound (anteromedially on the lower thigh). Drains are placed and sewn at their point of exit from the skin; resorbable (CaSO$_4$) antibiotic-impregnated (vancomycin + tobramycin) beads are placed (B) contiguous to the fracture [Biocomposites, Inc, Wilmington, NC, USA] and TNP was applied to each surgically closed wound. At 6 weeks, beads are still present on radiograph (C), and patient's ESR and CRP were normalizing. The patient's wounds and fracture fully healed, and a radiograph at 7 months is shown (D). The infection was completely resolved.

and retained implants, is problematic. Provided the patient is not a "C" host according to the Cierni Mader classification (patient with bone infection who is better off living with the infection vs undergoing the extensive treatment necessary to eradicate the disease),[41] the situation is often only remedied by removal of the involved implant or implants and resection of the nonviable bone and soft tissue. This resection is followed by staged reconstruction. Antibiotics should be directed by culture and sensitivity studies. The role of TNP here is ancillary and may be used to support or safeguard the reconstructive procedures as outlined in the earlier portions of this article.[47] Prosthetic joint infections are usually best managed with a 2-staged reconstruction.[48] Use of the TNP with instillation as pioneered by Fleischmann and colleagues[49–51] has had some favorable reports, but there is a lack of high-evidence studies with long-term follow-up.

ACKNOWLEDGMENTS

The assistance of Marian Baugh is greatly appreciated and acknowledged in the preparation of this article.

REFERENCES

1. Gustilo RB. Orthopaedic infection: diagnosis and treatment. Philadelphia: W. B. Saunders Company; 1989. Print.
2. Brumback RJ. Wound debridement. p79 in lower extremity salvage and reconstruction. New York: Elsevier; 1989.
3. Webb LX, Dedmond B, Schlatterer D, et al. The contaminated high-energy open fracture: a protocol to prevent and treat inflammatory mediator storm-induced soft-tissue compartment syndrome (IMSICS). J Am Acad Orthop Surg 2006;14:S82–6. Print.
4. Tejwani NC, Webb LX, Harvey EJ, et al. Soft-tissue management after trauma: initial management and wound coverage. AAOS Instructional Course Lectures 2011;60:15–25. Print.
5. Laverty D, Webb LX. Vacuum assisted closure: orthopaedic applications—surgery in wounds. Berlin: Springer-Verlag; 2004. p. 251–8. Print.
6. Morykwas MJ, David LR, Schneider AM, et al. Use of subatmospheric pressure to prevent progression of partial-thickness burns in a swine model. J Burn Care Rehabil 1999;20(1):15–21.
7. Langfitt M, Webb LX, Onwachuruba C, et al. Microvascular effects of subatmospheric pressure in striated muscle. J Reconstr Microsurg 2013;29(2):117–23.
8. Lindstedt S, Malmsjo M, Ingemansson R. Blood flow changes in normal and ischemic myocardium during topically applied negative pressure. Ann Thorac Surg 2007;84(2):568–73.
9. Argenta LC, Morykwas MJ, Mays JJ, et al. Reduction of myocardial ischemia-reperfusion injury by mechanical tissue resuscitation using subatmospheric pressure. J Cardiovasc Surg 2010;25(2):247–52.
10. Jordan JE, Mays JJ, Shelton JE, et al. Mechanical tissue resuscitation protects against myocardial ischemia-reperfusion injury. J Cardiovasc Surg 2014;29(1):116–23.
11. Argenta LC, Zheng Z, Bryant A, et al. A new method for modulating traumatic brain injury with mechanical tissue resuscitation. Neurosurgery 2012;70(5):1281–95.
12. Zheng ZL, Morykwas MJ, Tatter S, et al. Ameliorating spinal cord injury in an animal model with mechanical tissue resuscitation. Neurosurgery 2016;78(6):868–76.
13. Zheng ZL, Morykwas M, Campbell D, et al. Mechanical tissue resuscitation at the site of traumatic brain injuries reduces the volume of injury and hemorrhage in a swine model. Neurosurgery 2014;2(78):152–62.
14. Morykwas MJ, Argenta L, Shelton-Brown EI, et al. Vacuum-assisted closure: a new method for wound control and treatment: animal studies and basic foundation. Ann Plast Surg 1997;38(6):553–62.
15. Lindstedt S, Malmsjo M, Sjogren J, et al. Impact of different topical negative pressure levels on myocardial microvascular blood flow. Cardiovasc Revascularization Med 2008;9(1):29–35.
16. Peterson K, Riddle MD, Danko JR, et al. Trauma-related infections in battlefield casualties from Iraq. Ann Plast Surg 2007;245(5):803–11.
17. Osler W. Medical notes on England at war. JAMA 1914;63:2303–5.
18. Leininger BE, Rasmussen TE, Smith DL, et al. Experience with wound VAC and delayed primary closure of contaminated soft tissue injuries in Iraq. J Trauma 2006;61(5):1207–11.
19. DeFranzo AJ, Argenta LC, Marks MW, et al. The use of vacuum-assisted closure therapy for the treatment of lower-extremity wounds with exposed bone. Plast Reconstr Surg 2001;108(5):1184–91.
20. Schneider AM, Morykwas MJ, Argenta LC. A new and reliable method of securing skin grafts to the difficult recipient bed. Plast Reconstr Surg 1998;102(4):1195–8.
21. Morykwas MJ, Simpson J, Punger K, et al. Vacuum-assisted closure: state of basic research and physiologic foundation. Plast Reconstr Surg 2006;117(7 Suppl):121S–6S.
22. Yannas IV, Burke JF. Design of an artificial skin. I. Basic design principles. J Biomed Mater Res 1980;14(1):65–81.

23. Halim AS, Khoo TL, Mohd Yussof SJ. Biologic and synthetic skin substitutes: an overview. Indian J Plast Surg 2010;43(Suppl):S23–8.

24. Molnar JA, DeFranzo A, Hadaegh A, et al. Acceleration of integra incorporation in complex tissue defects with subatmospheric pressure. Plast Reconstr Surg 2004;113(5):1339–46.

25. DeFranzo A, Argenta L. Vacuum assisted closure in extremity trauma. In: Moran SL, Cooney WP, editors. Master techniques in orthopaedic surgery: soft tissue surgery. Philadelphia: Lippincott Williams & Wilkens + Walters Kluwer Baltimore; 2009. p. 49–60.

26. Godina M. Early microsurgical reconstruction of complex trauma of the extremities. Plast Reconstr Surg 1986;78(3):285–92.

27. Available at: http://news.mit.edu/2015/ioannis-yannas-to-be-inducted-national-inventors-hall-of-fame-0203. Accessed February 13, 2017.

28. Barnett TM, Shilt JS. Use of vacuum-assisted closure and a dermal regeneration template as an alternative to flap reconstruction in pediatric grade IIIB open lower-extremity injuries. Am J Orthop (Belle Mead NJ) 2009;38(6):301–5.

29. Schlatterer DR, Hirschfeld AG, Webb LX, et al. Negative pressure wound therapy in grade IIIB tibial fractures: fewer infections and fewer flap procedures? Clin Orthop Relat Res 2015;473(5):1802–11.

30. Stannard JP, Volgas DA, Stewart R, et al. Negative pressure wound therapy after severe open fractures: a prospective study. J Orthop Trauma 2009;23(8):552–7.

31. Reddix RN Jr, Leng XI, Woodall J, et al. The effect of incisional negative pressure therapy on wound complications after acetabular fracture surgery. J Surg Orthop Adv 2010;19(2):91–7.

32. Reddix RN Jr, Tyler HK, Kulp B, et al. Incisional vacuum-assisted wound closure in morbidly obese patients undergoing acetabular fracture surgery. Am J Orthop (Belle Mead NJ) 2009;38(9):446–9.

33. Porter SE, Russell GV, Dews RC, et al. Complications of acetabular fracture surgery in morbidly obese patients. J Orthop Trauma 2008;22(9):589–94.

34. Stannard JP, Volgas DA, McGwin G 3rd, et al. Incisional negative pressure wound therapy after high-risk lower extremity fractures. J Orthop Trauma 2012;26(1):37–42.

35. Scalise A, Calamita R, Tartaglione C, et al. Improving wound healing and preventing surgical site complications of closed surgical incisions: a possible role of incisional negative pressure wound therapy. A systematic review of the literature. Int Wound J 2015;13(6):1260–81.

36. Semsarzadeh NN, Tadisina KK, Maddox J, et al. Closed incision negative-pressure therapy is associated with decreased surgical-site infections: a meta-analysis. Plast Reconstr Surg 2015;136(3):592–602.

37. Sandy-Hodgetts K, Watts R. Effectiveness of negative pressure wound therapy/closed incision management in the prevention of post-surgical wound complications: a systematic review and meta-analysis. JBI Database Syst Rev Implement Rep 2015;13(1):253–303.

38. Timmers MS, Le Cessie S, Banwell P, et al. The effects of varying degrees of pressure delivered by negative-pressure wound therapy on skin perfusion. Ann Plast Surg 2005;55(6):665–71.

39. Kilpadi DV, Cunningham MR. Evaluation of closed incision management with negative pressure wound therapy (CIM): hematoma/seroma and involvement of the lymphatic system. Wound Repair Regen 2011;19(5):588–96.

40. Cierny G, Mader JT. Approach to adult osteomyelitis. Orthop Rev 1987;16(4):259–70.

41. Cierny G. Managing the debridement defect p123-121 in infection in the orthopaedic patient. In: Coombs R, Fitzgerald RH, editors. Orthopaedic infections. London: Butterworths; 1989. p. 123–31.

42. Miller MB, Bassler BL. Quorum sensing in bacteria. Annu Rev Microbiol 2001;55:165–99.

43. Romero D, Traxler MF, López D, et al. Antibiotics as signal molecules. Chem Rev 2011;111(9):5492–505.

44. Available at: https://www.ted.com/talks/bonnie_bassler_on_how_bacteria_communicate?language=en.

45. O'Louhlin C, Miller LC, Siryaporn A, et al. A quorum-sensing inhibitor blocks Pseudomonas aeruginosa virulence and biofilm formation. Proc Natl Acad Sci U S A 2013;110(44):17981–6.

46. Gristina AG, Webb LX, Hobgood CD, et al. Microbial adhesion, biofilms, and the pathophysiology of osteomyelitis. In: D'Ambrosia RD, Marier RL, editors. Orthopaedic infections. Thorofare (NJ): Slack; 1989. p. 49–69.

47. Cierny G, Mader JT. Adult chronic osteomyelitis: an overview. In: D'Ambrosia RD, Marier RL, editors. Orthopaedic infections. Thorofare (NJ): Slack; 1989. p. 31–47.

48. Zahar A, Gehrke TA. One-stage revision for infected total hip arthroplasty. Orthop Clin North Am 2016;47(1):11–8.

49. Fleischmann W, Strecker W, Bombelli M, et al. Vacuum sealing as treatment of soft tissue damage in open fractures. Unfallchirurgie 1993;96(9):488–92.

50. Fleischmann W, Russ M, Westhauser A, et al. Vacuum sealing as carrier system for controlled local drug administration in wound infection. Unfallchirurgie 1998;101(8):649–54.

51. Fleischmann W, Lang E, Russ M. Treatment of infection by vacuum sealing. Unfallchirurgie 1997;100(4):301–4.

Pediatrics

Double-Edged Sword
Musculoskeletal Infection Provoked Acute Phase Response in Children

Michael Benvenuti, MD[a,1], Thomas An, MD[a,1],
Emilie Amaro, BS[a], Steven Lovejoy, MD[b],
Gregory Mencio, MD[b], Jeffrey Martus, MD[b],
Megan Mignemi, MD[b],
Jonathan G. Schoenecker, MD, PhD[b,c,*]

KEYWORDS

• Musculoskeletal infection • Septic arthritis • Osteomyelitis • Pyomyositis
• Acute phase response

KEY POINTS

- The acute phase response is the physiologic reaction to tissue injury, such as musculoskeletal infection, trauma, and orthopedic surgery.
- Although trauma and orthopedic surgery are temporally isolated injuries, musculoskeletal infection is a continuous injury that leads to exuberant activation of the acute phase response that persists until the infection resolves.
- The acute phase response to musculoskeletal infection is paradoxic, as it is not only necessary to combat infection and repair damaged tissue, but also responsible for many of the associated complications.
- Given the interplay between musculoskeletal infection and the acute phase response, measuring positive and negatively regulated acute phase reactants has been useful in diagnosing and monitoring patients with musculoskeletal infection.
- Future strategies that modulate the acute phase response have the potential to improve treatment and prevent complications associated with musculoskeletal infection.

INTRODUCTION

Musculoskeletal infection represents a challenging disease process for orthopedic surgeons that poses significant health care costs and carries a high potential for morbidity and mortality. The most common pathogens of the musculoskeletal system express virulence factors that lead to a tropism, or selectivity, for damaged and regenerating tissue.[1] As developing and regenerative tissue share many overlapping features (eg, growth factors and angiogenesis), there is an increased prevalence of infection in children as compared with adults,

Funding provided by a research grant from Pediatric Orthopaedic Society of North America (JGS) and the Caitlyn Lovejoy Fund.
[a] Vanderbilt University School of Medicine, Nashville, TN, USA; [b] Department of Orthopaedics, Vanderbilt University Medical Center, Nashville, TN, USA; [c] Departments of Orthopaedics, Pharmacology, and Pathology, Microbiology and Immunology, Vanderbilt University Medical Center, Nashville, Tennessee
[1]Contributed equally.
* Corresponding author. 4202 Doctor's Office Tower, 2200 Children's Way, Nashville, TN 37232-9565.
E-mail address: jon.schoenecker@vanderbilt.edu

even in the absence of injury.[2] Only recently in orthopedics, the burden and mortality of musculoskeletal infection has been surpassed by other pathologies. In the pre-antibiotic era, the mortality rate of acute hematogenous osteomyelitis in children was upward of 50% due to overwhelming sepsis and metastatic abscesses.[3,4] The advent of antibiotics and the capacity to perform debridement of infected tissue has tremendously impacted the outcome of these patients and in the modern era mortality rates from pediatric musculoskeletal infection in the United States have dropped significantly.

Nevertheless, although most pediatric musculoskeletal infections are effectively treated and resolve without complications, severe infections continue to cause devastating complications.[5] For example, without timely treatment, septic arthritis of the hip and severe osteomyelitis may lead to avascular necrosis, pathologic fracture, growth arrest, and even amputation.[6–8] Disseminated infections have the potential to cause venous and arterial thromboembolic disease and septic shock.[9,10] In extreme infections, such as necrotizing fasciitis, mortality rates in epidemiologic studies have been recorded as high as 76%.[11,12] Moreover, the incidence of musculoskeletal infection has increased in recent years due to a number of factors, including the rising prevalence of diseases such as diabetes and obesity, which impair the immune system.[13,14]

In addition, the pharmacologic basis of antibiotic therapy is overwhelmingly based on disrupting microbial genetic machinery, such as cell wall and protein synthesis.[15] As microbial genetics evolve, drug-resistant pathogens, such as methicillin-resistant *Staphylococcus aureus* (MRSA), are increasingly common and often more difficult to treat.[16,17] Without the development of novel antibiotics capable of countering these organisms' genetic adaptations, the tremendous gains against musculoskeletal infection of the past century may be short-lived.

ACUTE PHASE RESPONSE: THE DOUBLE-EDGED SWORD IN ORTHOPEDICS

Damage to musculoskeletal tissue initiates a cascade of reactions that is collectively referred to as the acute phase response (Fig. 1). This dramatic physiologic response has far-reaching effects, affecting the activity of nearly all organ systems through coagulation, inflammatory, and regenerative processes. The acute phase response typically occurs over a 6-week process following an isolated injury, such as trauma or elective surgery (Fig. 2).[18] (The acute phase response in response to a total knee arthroplasty is used in this review as a point of reference of an elective surgical procedure. It is a procedure familiar to most orthopedic surgeons and stimulates a well-described acute phase response to the brink of developing acute phase response–related complications.)

The acute phase response is a critical mechanism for humans to survive and recover from injury. An insufficient response leads to hemorrhage, infection, and impaired tissue regeneration. *A decreased acute phase response may be observed in patients with cirrhosis, as the liver is the principal effector organ of the acute phase response.*[19,20] On the other hand, an excessive or prolonged acute phase response (see Fig. 2A, B) is a major cause of systemic complications observed in orthopedics (Fig. 3A), ranging from the relatively benign (nausea/pain) to more severe (coagulopathy, venous thromboembolism [VTE], systemic inflammatory response syndrome [SIRS]) and most severe (multiorgan failure [MOF] and death). As such, close monitoring of the acute phase response is the cornerstone concept of "damage control orthopedics."[21] Given that both trauma and orthopedic surgery elicit an acute phase response, the principle of damage control orthopedics is to perform more invasive surgical management such that their cumulative response does not push a patient into the threshold of more severe complications, such as SIRS, shock, MOF, or death (Fig. 3B, C). Furthermore, although this response has "acute" in the name, it is activated in the context of both acute and chronic inflammatory conditions. Chronic baseline activation of the acute phase response causes degeneration of musculoskeletal tissue in conditions such as osteoporosis.[22] Additionally, elevated baseline activity of the acute phase response amplifies the response to an elective or traumatic injury, increasing the risk of complications in those patients.[23] Therefore, the acute phase response as a whole may be viewed as a "double-edged sword," because a well-coordinated acute phase response is essential for survival and recovery from tissue injury, but an excessive response may lead to devastating complications.

When infectious pathogens invade the body, bacterial proliferation and virulence factor expression cause damage to surrounding tissues. However, injury caused by a developing infection is dramatically different from isolated surgery or trauma in that it is continuous (Fig. 4). As the infection propagates, tissue injury persists until it is resolved by the immune system, antibiotics, and/or surgical debridement

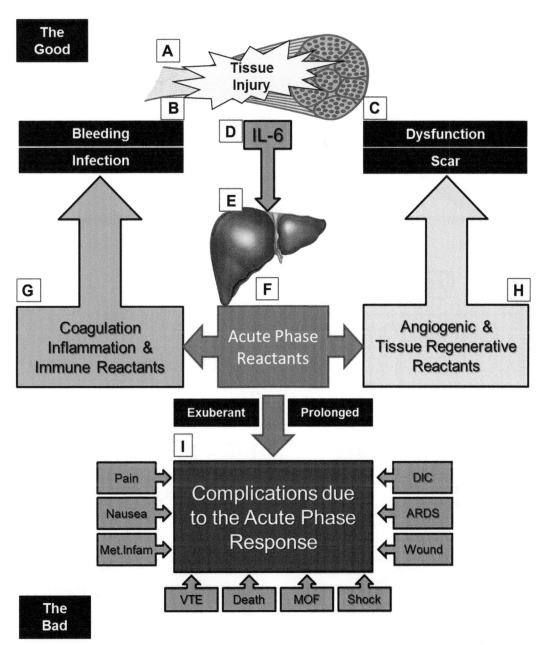

Fig. 1. Acute phase response overview. (*A*) Tissue injury inevitably causes (*B*) hemorrhage and an environment that supports infection and (*C*) tissue dysfunction and potential scar. The acute phase response is initiated by (*D*) systemic liberation of cytokines such as IL-6 that travel to effector organs, primarily the liver (*E*), and regulate thousands of genes. (*F*) These genes produce "acute phase reactants," most notably (*G*) clotting, inflammatory, and immune factors that resolve bleeding and fight potential infection associated with the tissue injury. (*H*) In later phases of the acute phase response, acute phase reactants promote angiogenesis and tissue regeneration to resolve tissue dysfunction and limit inflammatory scar tissue.[23] (*I*) Too exuberant (peak levels of acute phase reactants) or too prolonged (total amount of acute phase reactant over time) response leads to systemic complications.

(see Fig. 4B). In essence, musculoskeletal infection may be considered continuous activation of the acute phase response, only halted by initiation of antibiotic therapy or surgical debridement. Patients with musculoskeletal infection often suffer from both greater peak and total acute phase response than a patient with a singular injury (see Fig. 4C). This concept

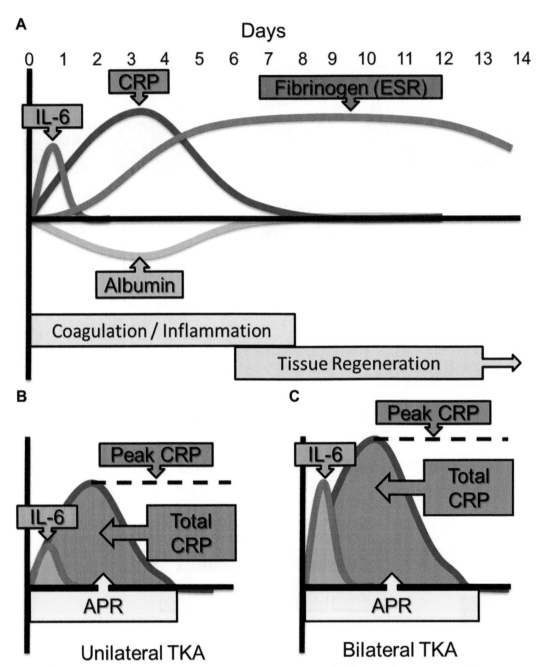

Fig. 2. Acute phase reactions: temporal and injury severity. (*A*) Levels of acute phase reactants following tissue injury change dramatically and rapidly. (*B*) The extent and duration of an acute phase response is dependent on the severity of a tissue injury. The magnitude of the acute phase reaction can be quantified by both the peak concentration of an acute phase reactant as well as the levels of that reactant over time (area under the curve). (*C*) A patient sustaining greater tissue damage, such as a bilateral TKA (Total knee arthoplasty) compared with a unilateral TKA, will experience both a greater peak and total acute phase reaction.

of continuous activation of the acute phase response provides rationale for why patients with musculoskeletal infection are at increased risk of suffering from clinical complications, such as thrombosis, and impaired tissue regeneration than those with an isolated, traumatic injury. Specifically, continuous activation of the acute phase response in patients with musculoskeletal infection leads to a markedly increased "area under the curve" for acute phase reactants such as C-reactive protein (CRP), which implies a significantly greater overall inflammatory

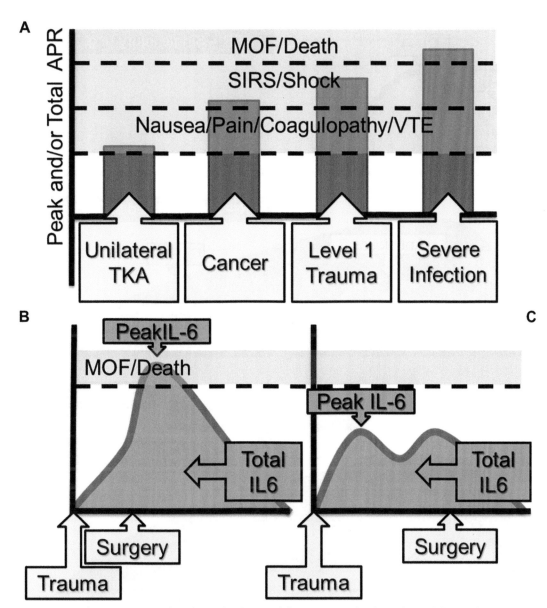

Fig. 3. Acute phase response induced complications and damage control orthopedics. (*A*) Too exuberant or prolonged (total) acute phase response can lead to systemic complications. Because the peak and duration of an acute phase response is directly proportional to the injury severity, duration and intensity of a tissue injury can predict these complications. The principle of damage control orthopedics: as surgical intervention elicits an acute phase response, untimely surgery (*B*) in reference to the acute phase response from a trauma can push a patient beyond a threshold of complications, whereas allowing the initial response to subside before surgical intervention (*C*) avoids this complication, despite both patients having the same total acute phase response, indicated here by level of IL-6. VTE, venous thromboembolism.

response (see Fig. 4C). As such, complications caused by musculoskeletal infection generally arise from either an excessive acute phase response (see Fig. 3A) or complete exhaustion of one or more elements of the acute phase response (eg, disseminated intravascular coagulation).[24]

In addition to systemic complications, an overly exuberant, or prolonged, acute phase response also has dire consequences on tissue regeneration. Tissue regeneration occurs in phases, beginning with coagulation to promote compartmentalization, followed by inflammation to kill pathogens, and finally progression to tissue

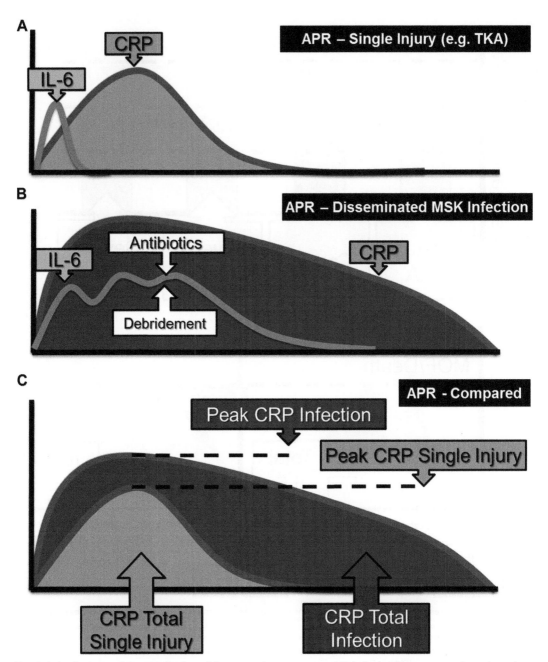

Fig. 4. Infection: a continuous activation of the acute phase response. (*A*) A single injury causes a dynamic and predictable acute phase response. (*B*) Musculoskeletal infection causes continuous tissue damage, activating the acute phase response (indicated by sustained release of IL-6, *blue line*). The infection provoked acute phase response subsides only once bacteria are killed by the immune system, antibiotics, and/or debridement. (*C*) The continuous activation of the acute phase response leads to a more exuberant (peak) and prolonged (total) acute phase response when compared with the single episode of tissue damage. APR, acute phase response.

proliferation and remodeling. The failure to proceed from one phase to the next prohibits normal tissue healing and recovery. For example, the failure to remove the coagulation matrix protein fibrin prevents angiogenesis and fracture repair.[25,26] As an infection persists, the dynamic and coordinated progression of the acute phase response is lost in continuous activation without resolution. Thus, the acute phase response during a musculoskeletal infection is drastically different from that of trauma or isolated surgery and has a greater propensity for morbidity and mortality.

THE PARADOX

Together, these concepts present a paradox for surgeons and health care providers caring for these patients. Many of the elements of the acute phase response are essential to combat and eliminate developing infections; however, in the process, this response may lead to many of the complications observed in patients suffering from infected musculoskeletal tissue (see Fig. 1).

BACTERIAL HIJACKING OF THE ACUTE PHASE RESPONSE

Pathogenic bacteria possess an arsenal of virulence factors that allow them to invade, persist, and disseminate within the human body (Fig. 5). Co-evolution between pathogens and the acute phase response has led to bacterial manipulation of specific elements of the acute phase reactants, thereby enabling them to hijack the response. For example, the coagulation system serves as one of the initial defense mechanisms against bacterial invasion by

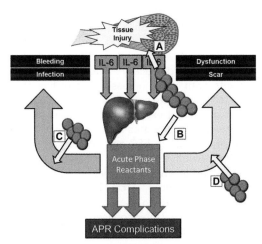

Fig. 5. Bacteria promote and hijack the acute phase response. Bacteria that cause musculoskeletal infections in humans have evolved to hijack specific elements of the acute phase response to allow them to colonize and disseminate.[1] For example, certain subspecies of S aureus (A) produce virulence factors that promote tissue injury and (B) production of the acute phase reactants. (C) They also produce factors that specifically interact with elements of the acute phase reaction, using proteins intended to eliminate pathogens and stop bleeding to instead support their survival. (D) Finally, bacteria have evolved to hijack factors essential for tissue regeneration. This combination of virulence factors promotes continuous, exuberant activation of the acute phase response, leading to severe complications.

immobilizing bacteria within clots and recruiting leukocytes to the site of infection through integrin expression on fibrin.[27–29] The most well-known of the S aureus virulence factors is coagulase (Coa), which is secreted into the extracellular environment and activates the conversion of prothrombin to thrombin.[30,31] This Coa-thrombin complex then catalyzes the cleavage of fibrinogen to fibrin, promoting the formation of protective abscess for the bacteria. This remarkable interaction between the host's acute phase response and infection pathogenesis is an evolutionary battle that continues to the present day. Importantly, virulence factor expression differs significantly not only between species (eg, S aureus vs Kingella kingae), but also among bacteria of a single species. In other words, a strain of S aureus with a greater arsenal of virulence factors should activate the acute phase response to a greater extent than a strain of S aureus with fewer virulence factors. Nevertheless, awareness of the interplay between the acute phase response and bacterial infection will aid in diagnosis, prognostication, and treatment of musculoskeletal infections.

PATIENT EVALUATION OVERVIEW

Acute Phase Reactants: Marker of Infection Severity

Monitoring acute phase reactants has become common practice in many diseases that cause tissue damage. Even chronic diseases that cause significantly less tissue injury than acute or surgical trauma lead to baseline alterations in acute phase reactants. For example, coronary artery disease has been correlated with elevated CRP and fibrinogen, whereas cirrhosis leads to an attenuated acute phase response and decreased levels of CRP and albumin due to impaired hepatic protein synthesis.[32] Acute phase reactants also correlate with prognosis in stroke and renal cell carcinoma.[33,34]

Disease severity in musculoskeletal infection is similarly associated with elevations in acute phase reactants, as numerous models for assessing disease severity have relied heavily on acute phase reactants, such as CRP and erythrocyte sedimentation rate (ESR) (Fig. 6). For example, CRP is included in prognostic and diagnostic models for patients with osteomyelitis.[35,36] In addition, the "Kocher criteria" include ESR as a factor for diagnosing septic arthritis.[37] Inflammatory markers have a crucial role in diagnosis, prognosis, and gauging response to treatment for musculoskeletal infections. Therefore, a deeper understanding of the acute phase response has the potential to improve

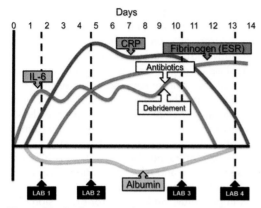

Fig. 6. Monitoring acute phase reactants to diagnose and monitor treatment in infection. Understanding the dynamic nature of the acute phase reactants allows for surgeons to diagnose and monitor the efficacy of treatment of patients with musculoskeletal infection.

orthopedic surgeons' ability to interpret these laboratory markers in clinical settings.

Acute Phase Reactants

Thousands of proteins are upregulated and downregulated with activation of the acute phase response. By definition, proteins may be considered acute phase reactants only if they increase or decrease in quantity by greater than 25%, with most fluctuations mediated by changes in hepatic synthesis.[38] The magnitude of change in serum concentration and time course for resolution for different acute phase reactants varies significantly, depending on their role in activating, sustaining, or resolving the acute phase response (see Fig. 4C). With specific acute phase reactants, understanding the temporal relationship between the specific acute phase reactant and the pathogen-induced injury provides considerable diagnostic utility. For example, understanding that CRP is produced more rapidly in the liver than fibrinogen explains the increased utility in monitoring CRP as opposed to fibrinogen (or ESR, see later in this article) in the early diagnosis of infection (see Fig. 6 "Lab 1") as compared with later in the infection (see Fig. 6 "Lab 2"). Additionally, serial monitoring acute phase reactants may provide valuable information regarding the efficacy of antibiotics and/or debridement by observing the change over time (see Fig. 6 compare "Lab 3" with "Lab 4").

Interleukin-6

Interleukin (IL)-6 is the principal initiating factor in the acute phase response and is released by damaged tissue during infection (see Fig. 1). It is stored in musculoskeletal tissue and released immediately after injury, and therefore provides the earliest measurable response to tissue damage.[39] IL-6 has been studied as a potential marker for assessing prognosis and guiding treatment in the setting of trauma, sepsis, and heart disease.[39–42] However, there is limited literature describing its use in the context of musculoskeletal infection, likely because measurement of IL-6 has associated challenges, such as limited availability for testing in the clinical setting, short half-life in plasma, and absence of standardization. Currently, its measurement for gauging musculoskeletal infection severity is limited mainly to research settings.

C-reactive protein

CRP is produced by the liver in response to IL-6 and other cytokines. The origin of the name derives from C polysaccharide of *Streptococcus pneumoniae*.[43] At a molecular level, CRP has several defined roles. For example, it has the capability to bind dying cells and/or bacterial pathogens and activate the complement system.[44] In addition, CRP is able to activate monocytes and induce the release of inflammatory cytokines.[45,46] In response to acute episodes of tissue injury, there are short but dramatic increases in the levels of serum CRP. In fact, it is one of the most drastically induced acute phase reactants, with levels increasing more than 100-fold in the immediate postinjury period.[47] In addition, as one might expect, the magnitude of the increase in CRP correlates with the scale of tissue injury. In contrast to ESR and fibrinogen, which have long half-lives, CRP has a half-life of only 17 hours and levels increase within 4 to 6 hours of injury.[48] Therefore, it can be used to track real-time responses to therapy and guide care for musculoskeletal infection (see Fig. 6).[49]

Mild baseline elevations in CRP are seen in the context of chronic diseases, such as coronary artery disease and diabetes. On the other hand, markedly elevated CRP levels are more indicative of an acute inflammatory process, such as bacterial infection.[50] Because of the correlation between CRP and tissue injury, CRP has been included in several prognostic and diagnostic models that help guide treatment in infection.[51,52] One of these is the scoring system for assessment of severity of illness in the context of pediatric acute hematogenous osteomyelitis.[35] In this model, osteomyelitis was stratified into mild, moderate, and severe categories based on objective clinical parameters. Not surprisingly, CRP values at admission, 48 hours, and 96 hours all significantly correlated with disease severity and outcomes, such as total length of stay. Other models have similarly used CRP as a marker of disease severity. For example, one prediction model that showed that children with a higher CRP at admission were more likely to develop complicated osteomyelitis[36] and another prognostic model for pediatric musculoskeletal infection is dominated by CRP.[53] CRP is also included in the Laboratory Risk Indicator for Necrotizing Fasciitis (LRINEC) score, as a CRP of greater than 150 mg/L in the system suggests an increased likelihood of necrotizing infection.[54] Overall, the marked elevation of CRP in the setting of acute inflammation and its short half-life make it an effective marker for gauging infection severity and monitoring response in clinical settings. Notably, the units for CRP measurement may vary by institution by a factor of 10, with some hospitals reporting CRP in units of mg/dL, whereas others report in units of mg/L.

Erythrocyte sedimentation rate/fibrinogen

The ESR is a simple, indirect measure for the acute phase response. The ESR measures the rate of descent of anticoagulated red blood cells in a vertical column in 1 hour. This measurement is influenced by numerous factors, the most important being the concentration of the acute phase reactant fibrinogen. Although ESR advanced medical science when introduced in the 1920s, it is often misleading because it is greatly influenced by immunoglobulins, plasma constituents, and changes to erythrocyte morphology and number. Thus, ESR is a less sensitive marker for the acute phase response than fibrinogen, an acute phase reactant.[23,55] Nevertheless, out of convention, most clinicians continue to monitor and report ESR in studies.

Currently, elevated ESR is a key diagnostic criterion for several noninfectious diseases, including polymyalgia rheumatic and temporal arteritis, and is often used as an adjunct "severity index" in the context of infection. However, there are also several noninflammatory etiologies of elevated ESR, including anemia, pregnancy, obesity, and old age, making it a less-specific marker for infection or inflammation.[56,57] Fibrinogen is a relatively late acute phase reactant with a long half-life. As such, ESR typically increases 24 to 48 hours after initiation of the acute phase response and decreases slowly with resolution of inflammation.

In the context of musculoskeletal infection, ESR has been used as a predictive marker for severity for several different disease processes. One study demonstrated an increased likelihood of diabetic foot osteomyelitis in the setting of appropriate symptoms and an ESR greater than 70 mm/h.[58] In addition, ESR levels remain elevated for a prolonged period postinfection (up to 3 months), which has led authors to suggest using ESR for monitoring long-term recovery.[59] In the context of pediatric musculoskeletal infections, ESR greater than 20 mm/h had 94% sensitivity for detecting musculoskeletal infection.[60] Based on these studies, it is evident that an elevated ESR has been used effectively as a marker of infection severity, with a relatively high sensitivity as a potential screening index for musculoskeletal infection.

Procalcitonin

Procalcitonin, a peptide precursor of calcitonin, is another acute phase reactant that has been studied for use in the diagnosis and treatment of musculoskeletal infection. Although calcitonin is typically secreted by the parafollicular cells of the thyroid in response to hypercalcemia, the biological function of procalcitonin is unknown. Procalcitonin is synthesized in the neuroendocrine cells of the lungs and intestine in response to cytokines including IL-1, IL-6, and tumor necrosis factor (TNF)-alpha. Serum concentrations are normally undetectable, but have been shown to increase 1000-fold in the setting of systemic bacterial infections.[61] In the setting of sepsis, procalcitonin has also been shown to be useful in measuring treatment response, with a decline in its levels expected within 72 to 96 hours of treatment initiation.[62]

Currently, there are few studies that examine the use of procalcitonin in the context of musculoskeletal infection. One meta-analysis based on these studies reports that a procalcitonin of less than 0.3 ng/mL suggests a low suspicion for infection, whereas a procalcitonin of greater than 0.5 ng/mL raises concern for infection.[63] Interestingly, current studies suggest that procalcitonin may have several advantages over CRP as a marker of musculoskeletal infection severity. It increases earlier than CRP in response to IL-6, reaching half of its maximum value in 8 hours compared with 20 hours for CRP.[64] It also has a shorter half-life, which means that its levels begin to fall earlier than CRP with the resolution of inflammation.[65,66] Additionally, procalcitonin does not increase significantly in the context of viral or noninfectious pathology, potentially making it a more specific test than CRP in the setting of bacterial infection.[67–69] In fact, Simon and colleagues[70] found that procalcitonin is more accurate than CRP in differentiating infection from noninfection and bacterial infection from viral infection. Overall, procalcitonin appears to be a promising inflammatory marker, but further research is necessary to characterize its response in the setting of musculoskeletal infection.

Additional acute phase reactants

There are thousands of additional proteins modulated by the acute phase response. In addition to IL-6, several other inflammatory cytokines also act as initiators of the acute phase response, including transforming growth factor beta, interferon gamma, and TNF-alpha.[71] These cytokines are produced predominantly by macrophages at sites of injury and inflammation, and have a similar role in stimulating the coagulant, inflammatory, and regenerative arms of the acute phase response.[23]

Given the wide range of proteins influenced by the acute phase response, the hepatic response to tissue injury has far-reaching physiologic effects. Studies have demonstrated that inflammatory cytokines significantly impact the hypothalamic-pituitary-adrenal axis, including leading to secretion of corticotropin-releasing hormone and increased cortisol production. This interaction with the body's central hormonal regulation contributes to many of the systemic symptoms that are typically associated with inflammatory conditions such as infection.[72]

Negatively regulated acute phase reactants

Although most proteins affected by the acute phase response are upregulated to propagate the acute phase response, there are many proteins whose production is inhibited in response to tissue injury. These are termed negative acute phase reactants, and include proteins such as albumin, transferrin, and transthyretin.[23] Decreased production of these proteins may serve to divert resources toward synthesis of proteins directly involved in the acute phase response. In addition, the decrease in level of certain proteins may also have a proinflammatory effect. For example, transthyretin has be shown to inhibit IL-1 production by monocytes.[73] Therefore, a decrease in production of transthyretin increases the inflammatory effects of IL-1, leading to fever and immune cell adhesion factor expression. Given their inverse relationship to the acute phase response, these proteins have the potential to be monitored as markers of the intensity of the acute phase response in the opposite manner of markers such as CRP and ESR. In the case of these negative acute phase reactants, marked decreases in plasma expression would be indicative of a more robust acute phase response.

Dysregulation of the Acute Phase Response

The acute phase response is crucial for clearing infection and healing damaged tissue through regulation of inflammatory, coagulant, and immune processes. However, dysregulation of the acute phase response has the potential to lead to severe complications related to these same processes, such as hypotension, septic shock, and coagulopathy (see Figs. 1 and 4). These complications are much more likely to occur in the context of severe, disseminated infections due to intense upregulation of the acute phase response.

Septic and toxin-mediated shock

One of the most severe complications of infection is shock, which carries a mortality of up to 20% in children.[74] In musculoskeletal infection, this may occur due to septic shock or toxic shock syndrome. Toxic shock syndrome is most often caused by S aureus and Streptococcus pyogenes production of super antigens, such as toxic shock syndrome toxin and streptococcal superantigens, respectively. These toxins produced by S aureus and S pyogenes are structurally related and act by binding major histocompatibility complex II and T-cell receptors, leading to the widespread activation of antigen-presenting cells and T cells.[75,76] This activation leads to the release of high systemic levels of cytokines such as TNF-alpha, TNF-beta, IL-1, and IL-2, thereby generating an overexuberant inflammatory response that is characterized by fever, hypotension, rash, and other systemic symptoms.[77,78] Of these cytokines, TNF-alpha has been shown to be the most significant mediator of the shock response, and its inhibition has been shown to improve mean arterial pressure and survival in animal studies.[79]

Septic shock results from a hyperinflammatory immune response due to overwhelming, systemic bacterial infection. Higher levels of acute phase reactants are indicative of worse prognosis and indicate the need for aggressive intervention. Interestingly, following intense activation of the acute phase response secondary to infection, many patients also experience a state of immunoparalysis due to a strong compensatory anti-inflammatory response.[80] Studies have demonstrated that people who die of sepsis and MOF sometimes have immunohistochemical evidence of immunosuppression, with CD4, CD8, and HLA-DR depletion and decreased levels of IL-6, IL-10, and interferon gamma.[81]

This immunosuppression associated with septic shock is due to increased apoptosis of immune system cells, T-cell exhaustion, monocyte deactivation, and the regulatory effect of the central nervous system immune system.[80] It is crucial to remember that acute phase response reactants and mediators are finite and may be depleted, leading to complications in the late stages of severe infections.

Coagulopathy

Severe cases of musculoskeletal infection have the potential to dysregulate the acute phase response, leading to systemic coagulopathy and disseminated intravascular coagulation (DIC).[82] Thrombosis is a common complication of musculoskeletal infection, and epidemiologic studies have detected venous thromboembolism in up to 10% of pediatric patients with hematogenous osteomyelitis.[9,10,83,84] Additional studies have shown that disseminated or musculoskeletal infection predisposes patients to developing severe coagulopathy.[82,85] This devastating complication has the potential to cause widespread thrombosis along with paradoxic bleeding, leading to mortality rates of approximately 50%.[86,87]

DIC is characterized by systemic activation of the coagulation system with deposition of fibrin and platelets throughout the vasculature.[24] The activation of the coagulation cascade is dependent on the activation of the tissue factor/factor VIIa pathway and the contact system. In addition to uncontrolled coagulation, anticoagulant pathways also become dysregulated in DIC, most notably the protein C, antithrombin, and tissue factor pathway inhibitor cascades.[88] Protein C levels are decreased by impaired synthesis, consumption, and degradation. In addition, its activation is decreased by proinflammatory cytokines.[89] Furthermore, sepsis leads to downregulation of endothelial protein C receptors and resistance to activated protein C via increased factor VIII levels.[90,91] Several clinical trials have attempted to improve sepsis outcomes by administering activated protein C, but these studies have failed to demonstrate benefit and actually identified an increased bleeding risk. Antithrombin, another anticoagulant, inhibits both thrombin and factor Xa to prevent hypercoagulability. However, during severe inflammation, antithrombin levels are decreased by impaired synthesis, neutrophil elastase degradation, and consumption.[92] Similar to protein C studies, trials investigating repletion of tissue factor pathway inhibitors, such as antithrombin, in clinical trials have demonstrated increased bleeding risks without improvement in mortality.[93]

Monitoring coagulation in the setting of coagulopathy

The combined hypercoagulable and hypocoagulable state of DIC due to widespread dysregulation of coagulation cascades poses a dilemma for both diagnosis and treatment.[24] Therefore, in the setting of severe infections, laboratory tests such as prothrombin time (PT), partial thromboplastin time, fibrinogen, and D-dimer may be warranted to detect early coagulopathic changes and allow for timely administration of clotting factors and platelets.

Critically ill patients with DIC often have platelet counts in the range of 50,000 to 100,000, if not lower.[94] Therefore, close monitoring of platelet count in the beginning stages of severe infection may allow for early transfusion and prevention of significant bleeding. PT/international normalized ratio is commonly used as a marker of a patient's coagulation status. Although this test was originally developed to measure the effects of warfarin on the clotting cascade, the accuracy, availability, and familiarity of the test has made it a widely used marker of coagulopathy.[95] Direct measurement of coagulation factors to assess for coagulopathy is not currently recommended, as the tests often have delayed turnaround times and most assays require factors to be less than 50% of their normal levels to be considered significant.

Fibrinogen, however, is a commonly measured coagulation factor, but is a nuanced marker in diagnosing DIC. Although it is an acute phase reactant that is dramatically upregulated in the setting of infection, it is also consumed rapidly in the setting of DIC. Therefore, a single measurement of fibrinogen in the setting of severe sepsis may be difficult to interpret accurately. However, a low fibrinogen level is suggestive of serious coagulopathy, with consumption outpacing the accelerated production caused by the acute phase response. Fibrin degradation products such as D-Dimer may be used as a proxy for the rate of fibrinogen consumption and clot formation. However, this test is dependent on the rate of fibrinolysis, which also can be variable in the setting of acute disease.

One test that offers a comprehensive picture of the coagulation and fibrinolytic systems is thromboelastography (TEG), which is a test that measures the speed and strength of clot formation from a sample of blood. It provides measurements of clot kinetics, strength, and lysis, allowing for a more comprehensive measurement of coagulation and fibrinolysis. Unfortunately, this test is not commonly used in the context of septic coagulopathy and DIC, but is gaining popularity in the setting of trauma.[96] However, a recent prospective observational study demonstrated that hypocoagulability identified with TEG correlated with increased bleeding and mortality in the context of severe sepsis.[97] Further studies are required to define the potential utility of this test in the context of DIC and musculoskeletal infection in pediatric patients.

FUTURE DIRECTIONS: MODULATING THE ACUTE PHASE DIRECTION

As discussed previously, exuberant activation acute phase response has the potential to lead to devastating complications. Therefore, prompt recognition and treatment of acute phase response dysregulation has the potential to prevent complications and improve morbidity and mortality related to musculoskeletal infection. The following section details several potential interventions that aim to modulate and correct dysregulation in the acute phase response.

Corticosteroids

Monitoring for adrenal insufficiency in the setting of severe musculoskeletal infection is crucial. Severe disease has the potential to overwhelm adrenal production of cortisol, which may lead to difficulty maintaining adequate blood pressure and preventing symptoms of shock. Although there is no evidence of an effective method for testing for acute adrenal insufficiency in the severely ill,[98] elevated cortisol levels and a poor response to a short corticotropin stimulation test have been shown to correlate with poor outcomes.[99,100] Therefore, the use of spot cortisol testing and corticotropin stimulation testing can help to guide care, with a poor response to stimulation testing indicating a poor prognosis and the need for cortisol supplementation. In patients in whom corticosteroids are indicated by a poor response to fluids and vasopressors, the Surviving Sepsis Campaign recommends 200 mg intravenous hydrocortisone daily.[101] In patients without adrenal insufficiency, steroids have also been shown to decrease the acute phase response and improve acute postoperative pain and decrease time to discharge in total joint replacement.[102,103] However, there is a higher threshold for administering systemic steroids in patients with known

infection because of their immunosuppressive effects.

Thromboprophylaxis

Despite the high incidence of deep vein thrombosis in children with musculoskeletal infection, such as osteomyelitis, thromboprophylaxis is not a regular part of their care. However, children with musculoskeletal infection are susceptible to all 3 elements of the Virchow triad, as they are hypercoagulable due to systemic inflammation, suffer from endothelial injury, and are often sedentary due to pain. As such, children with musculoskeletal infection may similarly benefit from some form of thromboprophylaxis (eg, low molecular weight heparin), especially those with more severe disease that is affecting the lower extremity.

Vitamin K Replacement

In the setting of infection-induced coagulopathy, repletion of platelets and fibrinogen is often performed. In addition, subcutaneous administration of vitamin K has potential to prevent development of coagulopathy through its role in coagulation factor synthesis. In case reports, prophylactic vitamin K administration effectively improved coagulopathy in the setting of both necrotizing fasciitis and osteomyelitis, and there have been no known adverse events associated with its administration.[82,104]

Protein C

The well-described dysregulation of protein C in acute infection has made it an appealing target for repletion in septic patients. However, recombinant activated protein C has been withdrawn from the market after phase II trials due to an increased risk of bleeding when administered.[105,106] Despite this setback, a small study of patients with coagulopathic pediatric sepsis who received nonactivated plasma-derived protein C has shown to reduce amputation rates without increased hemorrhagic events.[107] Small studies in adults with severe septic shock have also shown that protein C concentrate may be useful in controlling coagulopathy.[108,109] Further studies are required to determine the role for protein C repletion in septic patients with musculoskeletal infection.

SUMMARY

Overall, the acute phase response has a crucial role in mounting the body's response to infection. The different phases of the acute phase response have specific roles in coagulation, tissue repair, and remodeling following musculoskeletal infection. As demonstrated by this review, there exists abundant evidence that acute phase reactants are effective for monitoring infection severity and response to therapy in the setting of musculoskeletal infection. However, one must remember that the acute phase response is a double-edged sword, with the potential to cause significant complications in the context of an excessive response. Given that infection may be considered a continuous tissue injury that activates the acute phase response without any inhibition, children with musculoskeletal infections are at markedly increased risk for developing an exuberant acute phase response. Many of the serious complications associated with pediatric musculoskeletal infection, including venous thromboembolic disease and DIC, are the direct result of a dysregulated acute phase response. Monitoring of acute phase reactants is important for prompt recognition of dysregulation that may lead to devastating complications. Continued research is necessary to further delineate the role for acute phase reactants in guiding diagnosis and prognosis of musculoskeletal infections. In addition, there remains significant potential for manipulation of the acute phase response in the setting of infection to reduce and prevent complications related to hyperinflammation and dysregulation of the coagulation system.

REFERENCES

1. An TJ, Benvenuti MA, Mignemi ME, et al. Pediatric musculoskeletal infection: hijacking the acute phase response. JBJS Rev 2016;4(9).
2. Gafur OA, Copley LAB, Hollmig ST, et al. The impact of the current epidemiology of pediatric musculoskeletal infection on evaluation and treatment guidelines. J Pediatr Orthop 2008;28(7):777–85.
3. Song KM, Sloboda JF. Acute hematogenous osteomyelitis in children. J Am Acad Orthop Surg 2001;9(3):166–75.
4. Ciampolini J, Harding KG. Pathophysiology of chronic bacterial osteomyelitis. Why do antibiotics fail so often? Postgrad Med J 2000;76(898):479–83.
5. Frank G, Mahoney HM, Eppes SC. Musculoskeletal infections in children. Pediatr Clin North Am 2005;52(4):1083–106.
6. Forlin E, Milani C. Sequelae of septic arthritis of the hip in children: a new classification and a review of 41 hips. J Pediatr Orthop 2008;28(5):524–8.
7. Lew DP, Waldvogel FA. Osteomyelitis. Lancet 2004;364:369–79.
8. Maffulli N, Papalia R, Zampogna B, et al. The management of osteomyelitis in the adult. Surgeon 2015;14(6):345–60.
9. Bouchoucha S, Benghachame F, Trifa M, et al. Deep venous thrombosis associated with acute hematogenous osteomyelitis in children. Orthop Traumatol Surg Res 2010;96(8):890–3.
10. Mantadakis E, Plessa E, Vouloumanou EK, et al. Deep venous thrombosis in children with musculoskeletal infections: the clinical evidence. Int J Infect Dis 2012;16(4):e236–43.
11. Elliott DC, Kufera JA, Myers RA. Necrotizing soft tissue infections. Risk factors for mortality and strategies for management. Ann Surg 1996;224(5):672–83.
12. Espandar R, Sibdari SY, Rafiee E, et al. Necrotizing fasciitis of the extremities: a prospective study. Strateg Trauma Limb Reconstr 2011;6(3):121–5.
13. Falagas ME, Kompoti M. Obesity and infection. Lancet Infect Dis 2006;6(7):438–46.
14. Hobizal KB, Wukich DK. Diabetic foot infections: current concept review. Diabet Foot Ankle 2012;3:1–8.
15. Kohanski MA, Dwyer DJ, Collins JJ. How antibiotics kill bacteria: from targets to networks. Nat Rev Microbiol 2010;8(6):423–35.
16. Patel A, Calfee RP, Plante M, et al. Methicillin-resistant Staphylococcus aureus in orthopaedic surgery. J bone Joint Surg Br 2008;90:1401–6.
17. Martínez-Aguilar G, Avalos-Mishaan A, Hulten K, et al. Community-acquired, methicillin-resistant and methicillin-susceptible Staphylococcus aureus musculoskeletal infections in children. Pediatr Infect Dis J 2004;23(8):701–6.
18. An TJ, Engstrom SM, Oelsner WK, et al. Elevated d-Dimer is not predictive of symptomatic deep venous thrombosis after total joint arthroplasty. J Arthroplasty 2016;31(10):2269–72.
19. Borzio M, Salerno F, Piantoni L, et al. Bacterial infection in patients with advanced cirrhosis: a multicentre prospective study. Dig Liver Dis 2001;33(1):41–8.
20. Fiuza C, Salcedo M, Clemente G, et al. In vivo neutrophil dysfunction in cirrhotic patients with advanced liver disease. J Infect Dis 2000;182(2):526–33.
21. Roberts CS, Pape H-C, Jones AL, et al. Damage control orthopaedics. J Bone Joint Surg Am 2005;87(2):434–49.
22. Cole HA, Ohba T, Nyman JS, et al. Fibrin accumulation secondary to loss of plasmin-mediated fibrinolysis drives inflammatory osteoporosis in mice. Arthritis Rheumatol 2014;66(8):2222–33.
23. Gabay C, Kushner I. Acute-phase proteins and other systemic responses to inflammation. N Engl J Med 1999;340(6):448–54.
24. Stutz CM, O'Rear LD, O'Neill KR, et al. Coagulopathies in orthopaedics: links to inflammation and the potential of individualizing treatment strategies. J Orthop Trauma 2013;27(4):236–41.

25. Yuasa M, Mignemi NA, Nyman JS, et al. Fibrinolysis is essential for fracture repair and prevention of heterotopic ossification. J Clin Invest 2015; 125(8):3117–31.

26. O'Keefe RJ. Fibrinolysis as a target to enhance fracture healing. N Engl J Med 2015;373(18): 1776–8.

27. Krautgartner WD, Klappacher M, Hannig M, et al. Fibrin mimics neutrophil extracellular traps in SEM. Ultrastruct Pathol 2010;34(4):226–31.

28. Esmon C, Xu J, Lupu F. Innate immunity and coagulation. J Thromb Haemost 2011;9:182–8.

29. Loike JD, el Khoury J, Cao L, et al. Fibrin regulates neutrophil migration in response to interleukin 8, leukotriene B4, tumor necrosis factor, and formyl-methionyl-leucyl-phenylalanine. J Exp Med 1995; 181(5):1763–72. Availavle at: http://www.pubmed central.nih.gov/articlerender.fcgi?artid=2191980& tool=pmcentrez&rendertype=abstract. Accessed September 28, 2015.

30. Panizzi P, Friedrich R, Fuentes-Prior P, et al. The staphylocoagulase family of zymogen activator and adhesion proteins. Cell Mol Life Sci 2004; 61(22):2793–8.

31. Friedrich R, Panizzi P, Fuentes-Prior P, et al. Staphylocoagulase is a prototype for the mechanism of cofactor-induced zymogen activation. Nature 2003;425(6957):535–9.

32. Pellegrino PL, Brunetti ND, De Gennaro L, et al. Inflammatory activation in an unselected population of subjects with atrial fibrillation: links with structural heart disease, atrial remodeling and recent onset. Intern Emerg Med 2013;8(2):123–8.

33. Ljungberg B, Grankvist K, Rasmuson T. Serum acute phase reactants and prognosis in renal cell carcinoma. Cancer 1995;76(8):1435–9. Available at: http://www.ncbi.nlm.nih.gov/pub med/8620420. Accessed July 19, 2016.

34. Muir KW, Weir CJ, Alwan W, et al. C-reactive protein and outcome after ischemic stroke. Stroke 1999;30(5):981–5.

35. Copley LA, Barton T, Garcia C, et al. A proposed scoring system for assessment of severity of illness in pediatric acute hematogenous osteomyelitis using objective clinical and laboratory findings. Pediatr Infect Dis J 2014;33(1):35–41.

36. Martin AC, Anderson D, Lucey J, et al. Predictors of outcome in pediatric osteomyelitis. Pediatr Infect Dis J 2016;35(4):387–91.

37. Kocher MS, Zurakowski D, Kasser JR. Differentiating between septic arthritis and transient synovitis of the hip in children: an evidence-based clinical prediction algorithm. J Bone Joint Surg Am 1999;81(12):1662–70.

38. Morley JJ, Kushner I. Serum C-reactive protein levels in disease. Ann N Y Acad Sci 1982;389(1 C-Reactive Pr):406–18.

39. Wirtz DC, Heller KD, Miltner O, et al. Interleukin-6: a potential inflammatory marker after total joint replacement. Int Orthop 2000;24(4):194–6. Available at: http://www.ncbi.nlm.nih.gov/pubmed/11081839. Accessed June 21, 2016.

40. Oda S, Hirasawa H, Shiga H, et al. Sequential measurement of IL-6 blood levels in patients with systemic inflammatory response syndrome (SIRS)/sepsis. Cytokine 2005;29(4):169–75.

41. Ridker PM, Rifai N, Stampfer MJ, et al. Plasma concentration of interleukin-6 and the risk of future myocardial infarction among apparently healthy men. Circulation 2000;101(15):1767–72.

42. Pape HC, van Griensven M, Rice J, et al. Major secondary surgery in blunt trauma patients and perioperative cytokine liberation: determination of the clinical relevance of biochemical markers. J Trauma 2001;50(6):989–1000. Available at: http://www.ncbi.nlm.nih.gov/pubmed/11426112. Accessed June 21, 2016.

43. Tillett WS, Francis T. Serological reactions in pneumonia with a non-protein somatic fraction of pneumococcus. J Exp Med 1930;52(4): 561–71.

44. Thompson D, Pepys MB, Wood SP. The physiological structure of human C-reactive protein and its complex with phosphocholine. Structure 1999;7(2):169–77.

45. Ballou SP, Lozanski G. Induction of inflammatory cytokine release from cultured human monocytes by C-reactive protein. Cytokine 1992;4(5): 361–8.

46. Cermak J, Key NS, Bach RR, et al. C-reactive protein induces human peripheral blood monocytes to synthesize tissue factor. Blood 1993;82(2): 513–20.

47. Markanday A. Acute phase reactants in infections: evidence-based review and a guide for clinicians. Open Forum Infect Dis 2015;2(3):ofv098.

48. Kamath S, Lip GYH. Fibrinogen: biochemistry, epidemiology and determinants. QJM 2003; 96(10):711–29.

49. Vigushin DM, Pepys MB, Hawkins PN. Metabolic and scintigraphic studies of radioiodinated human C-reactive protein in health and disease. J Clin Invest 1993;91(4):1351–7.

50. Vanderschueren S, Deeren D, Knockaert DC, et al. Extremely elevated C-reactive protein. Eur J Intern Med 2006;17(6):430–3.

51. Mignemi ME, Benvenuti MA, An TJ, et al. A novel classification system based on dissemination of musculoskeletal infection is predictive of hospital outcomes. J Pediatr Orthop 2016;1.

52. Mignemi ME, Menge TJ, Cole HA, et al. Epidemiology, diagnosis, and treatment of pericapsular pyomyositis of the hip in children. J Pediatr Orthop 2014;34(3):316–25.

53. Benvenuti MA, An TJ, Mignemi ME, et al. A clinical prediction algorithm to stratify pediatric musculoskeletal infection by severity. J Pediatr Orthop 2016. [Epub ahead of print].

54. Borschitz T, Schlicht S, Siegel E, et al. Improvement of a clinical score for necrotizing fasciitis: "Pain Out of Proportion" and high CRP levels aid the diagnosis. PLoS One 2015;10(7):e0132775.

55. Oelsner WK, Engstrom SM, Benvenuti MA, et al. Characterizing the acute phase response in healthy patients following total joint arthroplasty: predictable and consistent. J Arthroplasty 2016; 32(1):309–14.

56. Böttiger LE, Svedberg CA. Normal erythrocyte sedimentation rate and age. Br Med J 1967; 2(5544):85–7.

57. Sox HC, Liang MH. The erythrocyte sedimentation rate. Guidelines for rational use. Ann Intern Med 1986;104(4):515–23.

58. Markanday A. Diagnosing diabetic foot osteomyelitis: narrative review and a suggested 2-step score-based diagnostic pathway for clinicians. Open Forum Infect Dis 2014;1(2):ofu060.

59. Michail M, Jude E, Liaskos C, et al. The performance of serum inflammatory markers for the diagnosis and follow-up of patients with osteomyelitis. Int J Low Extrem Wounds 2013;12(2):94–9.

60. Pääkkönen M, Kallio MJT, Kallio PE, et al. Sensitivity of erythrocyte sedimentation rate and C-reactive protein in childhood bone and joint infections. Clin Orthop Relat Res 2010;468(3):861–6.

61. Hausfater P, Garric S, Ben Ayed S, et al. Usefulness of procalcitonin as a marker of systemic infection in emergency department patients: a prospective study. Clin Infect Dis 2002;34(7): 895–901.

62. Poddar B, Gurjar M, Singh S, et al. Procalcitonin kinetics as a prognostic marker in severe sepsis/septic shock. Indian J Crit Care Med 2015;19(3): 140–6.

63. Shen C-J, Wu M-S, Lin K-H, et al. The use of procalcitonin in the diagnosis of bone and joint infection: a systemic review and meta-analysis. Eur J Clin Microbiol Infect Dis 2013;32(6):807–14.

64. Nijsten MW, Olinga P, The TH, et al. Procalcitonin behaves as a fast responding acute phase protein in vivo and in vitro. Crit Care Med 2000;28(2): 458–61.

65. Meisner M. Pathobiochemistry and clinical use of procalcitonin. Clin Chim Acta 2002;323(1–2): 17–29. Available at: http://www.ncbi.nlm.nih.gov/pubmed/12135804. Accessed June 21, 2016.

66. Monneret G, Labaune JM, Isaac C, et al. Procalcitonin and C-reactive protein levels in neonatal infections. Acta Paediatr 1997;86(2):209–12. Available at: http://www.ncbi.nlm.nih.gov/pubmed/9055895. Accessed June 21, 2016.

67. Assicot M, Gendrel D, Carsin H, et al. High serum procalcitonin concentrations in patients with sepsis and infection. Lancet 1993;341(8844): 515–8. Available at: http://www.ncbi.nlm.nih.gov/pubmed/8094770. Accessed June 21, 2016.

68. Davidson J, Tong S, Hauck A, et al. Kinetics of procalcitonin and C-reactive protein and the relationship to postoperative infection in young infants undergoing cardiovascular surgery. Pediatr Res 2013;74(4):413–9.

69. Theodorou VP, Papaioannou VE, Tripsianis GA, et al. Procalcitonin and procalcitonin kinetics for diagnosis and prognosis of intravascular catheter-related bloodstream infections in selected critically ill patients: a prospective observational study. BMC Infect Dis 2012;12(1):247.

70. Simon L, Gauvin F, Amre DK, et al. Serum procalcitonin and C-reactive protein levels as markers of bacterial infection: a systematic review and meta-analysis. Clin Infect Dis 2004;39(2):206–17.

71. Kushner I. Regulation of the acute phase response by cytokines. Perspect Biol Med 1993;36(4): 611–22.

72. Chrousos GP. The hypothalamic-pituitary-adrenal axis and immune-mediated inflammation. N Engl J Med 1995;332(20):1351–62.

73. Borish L, King MS, Mascali JJ, et al. Transthyretin is an inhibitor of monocyte and endothelial cell interleukin-1 production. Inflammation 1992; 16(5):471–84.

74. Schlapbach LJ, Straney L, Alexander J, et al. Mortality related to invasive infections, sepsis, and septic shock in critically ill children in Australia and New Zealand, 2002-13: a multicentre retrospective cohort study. Lancet Infect Dis 2015; 15(1):46–54.

75. Herman A, Kappler JW, Marrack P, et al. Superantigens: mechanism of T-cell stimulation and role in immune responses. Annu Rev Immunol 1991;9: 745–72.

76. Kotzin BL, Leung DY, Kappler J, et al. Superantigens and their potential role in human disease. Adv Immunol 1993;54:99–166. Available at: http://www.ncbi.nlm.nih.gov/pubmed/8397479. Accessed July 19, 2016.

77. Hackett SP, Stevens DL. Streptococcal toxic shock syndrome: synthesis of tumor necrosis factor and interleukin-1 by monocytes stimulated with pyrogenic exotoxin A and streptolysin O. J Infect Dis 1992;165(5):879–85. Available at: http://www.ncbi.nlm.nih.gov/pubmed/1569337. Accessed July 19, 2016.

78. Fast DJ, Schlievert PM, Nelson RD. Toxic shock syndrome-associated staphylococcal and streptococcal pyrogenic toxins are potent inducers of tumor necrosis factor production. Infect Immun 1989;57(1):291–4. Available at: http://www.ncbi.

nlm.nih.gov/pubmed/2642470. Accessed July 19, 2016.

79. Stevens DL, Bryant AE, Hackett SP, et al. Group A streptococcal bacteremia: the role of tumor necrosis factor in shock and organ failure. J Infect Dis 1996;173(3):619–26. Available at: http://www.ncbi. nlm.nih.gov/pubmed/8627025. Accessed July 19, 2016.

80. Prucha M, Bellingan G, Zazula R. Sepsis biomarkers. Clin Chim Acta 2015;440:97–103.

81. Boomer JS, To K, Chang KC, et al. Immunosuppression in patients who die of sepsis and multiple organ failure. JAMA 2011;306(23):2594–605.

82. Mignemi ME, Langdon N, Schoenecker J. Vitamin K-dependent coagulopathy in pediatric osteomyelitis. JBJS Case Connect 2013;3(21):1–6.

83. Gonzalez BE, Teruya J, Mahoney DH, et al. Venous thrombosis associated with staphylococcal osteomyelitis in children. Pediatrics 2006; 117(5):1673–9.

84. Hollmig ST, Copley LA, Browne RH, et al. Deep venous thrombosis associated with osteomyelitis in children. J Bone Joint Surg 2007;89(7):1517–23.

85. Gonzalez BE. Severe staphylococcal sepsis in adolescents in the era of community-acquired methicillin-resistant Staphylococcus aureus. Pediatrics 2005;115(3):642–8.

86. Semeraro N, Ammollo CT, Semeraro F, et al. Sepsis-associated disseminated intravascular coagulation and thromboembolic disease. Mediterr J Hematol Infect Dis 2010;2(3):e2010024.

87. Fourrier F, Chopin C, Goudemand J, et al. Septic shock, multiple organ failure, and disseminated intravascular coagulation: compared patterns of antithrombin III, protein C, and protein S deficiencies. Chest 1992;101(3):816–23.

88. Levi M, van der Poll T. The role of natural anticoagulants in the pathogenesis and management of systemic activation of coagulation and inflammation in critically ill patients. Semin Thromb Hemost 2008;34(5):459–68.

89. Levi M, van der Poll T. A short contemporary history of disseminated intravascular coagulation. Semin Thromb Hemost 2014;40(08):874–80.

90. de Pont A-CJM, Bakhtiari K, Hutten BA, et al. Endotoxaemia induces resistance to activated protein C in healthy humans. Br J Haematol 2006;134(2):213–9.

91. Taylor FB, Stearns-Kurosawa DJ, Kurosawa S, et al. The endothelial cell protein C receptor aids in host defense against Escherichia coli sepsis. Blood 2000;95(5):1680–6. Available at: http://www.ncbi. nlm.nih.gov/pubmed/10688824. Accessed July 17, 2016.

92. Levi M, van der Poll T, Büller HR. Bidirectional relation between inflammation and coagulation. Circulation 2004;109(22):2698–704.

93. Abraham E, Reinhart K, Opal S, et al. Efficacy and safety of tifacogin (recombinant tissue factor pathway inhibitor) in severe sepsis: a randomized controlled trial. JAMA 2003;290(2):238–47.

94. Stéphan F, Hollande J, Richard O, et al. Thrombocytopenia in a surgical ICU. Chest 1999;115(5): 1363–70. Available at: http://www.ncbi.nlm.nih. gov/pubmed/10334154. Accessed June 21, 2016.

95. Keeling D. International normalized ratio in patients not on vitamin K antagonists. J Thromb Haemost 2007;5(1):188–9.

96. Park MS, Martini WZ, Dubick MA, et al. Thromboelastography as a better indicator of hypercoagulable state after injury than prothrombin time or activated partial thromboplastin time. J Trauma 2009;67(2):266–75 [discussion: 275–76].

97. Haase N, Ostrowski SR, Wetterslev J, et al. Thromboelastography in patients with severe sepsis: a prospective cohort study. Intensive Care Med 2015;41(1):77–85.

98. Dellinger RP, Levy MM, Carlet JM, et al. Surviving Sepsis Campaign: international guidelines for management of severe sepsis and septic shock: 2008. Crit Care Med 2008;36(1):296–327.

99. Annane D. A 3-level prognostic classification in septic shock based on cortisol levels and cortisol response to corticotropin. JAMA 2000;283(8):1038.

100. Sam S, Corbridge TC, Mokhlesi B, et al. Cortisol levels and mortality in severe sepsis. Clin Endocrinol (oxf) 2004;60(1):29–35. Available at: http://www.ncbi. nlm.nih.gov/pubmed/14678284. Accessed June 14, 2016.

101. Dellinger RP, Levy MM, Rhodes A, et al. Surviving Sepsis Campaign: international guidelines for management of severe sepsis and septic shock, 2012. Intensive Care Med 2013;39(2):165–228.

102. Kardash KJ, Sarrazin F, Tessler MJ, et al. Single-dose dexamethasone reduces dynamicpain after total hip arthroplasty. Anesth Analg 2008;106(4): 1253–7.

103. Backes JR, Bentley JC, Politi JR, et al. Dexamethasone reduces length of hospitalization and improves postoperative pain and nausea after total joint arthroplasty: a prospective, randomized controlled trial. J Arthroplasty 2013;28(8 Suppl):11–7.

104. Micronutrients I of M (US) P on. Dietary reference intakes for vitamin A, vitamin K, arsenic, boron, chromium, copper, iodine, iron, manganese, molybdenum, nickel, silicon, vanadium, and zinc. Natl Academies Press; 2001. Available at: http://www.ncbi.nlm.nih.gov/pubmed/25057538. Accessed June 21, 2016..

105. Ranieri VM, Thompson BT, Barie PS, et al. Drotrecogin alfa (activated) in adults with septic shock. N Engl J Med 2012;366(22):2055–64.

106. Bernard G, Vincent J, Laterre P, et al. Efficacy and safety of recombinant human activated protein C

for severe sepsis. N Engl J Med 2001;345(3):
219–25.

107. Piccin A, O' Marcaigh A, Mc Mahon C, et al. Non-activated plasma-derived PC improves amputation rate of children undergoing sepsis. Thromb Res 2014;134(1):63–7.

108. Baratto F, Michielan F, Meroni M, et al. Protein C concentrate to restore physiological values in adult septic patients. Intensive Care Med 2008; 34(9):1707–12.

109. Baratto F, Michielan F, Gagliardi G, et al. Use of protein C concentrate in adult patients with severe sepsis and septic shock. Minerva Anestesiol 2004;70(5):351–6 [article in Italian]. Available at: http://www.ncbi.nlm.nih.gov/pubmed/15181415. Accessed July 19, 2016.

Acute Hematogenous Osteomyelitis in Children
Pathogenesis, Diagnosis, and Treatment

Shawn S. Funk, MD[a], Lawson A.B. Copley, MD[b],*

KEYWORDS

• Acute hematogenous osteomyelitis • Children • Pathogenesis • Diagnosis • Treatment

KEY POINTS

- Proper care for children with AHO is inherently a multidisciplinary and collaborative process that should be guideline driven and evidence based.
- AHO is the most difficult condition to understand in the realm of pediatric musculoskeletal infection and continues to present a significant clinical challenge due to the evolving epidemiology and complex pathogenesis.
- A lack of institutional consensus as to the most effective evaluation and management strategies may lead to variation in care, which in turn may have an adverse impact on clinical outcomes. Such variability, which may easily occur in large pediatric medical centers, can make coordination of care extremely difficult.
- Despite these challenges, a guideline-driven, multidisciplinary approach has been introduced and shown to effectively reduce hospital stay, improve the timing and selection of empirical antibiotic administration, reduce delay to initial MRI, reduce the rate of readmission, and shorten antibiotic duration.
- Carefully monitoring regional trends in microbiologic epidemiology and applying a guideline-driven approach for evaluation and treatment will improve care for children with AHO and, inevitably, those with other forms of musculoskeletal infection as well.

INTRODUCTION

Musculoskeletal infection in children is a broad topic covering an array of conditions that may occur in isolation or in combination, including complex or systemic forms. These conditions include osteomyelitis (acute, subacute, and chronic), discitis, septic arthritis, pyomyositis, abscess (superficial or deep), cellulitis, fasciitis (including necrotizing fasciitis), lymphangitis, and lymphadenitis. Children with musculoskeletal infection may have additional involvement of other systems, including deep vein thrombosis (DVT), septic pulmonary embolism, pneumonia, empyema, endocarditis, bacteremia, and septic shock. The clinical presentation of children with any of these conditions may have sufficiently similar features to create an initial diagnostic dilemma until thorough history, physical examination, laboratory tests, plain radiographs, and advanced imaging can be performed. A variety of disciplines and hospital services are usually involved in the evaluation process, including emergency medicine,

The authors have nothing to disclose.
[a] Department of Orthopaedic Surgery, The Children's Hospital of San Antonio, Baylor College of Medicine, 315 North San Saba Street, Suite 1135, San Antonio, TX 78207, USA; [b] Department of Orthopaedic Surgery, Children's Medical Center of Dallas, University of Texas Southwestern, 1935 Medical District Drive, Dallas, TX 75235, USA
* Corresponding author.
E-mail address: lawson.copley@childrens.com

Orthop Clin N Am 48 (2017) 199–208
http://dx.doi.org/10.1016/j.ocl.2016.12.007
0030-5898/17/© 2016 Elsevier Inc. All rights reserved.

pediatrics, infectious disease, orthopedic surgery, intensive care, radiology, anesthesiology, laboratory, nursing, and pharmacy. Because of this, the care of children with musculoskeletal infection inevitably requires an organized, interdisciplinary approach to reach timely, comprehensive, and accurate diagnoses. From that point forward, effective treatment may be carefully planned and enacted with subsequent monitoring of the child until clinical resolution is achieved. Ideally, clinical practice guidelines should be established to help orchestrate the complex array of events that are necessary to reach the point of resolution with the best outcomes. Unfortunately, this is not a simple undertaking. There is a paucity of high-quality evidence to guide care. There are substantial regional variations in the incidence and severity of illness of children with these conditions. There is also moderate disagreement as to the categorical differentiation of the array of conditions that comprise musculoskeletal infection in children, which can confuse recommendations of evaluation and treatment at regional and institutional levels. Of even greater relevance, however, is the wide range of individual practice preferences, knowledge limitations, and institutional workflows that lead to variation in understanding and treating these conditions. To overcome these limitations, it is necessary to focus on foundational disorders and develop sound principles to guide awareness of pathophysiology, diagnosis, and treatment that serve to guide care for the wide array of disorders that comprise pediatric musculoskeletal infection. AHO is the principal disorder that enables establishing this foundation. Developing rational, evidence-based clinical practice guidelines for this one condition will effectively support the evaluation and management of the full spectrum of pediatric musculoskeletal infections because children with AHO represent the entire gamut of illness from mild to severe, simple to complex, and focal to systemic. For these reasons, this review is devoted exclusively to AHO in children, with the intent to provide an update on the current understanding of existing evidence and future directions, which should be explored to improve care for those with any form of musculoskeletal infection.

EPIDEMIOLOGY

The incidence of AHO varies by region and time.[1] The authors reported a 600% increase in pediatric osteomyelitis over a 2-decade period within a community.[1] During that time, the local population had increased by 220%.[1] The relative virulence of the infections has seemingly increased, a concern attributed to the causative organism. The Agency for Healthcare Research and Quality provides national estimates on hospital discharges for children ages 0 to 17 years from the Healthcare Cost and Utilization Project (HCUP) Kids' Inpatient Database (KID). Trends between 1997 and 2012 suggest that the incidence of AHO has varied regionally, with the highest percentage currently reported the southern region (Fig. 1). Surveillance data from specific communities have reported varying incidence rates over time, with 1 report indicating a 600% increase in the incidence of osteomyelitis when comparison was made to the experience of the same organization 2 decades prior.[1] The incidence of AHO also varies according to the age and gender of the child due to processes of skeletal and vascular development.[2,3] The reported rate of AHO varies between 1:5000 and 1:10,000, with boys having a rate twice that of girls.[4–7]

PATHOGENESIS

AHO is caused by bacterial seeding that is thought to develop due to transient bacteremia, which can result from otitis media, pharyngitis, and daily activities, such as brushing teeth.[8] A transient bacteremia alone is thought insufficient for the development of AHO due to the lack of available free iron in human blood to sustain the bacteria. Bacterial genetic up-regulation of virulence and iron metabolism genes or regional bone trauma are postulated to predispose to infection.[3] In rabbits, bacterial inoculation associated with bone trauma had a higher rate of osteomyelitis than those without injury.[9,10]

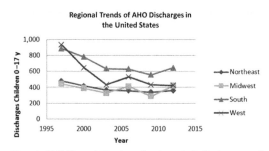

Fig. 1. HCUPnet KID data for hospital discharges of children 0 to 17 years by regions of the United States from 1997 to 2012. (*Data from* HCUP Kids' Inpatient Database (KID). Healthcare cost and utilization project (HCUP). Rockville (MD): Agency for Healthcare Research and Quality; 2015.)

Osteomyelitis typically develops in the metaphyseal region of long bones (or long bone equivalent areas, such as the calcaneal apophysis or inferior pubic ramus). It is surmised that the bacteria aggregate in these areas due to the tortuous blood flow, where the dilated capillaries make a sharp turn at the physis.[2,4,8] Once infection is established, it may expand and evolve to intraosseous, subperiosteal, or extraperiosteal abscesses or extend into an adjacent joint space, particularly if the metaphysis is intracapsular, resulting in contiguous septic arthritis.[2,8] The rate of adjacent septic arthritis and osteomyelitis is 33%.[6] Historically, the sequela-prone child was suspected of having contiguous osteomyelitis and septic arthritis due to persistent elevation of inflammatory markers after initial drainage of septic arthritis and considered to have a poor prognosis compared with those who had isolated septic arthritis.[7,11,12]

The microbiologic epidemiology of AHO has remained relatively consistent over time, with *Staphylococcus aureus* accounting for a majority of cases.[13] Regional variation of antibiotic resistance of *S aureus* has occurred in several communities within the United States. In south Texas, rates of methicillin-resistant *S aureus* (MRSA) (30.4%), methicillin-sensitive *S aureus* (28.6%), other organisms (19.6%), and no growth (21.4%) have been reported.[1,14] Identifying a causative organism may be a challenge, with rates of culture-negative osteomyelitis from 16% to 42%.[15] Supplemental techniques may enhance bacterial identification and include inoculation of blood or chocolate agar plates intraoperatively or the utilization of polymerase chain reaction (PCR) to identify *Kingella kingae* in children between the ages of 6 months and 4 years.[13,16] An organized approach to specimen acquisition and laboratory processing may improve utilization of resources (Table 1).[13] It is important to attempt to identify the causative organism whenever possible to effectively guide specific antibiotic therapy.[15,17,18]

Recent basic science research has explored the genome of *S aureus* and the virulence factors that may underlie the variability of illness severity seen among children with AHO.[13,19,20] A better understanding of the genetically encoded virulence capability of the bacteria may help to improve early recognition of children who are prone to develop severe illness and encourage a more aggressive initial treatment strategy in those cases.

CLINICAL PRESENTATION

Children with AHO typically have symptoms 3 to 4 days prior to presentation.[5,21] Infection is more common in lower extremities than upper extremities, with the 3 most common sites the

Table 1		
Culture recommendations in the setting of acute hematogenous osteomyelitis in children		
Source	**Host Factors**	**Culture Recommendations**
Blood		Aerobic blood culture obtained prior to antibiotic administration.
		If positive, repeat daily until 2 consecutive negative cultures.
		If peripherally inserted central catheter or central line is placed, obtain surveillance cultures when febrile.
Bone	Healthy	Aerobic culture (only) obtained from the site of infection whenever possible.
		Can be performed after antibiotic administration; do not withhold antibiotic if child is septic.
	Immunocompromise	Aerobic, anaerobic, fungal, and acid-fast bacilli cultures; consider 16S or fungal PCR.
	Penetrating inoculation	
	Failed primary treatment	
	Age 6 mo to 4 y	Consider *K kingae*; swab to blood or chocolate agar plate in operating room.
Joint fluid		Assess for contiguous septic arthritis using cell count and aerobic culture.
Abscess		Aerobic culture; consider *Bartonella* PCR if cat-scratch disease is suspected.

femur (27%), tibia (22%), and humerus (12%).[7] Single-bone involvement is more common than multifocal infection.[4,5,7] More than 50% of cases occur in children under the age of 5 years.[7]

Radiology

Evaluation of a child with concern for infection requires a thorough history and physical examination to be able to guide the appropriate selection of body area to be imaged and imaging modality.

Conventional Radiography

Imaging always starts with conventional radiographs due to their low cost, availability, and ability suggest correct diagnosis and exclude other diagnoses.[22] High-quality plain radiographs demonstrate local bony changes, periosteal reaction, deep soft tissue involvement, and may identify concerning features suggestive of neoplasm or fracture which might have otherwise been overlooked. The first radiographic sign of AHO is deep soft tissue swelling with.[23,24] Lytic changes in the bone require 50% to -75% of the bone mineral density to be depleted before becoming evident on plain radiographs.[24] These more definitive signs of bone destruction and periosteal reaction may not occur until 1 to -2 weeks after the infection has been present.[23–25]

Advanced Imaging

There are advantages and disadvantages with the use of advanced imaging modalities in the evaluation of children who present with signs and symptoms of possible deep infection (Table 2). Clinicians must carefully consider the issues of cost, diagnostic accuracy, timeliness of diagnosis, and potential delay in treatment with or without the use of these modalities. Additional imaging for osteomyelitis may include ultrasound (US), CT, and MRI. US is commonly used to evaluate hips for effusion and possible septic arthritis as well as screen for DVT in the setting of MRSA osteomyelitis. This imaging modality also is used to assess for psoas and subperiosteal abscesses.[26] US may demonstrate early changes of osteomyelitis with findings of deep soft tissue swelling.[26] Advantages include the noninvasive nature of the study and the ability to acquire the information without sedation.

CT is excellent for defining bony pathology.[23] This method has limited application, however, in the diagnosis and management of osteomyelitis in children due to radiation exposure and limited visualization of the anatomic and spatial extent of tissue inflammation. CT has demonstrated a sensitivity for osteomyelitis of 66% and specificity of 97%.[27] CT can provide detail about sequestration and large abscess formation, so

Table 2 Imaging modalities for acute hematogenous osteomyelitis		
	Advantages	**Disadvantages**
Radiograph	• Low cost • No need for sedation • Readily available • High sensitivity, late	• Delayed appearance on radiograph • Under-represents extent of disease
US	• Low cost • Absence of radiation exposure • No need for sedation • Ability to detect and localize fluid collections for aspiration	• Technique dependent • Depth of visualization • Unable to penetrate bone
CT	• Higher cost • Rare need for sedation • Fast • Excellent bony detail • Ability to detect and localize fluid collections for aspiration	• Radiation exposure • Uses CT resources • Not great soft tissue visualization • Does not distinguish inflammation in tissues • Scatter from nearby metal
MRI	• No radiation exposure • Uses MRI resources • Excellent soft tissue visualization • Distinguishes inflammation in tissues • Ability to detect and localize fluid collections for aspiration	• Radiation exposure • Uses CT resources • Not great soft tissue visualization • Does not distinguish inflammation in tissues • Scatter from nearby metal

it may play a role in monitoring disease progression after initial MRI acquisition. This may be a useful tool for the evaluation of AHO in resource constrained settings but the sensitivity is not nearly as high as that of MRI.[23,25,27]

MRI is excellent at soft tissue characterization at high resolution. It offers improved sensitivity and specificity over CT and the advantage of identifying marrow inflammation.[27,28] A multidisciplinary approach has been shown to decrease the time to MRI and surgery and demonstrated that continuation to the operating room from MRI can be safely performed as a single anesthetic event.[29,30] Earlier MRI and surgery leads to decreased hospital stay.[29,30] Interdisciplinary MRI protocols have been shown to reduce scan duration by limiting the number of body areas imaged and the number of MRI sequences performed.[30] MRI provides powerful information but the cost and resource utilization must be justified. In 1 study, only 16% of repeat MRIs demonstrated new findings and did not necessarily result in a change in intervention.[31] MRI has great utility as an initial screening test and has been recommended in cases of septic arthritis to identify adjacent bone infection prior to arthrotomy.[32] A particularly challenging area for which MRI has proved useful is the assessment of deep musculoskeletal infection in the pelvis.[33–35]

Laboratory Studies

In the acquisition of blood and local tissue cultures for microbiology processing, additional laboratory studies can guide efficient and appropriate treatment of children with AHO. Multiple acute-phase reactants have been described and evaluated for their utility diagnosing infection, including C-reactive protein (CRP), erythrocyte sedimentation rate (ESR), white blood cell count (WBC), interleukin 6, and D-dimer.[11,36–38] CRP and ESR have been demonstrated the most useful in evaluating AHO. CRP rises rapidly and is useful in monitoring disease resolution during the acute hospitalization phase, because it normalizes 7 days after the initiation of effective treatment.[11] ESR rises more slowly and gradually declines over 2 weeks to 3 weeks. This marker often helps ensure that the standard treatment duration is appropriate to resolve the infection. Initial blood cultures are positive in approximately 30% of children with AHO.[13] This rate may have an adverse impact from prior administrative of antibiotics.[13] It is, therefore, essential to obtain blood cultures from all children in whom there is legitimate concern of possible bone infection.

Prognosis

Prognosis of osteomyelitis has yet to be carefully studied through longitudinal, prospective clinical outcomes research. Risks for poor outcome, however, generally include delay in diagnosis and contiguous involvement of bone and joint in areas of tenuous blood supply, such as the proximal hip or femur. A multidisciplinary approach to the evaluation and treatment of AHO, involving orthopedic surgeons, pediatricians, infectious disease specialists, and ancillary services, has resulted in a trend to decrease hospital length of stay and decrease delay to initial MRI.[29] Evidence-based algorithms for treatment may be used to guide decision making.[7,29] Although these improvements in process measures and intermediate outcomes have been demonstrated, it is still unclear whether these initiatives will ultimately improve the long-term clinical outcomes of children with AHO.

Classification

To discuss and treat any disease, a classification system can help improve communication with other practitioners. Classification systems are only of utility, however, if they are reproducible and predict prognosis or guide treatment. Cierny and colleagues[39] developed a classification system for osteomyelitis and proposed treatment strategies based on this system. This classification was developed, however, for adults who often have underlying comorbidities.[39] The utility of Cierny's classification has not been validated for children who are typically healthy, with normal immune function at the time of infection. Pediatric AHO has traditionally been classified by age of onset and circumstance that are relevant to the most likely causative organisms. From this classification scheme, a proposal of empirical antibiotic therapy has been established (Table 3).[7,8]

More recently, a classification system has been proposed to assess the relative severity of illness of children with AHO as a guide to prognosis and risk of complications. A simple system to score illness severity using clinical, radiologic, and laboratory parameters, which are available during the first 4 days to 5 days of hospitalization, has been used to guide decisions for early hospital discharge in children with low severity scores.[14] This scoring system is heavily tied to the laboratory trending of the CRP, which has often been used to monitor recovery in children with AHO.[11,36]

Using a classification to guide decision making in the scheme of a clinical practice guideline, as seen in Table 4, can guide treatment,

Table 3
Classification of acute hematogenous osteomyelitis by age and factors of onset (nosocomial vs community acquired)

Patient Characteristics	Causative Organisms	Empirical Antibiotics
Nosocomial infection	*S aureus*, Streptococci species, Enterobacteriaceae, Candida species	Nafcillin or oxacillin plus gentamicin or cefotaxime (or cetriaxone) plus gentamicin
Community-acquired infection	*S aureus*, group B Streptococcus, *Escherichia coli*, Klebsiella species	Nafcillin or oxacillin plus gentamicin or cefotaxime (or cetriaxone) plus gentamicin
Infantile (2–18 mo)	*S aureus, K kingae, Streptococcus pneumoniae, Neisseria meningitidis, Haemophilus influenzae* type b (nonimmunized)	Immunized: nafcillin, oxacillin, or cefazolin Nonimmunized: nafcillin, oxacillin plus cefotaxime, or cefuroxime
Early childhood (18 mo to 3 y)	*S aureus, K kingae, Streptococcus pneumoniae, Neisseria meningitidis, Haemophilus influenzae* type b (nonimmunized)	Immunized: nafcillin, oxacillin, or cefazolin Nonimmunized: nafcillin, oxacillin plus cefotaxime, or cefuroxime
Childhood (3–12 y)	*S aureus*, group A β-hemolytic streptococcus	Nafcillin, oxacillin, or cefazolin
Adolescent (12–18 y)	*S aureus*, group A β-hemolytic streptococcus, *Neisseria gonorrhoeae*	Nafcillin, oxacillin, or cefazolin; ceftriaxone and doxycycline for disseminated gonococcal infection

Table 4
Modified severity of illness scoring system for acute hematogenous osteomyelitis

Scoring Parameter	Criteria	Points	Total
Initial CRP mg/dL)	>15	2	0–2
	10–15	1	
	<10	0	
CRP hospital day 4–5 (mg/dL)	>10	2	0–2
	5–10	1	
	<5	0	
CRP hospital day 2–3 (mg/dL)	>10	2	0–2
	5–10	1	
	<5	0	
Band percentage of WBC	≥1.5%	1	0–1
	<1.5%	0	
Febrile days on antibiotic	≥2	1	0–1
	<2	0	
Intensive care unit admission	Yes	1	0–1
	No	0	
Disseminated disease[a]	Yes	1	0–1
	No	0	
Total			0–10

[a] Examples of disseminated disease include: deep venous thrombosis, septic pulmonary embolism, pneumonia, endocarditis, and multifocal osteomyelitis.

reduce variability of care, and result in more effective treatment.[29] The severity of illness score for AHO can be determined within the first 4 days to 5 days of hospitalization. In general, children with mild (0–3) or moderate (4–7) scores can be considered for early discharge, whereas children with severe scores (8–10) typically require ongoing intensive evaluation and may require multiple surgical procedures or additional advanced imaging. This essentially enables a provider to objectively stratify a disease with a wide spectrum of clinical presentation. Using a guideline improves communication and decreases delay of necessary therapy.[29]

TREATMENT
Antibiotic Therapy
Management of AHO requires appropriate antimicrobial treatment to eradicate the infection. This typically begins with intravenous (IV) antibiotics to cover the most likely causative organism until culture or sensitivity data are available. Many cases of AHO are treated empirically either due to not obtaining a culture or a culture negative sample. In these cases, antibiotic selection is made from regional data about most common causative organism and rate of community-associated (CA)-MRSA, often with recommendations from pediatric infectious disease specialists.[18] Antibiotic selection is

essentially a community-based endeavor that requires knowledge of the local microbiologic epidemiology and antibiotic resistance patterns within each institution to guide effective empirical antibiotic selection. Culture-negative AHO has been successfully treated using clindamycin in communities with high rates of CA-MRSA.[15,17,18]

There has not been a consensus on antibiotic duration or route. A historical routine treatment, however, often consisted of 6 weeks of IV antibiotics. Better classification and monitoring of AHO have ultimately led to a reduction of the practice of prolonged IV antibiotic treatment, which has been shown to have a high complication rate of 25% to 38% and a 19% to 27% rehospitalization rate.[40]

Currently, the treatment of AHO involves sequential parenteral to oral antibiotic therapy for 4 weeks with a demonstrated efficacy similar to that of prolonged IV antibiotics.[41,42] Oral antibiotics offer an attractive alternative due to the reduction of cost and complications and should be considered in all appropriate cases.[43,44]

Surgical Treatment

Surgical indications and specific guidance as to the specific technique or extent of surgery for AHO have not been studied extensively or clearly defined.[45] Surgical intervention and drainage have been reported as a necessity to avoid progression of disease.[46] Timely initiation of antibiotics may prevent progression, however, to the development of subperiosteal or intraosseous abscess formation that might otherwise require surgical intervention.[47] Imaging and laboratory data can help guide decisions regarding surgery. The specific surgical procedure performed may range in extent from simple (eg, 11-gauge needle biopsy of bone accompanied by aspiration of a subperiosteal abscess) to complex (eg, creation of a corical window with extensive débridement of metaphyseal cancellous bone). Children with moderately large abscesses or those who fail to respond to antibiotic therapy after 48 hours to 72 hours should be considered candidates for surgery.[45] When surgical intervention is performed, appropriate cultures should be sent and a bone biopsy should always be obtained to assess for infiltrative or malignant processes that may mimic infection. Some children may require more than 1 surgical procedure to help decrease the local burden of infection and improve their response to ongoing antibiotic administration. This decision is typically guided by the trends in a child's temperature (fever curve) and CRP. In general, if the CRP is static or rising and the child remains febrile, a surgeon is called on to determine if additional surgical débridement may be beneficial. This is typically a decision that must be made on a case-by-case basis (**Fig. 2**).

Complications

Complications of AHO are reported in approximately 6% of children and include chronic infection, avascular necrosis, growth disturbance, pathologic fractures, DVT, and sepsis.[8,45,48,49] The rate of chronic osteomyelitis have been estimated to be 1.7% overall and the rate of recurrent infection has been reported as high as 6.8%.[45,50] Clinically significant DVT occurs between 0.4% and 6%, with a higher rate in children with MRSA.[45,49] Higher rates of DVT have been reported with routine DVT-US screening.[51] Growth disturbance occurs in 1.8% of children and presents a challenging problem that may not be evident for years after resolution of infection.[45,52] Pathologic fracture occurs in 1.7% of patients, typically occurring in those with who had more severe infections and who underwent surgical débridement.[45,53]

DISCUSSION

AHO in children is an ideal condition to study due to its representation of a wide spectrum of disorders that comprise pediatric musculoskeletal infection. Proper care for children with AHO is inherently a multidisciplinary and collaborative process that should be guideline driven and evidence based. AHO is the most difficult condition to understand in the realm of pediatric musculoskeletal infection and continues to present a significant clinical challenge due to the evolving epidemiology and complex pathogenesis. A lack of institutional consensus as to the most effective evaluation and management strategies may lead to variation in care, which, in turn, may have an adverse impact on clinical outcomes. Such variability, which may easily occur in large pediatric medical centers, can make coordination of care extremely difficult. Despite these challenges, a guideline-driven, multidisciplinary approach has been introduced and shown to effectively reduce hospital stay, improve the timing and selection of empirical antibiotic administration, reduce delay to initial MRI, reduce the rate of readmission, and shorten antibiotic duration.[21] Carefully monitoring regional trends in microbiologic epidemiology and applying a guideline-driven approach for evaluation and treatment improve care for children with AHO

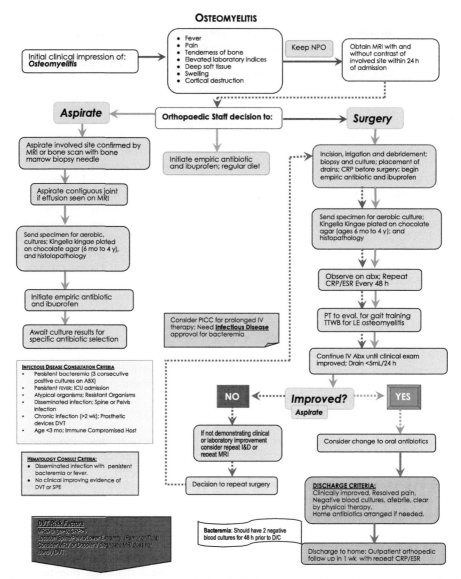

Fig. 2. Osteomyelitis treatment diagram. Abx, Antibiotic; D/C, discharge; DVT, deep venous thrombosis; eval., evaluation; I&D, irrigation and debridement; ICU, intensive care unit; LE, lower extremity; PICC, peripherally inserted central catheter; PT, physical therapy; SPE, septic pulmonary emboli; TTWB – toe touch weight bearing. (*Courtesy of* Children's Medical Center of Dallas, Dallas, TX; with permission.)

and, inevitably, those with other forms of musculoskeletal infection as well.

REFERENCES

1. Gafur OA, Copley LA, Hollmig ST, et al. The impact of the current epidemiology of pediatric musculoskeletal infection on evaluation and treatment guidelines. J Pediatr Orthop 2008;28(7): 777–85.

2. Trueta J. The 3 types of acute hematogenous osteomyelitis. Schweiz Med Wochenschr 1963;93: 306–12 [in German].

3. Kahn DS, Pritzker KP. The pathophysiology of bone infection. Clin Orthop 1973;96:12–9.

4. Weichert S, Sharland M, Clarke NM, et al. Acute haematogenous osteomyelitis in children: is there any evidence for how long we should treat? Curr Opin Infect Dis 2008;21(3): 258–62.

5. Dahl LB, Høyland AL, Dramsdahl H, et al. Acute osteomyelitis in children: a population-based retrospective study 1965 to 1994. Scand J Infect Dis 1998;30(6):573–7.

6. Perlman MH, Patzakis MJ, Kumar PJ, et al. The incidence of joint involvement with adjacent

osteomyelitis in pediatric patients. J Pediatr Orthop 2000;20(1):40–3.

7. Song KM, Sloboda JF. Acute hematogenous osteomyelitis in children. J Am Acad Orthop Surg 2001; 9(3):166–75.

8. Herring JA, Tachdjian MO, Texas Scottish Rite Hospital for Children. Tachdjian's Pediatric Orthopaedics: From the Texas Scottish Rite Hospital for Children. 2014. Available at: http://www.clinical-key.com/dura/browse/bookChapter/3-s2.0-C20091 59017X. Accessed April 19, 2016.

9. Morrissy RT, Haynes DW. Acute hematogenous osteomyelitis: a model with trauma as an etiology. J Pediatr Orthop 1989;9(4):447–56.

10. Whalen JL, Fitzgerald RH, Morrissy RT. A histological study of acute hematogenous osteomyelitis following physeal injuries in rabbits. J Bone Joint Surg Am 1988;70(9):1383–92.

11. Unkila-Kallio L, Kallio MJ, Peltola H. The usefulness of C-reactive protein levels in the identification of concurrent septic arthritis in children who have acute hematogenous osteomyelitis. A comparison with the usefulness of the erythrocyte sedimentation rate and the white blood-cell count. J Bone Joint Surg Am 1994;76(6):848–53.

12. Peltola H, Pääkkönen M, Kallio P, et al. Short-versus long-term antimicrobial treatment for acute hematogenous osteomyelitis of childhood: prospective, randomized trial on 131 culture-positive cases. Pediatr Infect Dis J 2010;29(12):1123–8.

13. Section J, Gibbons SD, Barton T, et al. Microbiological culture methods for pediatric musculoskeletal infection: a guideline for optimal use. J Bone Joint Surg Am 2015;97(6):441–9.

14. Roine I, Arguedas A, Faingezicht I, et al. Early detection of sequela-prone osteomyelitis in children with use of simple clinical and laboratory criteria. Clin Infect Dis 1997;24(5):849–53.

15. Floyed RL, Steele RW. Culture-negative osteomyelitis. Pediatr Infect Dis J 2003;22(8):731–6.

16. Gené A, García-García J-J, Sala P, et al. Enhanced culture detection of Kingella kingae, a pathogen of increasing clinical importance in pediatrics. Pediatr Infect Dis J 2004;23(9):886–8.

17. Martínez-Aguilar G, Hammerman WA, Mason EO, et al. Clindamycin treatment of invasive infections caused by community-acquired, methicillin-resistant and methicillin-susceptible Staphylococcus aureus in children. Pediatr Infect Dis J 2003;22(7): 593–8.

18. Afghani B, Kong V, Wu FL. What would pediatric infectious disease consultants recommend for management of culture-negative acute hematogenous osteomyelitis? J Pediatr Orthop 2007;27(7):805–9.

19. Gaviria-Agudelo C, Carter K, Tareen N, et al. Gene expression analysis of children with acute hematogenous osteomyelitis caused by methicillin-resistant staphylococcus aureus: correlation with clinical severity of illness. Smith TC. PLoS One 2014;9(7): e103523.

20. Gaviria-Agudelo C, Aroh C, Tareen N, et al. Genomic heterogeneity of methicillin resistant staphylococcus aureus associated with variation in severity of illness among children with acute hematogenous osteomyelitis. Becker K. PLoS One 2015; 10(6):e0130415.

21. Malcius D, Trumpulyte G, Barauskas V, et al. Two decades of acute hematogenous osteomyelitis in children: are there any changes? Pediatr Surg Int 2005;21(5):356–9.

22. Wu JS, Gorbachova T, Morrison WB, et al. Imaging-guided bone biopsy for osteomyelitis: are there factors associated with positive or negative cultures? AJR Am J Roentgenol 2007;188(6):1529–34.

23. Restrepo S, Vargas D, Riascos R, et al. Musculoskeletal infection imaging: past, present, and future. Curr Infect Dis Rep 2005;7(5):365–72.

24. Lazzarini L, Mader JT, Calhoun JH. Osteomyelitis in long bones. J Bone Joint Surg Am 2004;86(10): 2305–18.

25. Malcius D, Jonkus M, Kuprionis G, et al. The accuracy of different imaging techniques in diagnosis of acute hematogenous osteomyelitis. Medicina (Kaunas) 2009;45(8):624–31.

26. Mah ET, LeQuesne GW, Gent RJ, et al. Ultrasonic features of acute osteomyelitis in children. J Bone Joint Surg Br 1994;76(6):969–74.

27. Chandnani VP, Beltran J, Morris CS, et al. Acute experimental osteomyelitis and abscesses: detection with MR imaging versus CT. Radiology 1990; 174(1):233–6.

28. Averill LW, Hernandez A, Gonzalez L, et al. Diagnosis of osteomyelitis in children: utility of fat-suppressed contrast-enhanced MRI. Am J Roentgenol 2009;192(5):1232–8.

29. Copley LAB, Kinsler MA, Gheen T, et al. The impact of evidence-based clinical practice guidelines applied by a multidisciplinary team for the care of children with osteomyelitis. J Bone Joint Surg Am 2013;95(8):686.

30. Mueller AJ, Kwon JK, Steiner JW, et al. Improved magnetic resonance imaging utilization for children with musculoskeletal infection. J Bone Joint Surg Am 2015;97(22):1869–76.

31. Courtney PM, Flynn JM, Jaramillo D, et al. Clinical indications for repeat MRI in children with acute hematogenous osteomyelitis. J Pediatr Orthop 2010; 30(8):883–7.

32. Rosenfeld S, Bernstein DT, Daram S, et al. Predicting the presence of adjacent infections in septic arthritis in children. J Pediatr Orthop 2016;36(1):70–4.

33. Weber-Chrysochoou C, Corti N, Goetschel P, et al. Pelvic osteomyelitis: a diagnostic challenge in children. J Pediatr Surg 2007;42(3):553–7.

34. Kumar J, Ramachandran M, Little D, et al. Pelvic osteomyelitis in children. J Pediatr Orthop B 2010;19(1):38–41.

35. Mignemi ME, Menge TJ, Cole HA, et al. Epidemiology, diagnosis, and treatment of pericapsular pyomyositis of the hip in children. J Pediatr Orthop 2014;34(3):316–25.

36. Roine I, Faingezicht I, Arguedas A, et al. Serial serum C-reactive protein to monitor recovery from acute hematogenous osteomyelitis in children. Pediatr Infect Dis J 1995;14(1):40–4.

37. Rodelo JR, De la Rosa G, Valencia ML, et al. d-dimer is a significant prognostic factor in patients with suspected infection and sepsis. Am J Emerg Med 2012;30(9):1991–9.

38. Buck C, Bundschu J, Gallati H, et al. Interleukin-6: a sensitive parameter for the early diagnosis of neonatal bacterial infection. Pediatrics 1994;93(1):54–8.

39. Cierny G, Mader JT, Penninck JJ. The classic: a clinical staging system for adult osteomyelitis. Clin Orthop 2003;414:7–24.

40. Gomez M, Maraqa N, Alvarez A, et al. Complications of outpatient parenteral antibiotic therapy in childhood. Pediatr Infect Dis J 2001;20(5):541–3.

41. Bachur R, Pagon Z. Success of short-course parenteral antibiotic therapy for acute osteomyelitis of childhood. Clin Pediatr (Phila) 2007;46(1):30–5.

42. Lazzarini L, Lipsky BA, Mader JT. Antibiotic treatment of osteomyelitis: what have we learned from 30 years of clinical trials? Int J Infect Dis 2005;9(3):127–38.

43. Bernard L, Pron B, Lotthé A, et al. Outpatient parenteral antimicrobial therapy (OPAT) for the treatment of osteomyelitis: evaluation of efficacy, tolerance and cost. J Clin Pharm Ther 2001;26(6):445–51.

44. Maraqa NF, Gomez MM, Rathore MH. Outpatient parenteral antimicrobial therapy in osteoarticular infections in children. J Pediatr Orthop 2002;22(4):506–10.

45. Street M, Puna R, Huang M, et al. Pediatric acute hematogenous osteomyelitis. J Pediatr Orthop 2015;35(6):634–9.

46. Danielsson LG, Düppe H. Acute hematogenous osteomyelitis of the neck of the femur in children treated with drilling. Acta Orthop Scand 2002;73(3):311–6.

47. Cole WG, Dalziel RE, Leitl S. Treatment of acute osteomyelitis in childhood. J Bone Joint Surg Br 1982;64(2):218–23.

48. Copley LA, Barton T, Garcia C, et al. A proposed scoring system for assessment of severity of illness in pediatric acute hematogenous osteomyelitis using objective clinical and laboratory findings. Pediatr Infect Dis J 2014;33(1):35–41.

49. Hollmig ST. Deep venous thrombosis associated with osteomyelitis in children. J Bone Joint Surg Am 2007;89(7):1517.

50. Ramos OM. Chronic osteomyelitis in children. Pediatr Infect Dis J 2002;21(5):431–2.

51. Crary SE, Buchanan GR, Drake CE, et al. Venous thrombosis and thromboembolism in children with osteomyelitis. J Pediatr 2006;149(4):537–41.

52. Peters W, Irving J, Letts M. Long-term effects of neonatal bone and joint infection on adjacent growth plates. J Pediatr Orthop 1992;12(6):806–10.

53. Belthur MV, Birchansky SB, Verdugo AA, et al. Pathologic fractures in children with acute *Staphylococcus aureus* osteomyelitis. J Bone Joint Surg Am 2012;94(1):34–42.

Pediatric Septic Arthritis

Nicole I. Montgomery, MD[a],*, Howard R. Epps, MD[b]

KEYWORDS

• Septic arthritis • Pyogenic arthritis • Osteoarticular infection • Acute inflammation

---

KEY POINTS

- Septic arthritis requires urgent recognition and treatment to avoid joint destruction.
- The most common pathogen responsible for septic arthritis in children remains *Staphylococcus aureus*.
- Our understanding of pathogens continues to evolve as detection methods, such as targeted real-time polymerase chain reaction, continue to improve. MRI has improved our ability to detect concurrent infections and is a useful clinical tool where readily available.
- The treatment course involves intravenous antibiotics followed by transition to oral antibiotics when clinically appropriate.
- The recommended surgical treatment of septic arthritis is open arthrotomy with decompression of the joint, irrigation, and debridement as well as treatment of any concurrent infections.

INTRODUCTION

Septic arthritis is a bacterial joint infection that can result in significant acute and chronic disability. This condition requires urgent identification and treatment. In many cases acute bacterial arthritis may be associated with infection at other sites and in other tissue types.[1] The overall incidence of acute septic arthritis is estimated to be 4 to 10 per 100,000 children in well-resourced countries.[2] The most commonly affected joints are in the lower extremities: knees, hips, and ankles account for up to 80% of the cases.[3]

Pathophysiology

The joint can become infected via hematogenous inoculation through the transphyseal vessels, spread of infection of the adjacent metaphysis, or direct inoculation from trauma or surgery.[4,5] The inflammatory response to septic arthritis leads to high local cytokine concentrations, which increase the release of host matrix metalloproteinases and other collagen-degrading enzymes. Direct release of bacterial toxins and lysosomal enzymes further damages the articular surfaces.[6] Joint destruction may start as soon as 8 hours following inoculation.[7] In addition, increased intracapsular pressure in the hip joint may lead to compressive ischemia and avascular necrosis of the femoral head if not promptly addressed.

Bacteriology

The organisms most likely to cause bacteremia in a child are the organisms most likely responsible for acute bacterial arthritis. *Staphylococcus aureus*, both methicillin sensitive and methicillin resistant, is the most commonly cultured organism.[8] In the past 10 years studies have identified an increasing prevalence of community-associated methicillin-resistant *S aureus* (CA-MRSA) as an isolate in 26% to 63% of cases of septic arthritis.[9] Some strains of CA-MRSA contain a gene encoding for the cytotoxin Panton-Valentine leukocidin (PVL).[10] PVL-positive CA-MRSA strains are associated with complex infections with higher rates of septic shock, longer hospital stays, greater

---

Disclosure Statement: The authors have nothing to disclose.
[a] Pediatric Orthopedics, Baylor College of Medicine, Houston, TX 77030, USA; [b] Orthopedic Surgery, Baylor College of Medicine, 6701 Fannin street, Ste. 660, Houston, TX 77030, USA
* Corresponding author. 1 Baylor Plaza, Houston, TX 77030.
E-mail address: NMontgomery@mdanderson.org

number of surgical interventions, and prolonged antibiotic therapy.

One organism that has increasing prevalence in the population less than 4 years of age is *Kingella kingae*. *K kingae* is a fastidious oral gram-negative bacterium. With *K kingae* septic arthritis there may be a history of a preceding upper respiratory tract infection.[11] Overall, these patients have a different presentation than the typical *S aureus* septic arthritis. Patients with *K kingae* septic arthritis tend to present with a milder clinical picture. Most patients do still present with an elevated erythrocyte sedimentation rate (ESR) and C-reactive protein (CRP) but less likely to be febrile and have normal white blood cell (WBC) counts.[12–14]

Other frequently isolated species include group A beta-hemolytic *Streptococcus* as well as *Streptococcus pneumoniae*. In neonates, *S aureus* remains a common organism but group B *Streptococcus* is also isolated. Neonates are also at risk for infection with gram-negative enteric organisms.[15] Because of widespread vaccination against *Haemophilus influenza* type B, the organism is now an unusual cause of septic arthritis. It should remain on the differential for septic arthritis in a child with unknown or unvaccinated status.[16] Neonates and sexually active adolescents are at risk for infection by *Neisseria gonorrhoeae*.[17] Patients with sickle cell disease are at risk for septic arthritis caused by *Salmonella* species in addition to the more common organisms. *Neisseria meningitides* may either cause a septic or reactive arthritis.

DIAGNOSIS

Acute septic arthritis carries the potential for joint destruction, avascular necrosis, bacteremia, and sepsis. Because acute bacterial septic arthritis is a surgical emergency, expedient and accurate diagnosis is of the utmost importance. Diagnosis is made by history and physical examination coupled with laboratory studies, imaging studies, and arthrocentesis. There are a few conditions to be aware of that may mimic the clinical presentation of acute bacterial septic arthritis. Diagnoses that may be confused with septic arthritis include trauma, hemarthrosis, reactive effusion, juvenile rheumatoid arthritis, arthritis of acute rheumatic fever, osteomyelitis, pyomyositis, septic bursitis, tumor, leukemia, slipped capital femoral epiphysis, Legg-Calvé-Perthes disease, Lyme arthritis, Henoch-Schönlein purpura, sickle cell anemia, and transient or toxic synovitis.

History and Physical

Children typically present with a combination of immobility and dysfunction of the involved joint, fever, malaise, and pain. The child may have a history of antecedent mild trauma, concurrent infection, or illness. Around 20% of children have a history of injury to the affected extremity or a nonspecific fall before presentation.[18] Supporting history is important in raising suspicion for more rare infections. Travel history, sick contacts, immunization status, recent illnesses, animal exposures, exposure to unpasteurized dairy products, and family history should be ascertained. Clinical findings may include swelling, erythema, tenderness to palpation, limited joint range of motion, and gait disturbance. Patients may or may not appear acutely ill or toxic. Some infections are life threatening and associated with deep vein thrombosis, septic emboli, and a diathesis of septic shock and multisystem organ failure.[19]

Laboratory Studies

Initial studies for a child with septic arthritis should include a complete blood count with differential, CRP, ESR, and blood cultures. Although these studies are helpful in the workup, they alone cannot make a definitive diagnosis. Some children will have minimally elevated or even normal laboratory values in septic arthritis. Meanwhile some patients with other diagnoses, like toxic synovitis, may have moderately elevated laboratory values.[20] In comparison with ESR, CRP has been shown to be a better independent predictor of infection. In addition, CRP is a better negative predictor than a positive predictor of disease. If the CRP is less than 1.0 mg/dL, the probability that patients do not have septic arthritis is 87%.[21] Some children who are ultimately found to have deep musculoskeletal infections may present with laboratory indices that are within the spectrum of normal; some children who do not have an infection, such as those with transient synovitis or reactive arthritis, may have moderately elevated laboratory indices.[22] A child with superficial infection, such as cellulitis, may have markedly elevated laboratory indices that suggest an underlying deep infection, which may ultimately be excluded after further imaging with MRI. It is important to consider each case as being unique and to seek to establish an early, accurate diagnosis with all of the available information.

Imaging

Imaging of the affected joint should start with plain radiographs. In the setting of isolated acute septic arthritis, radiographs will likely be negative aside from soft tissue swelling. Radiographic changes indicating a more chronic process do not become apparent until 7 to 10 days after the infection has commenced. In advanced infection, the destruction of the articular cartilage will manifest in joint space narrowing and subchondral erosion. Cortical or metaphyseal bone destruction may be seen in chronic concurrent osteomyelitis.

Ultrasound is a rapid, noninvasive, no-radiation test that is helpful in detecting the presence of a joint effusion (Fig. 1). It is particularly helpful in the shoulder and hip where palpation cannot reliably detect the presence of an effusion. A negative ultrasound of the hip with absence of fluid generally rules out septic arthritis. A positive ultrasound in the setting of supportive history, physical, and laboratory studies is enough evidence to warrant surgical intervention without obtaining more advanced imaging.[23] However, in cases with no hip effusion, there may be nearby osteomyelitis or pyogenic myositis causing the symptoms and advanced imaging with MRI is warranted.[24]

Between 15% and 50% of osteoarticular infections involve the joint and the bone.[4,25] MRI with contrast has the ability to reveal the full extent of these infections.[26] MRI should be ordered with and without gadolinium contrast as the dye aids in identification of concurrent infections as well as gives information related to the perfusion of the femoral head in cases of septic arthritis of the hip (Fig. 2).[22] Identifying concurrent infections aids the surgeon in planning the approach for surgery and also helps ensure that all areas requiring drainage are addressed. A recent algorithm was proposed to help identify the patients at risk for adjacent infection who would benefit from MRI to identify the additional sites of infection: Five variables (older than 3.6 years, CRP>13.8 mg/L, duration of symptoms >3 days, platelets <314 × 10 cells per muL (microliter), and ANC (absolute neutrophil count) >8.6 × 10 cells per muL) were found to be predictive of adjacent infection and were included in the algorithm. Patients with 3 or more risk factors were classified as high risk for having an adjacent infection and, thus, would benefit from MRI.[27] Patients with septic arthritis of the shoulder or elbow would also benefit from routine MRI, as it is associated with a high rate of concurrent osteomyelitis.[28,29]

Arthrocentesis

The cornerstone of the diagnosis of acute septic arthritis is the evaluation of aspirated synovial fluid sent for gram stain, aerobic and anaerobic culture, and cell count with differential.[30]

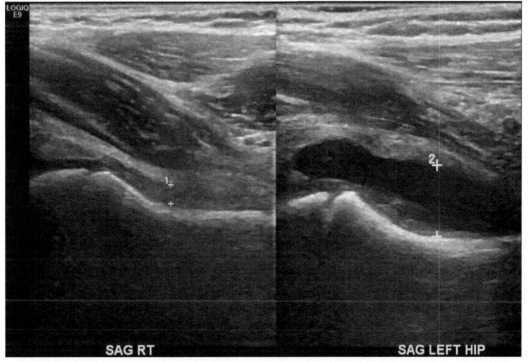

Fig. 1. Ultrasounds of a normal right hip and affected left hip showing a large effusion of the left hip and capsular distention.

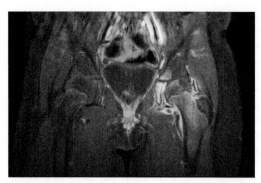

Fig. 2. MRI of the left hip demonstrates an enhancing effusion, synovitis, and enhancement of the left ischium suggestive of osteomyelitis. Additionally, there is decreased signal in the lateral femoral epiphysis suggesting diminished blood flow to this region likely due to increased intracapsular pressure from the septic effusion.

Typically the fluid aspirate in septic arthritis is turbid with a WBC count of greater than 50,000/mm³ with greater than 75% polymorphonuclear neutrophils and glucose less than 40 mg/dL. Synovial fluid should be obtained in a heparinized syringe if available to prevent clotting. Inoculating the fluid directly into blood culture bottles can increase the yield of fastidious organisms.[11] Several synovial fluid samples may remain culture negative,[31] but new technology promises to increase yield from synovial fluid samples.

The use of polymerase chain reaction (PCR) on synovial fluid or tissue samples has the potential to speed the time to identification of the responsible pathogen as well as enhance the identification of more fastidious organisms. One study found that real-time PCR was 100% accurate in differentiating between gram-negative and gram-positive organisms.[32] In addition, PCR can be used to target sequences unique to particular organisms. This ability is particularly pertinent to notoriously difficult-to-culture organisms, such as *K kingae*. Detection of *K kingae* has markedly improved with the advent of PCR over cultures.[33] The RTX toxin of *K kingae* has been identified as a high-yield target of PCR. The toxin can be identified from either a synovial fluid sample or a simple oropharyngeal swab in infected patients with high sensitivity and specificity.[12,34]

Distinguishing from Transient Synovitis

Transient synovitis of the hip is a relatively benign condition that can be treated with antiinflammatory medications and usually improves in 24 to 48 hours. Both transient synovitis and septic arthritis of the hip may present with acute onset of pain, hip flexion, abduction and external rotation, and refusal to bear weight. Transient synovitis is most common in children aged 4 to 8 years, with a male to female ratio of 2:1. Kocher and colleagues[35] proposed a clinical algorithm in 1999 to help distinguish septic arthritis from transient synovitis. The 4 clinic predictors were history of fever, non–weight bearing, ESR of greater than 40 mL/h, and serum WBC count of greater than 12,000 cells per milliliter. The probability of septic arthritis exceeded 99% when all 4 criteria were met.[35] These results have not as been reproducible at other institutions.[36,37] A more recent study has demonstrated an elevation in CRP to be an independent risk factor for septic arthritis.[38]

Distinguishing from Lyme Disease

Acute bacterial septic arthritis of the knee and acute knee swelling due to Lyme disease can have considerable similarities in clinical presentation. Lyme disease is endemic in the Northeast and Midwest United States. The clinical presentation of both conditions can be very similar. Laboratory studies including ESR, CRP, and peripheral and synovial WBC counts may be elevated in both conditions.[39,40] Definitive diagnosis for Lyme disease is usually made using Western blot to Lyme immunoglobulin G, which can take several days to finalize. Baldwin and colleagues[41] found that patients older than 2 years without history of fever, without limitation of motion, and a CRP of less than 4 mg/L may be safely observed in anticipation of serologic studies. It should be noted that other potential diagnoses should be considered in the interim.[41]

TREATMENT

The treatment of children with septic arthritis is often multidisciplinary involving the orthopedic surgeon, pediatrician, infectious disease specialist, anesthesiology, radiologist, nurses, and physical therapists. Institutional clinical diagnostic and treatment guidelines are useful in establishing systematic patient-centered care.[36] The first priority, along with obtaining the correct diagnosis, should be making the child comfortable. Nonsteroidal antiinflammatory medications can aid in pain relief and fever reduction.[42,43] Additionally, a 4-day course of low-dose dexamethasone can provide some symptomatic relief without evidence of deleterious side effects.[44–46]

Antibiotics

Empirical antibiotic coverage should start in suspected cases as soon as blood cultures and synovial fluid samples are collected. Ideally, antibiotic treatment is coordinated with an infectious disease specialist. Antibiotics have good penetrance into the joint, and synovial fluid concentrations are equivalent to serum concentrations 1 hour after initiation.[47] The gram stain of synovial fluid can provide information to help guide antibiotic administration, but the result should not delay the initiation of antibiotics. For gram-positive cocci, initial therapy is a penicillinase-resistant penicillin. In areas with a high rate of MRSA, initial therapy should include either vancomycin or clindamycin. A third-generation cephalosporin is added for gram-negative coverage if the gram stain reveals these organisms or if the initial studies are indeterminate. A third-generation cephalosporin like cefotaxime or ceftriaxone will cover K kingae, Gonococcus, and Salmonella species. Of note, K kingae is resistant to clindamycin and vancomycin.[12] Patients in countries where H influenza B is common and children who are unvaccinated should receive additional coverage with ampicillin or amoxicillin until culture results are back.[48] Recent evidence supports a shorter duration of intravenous antibiotics before switching to oral administration given improvement in clinical symptoms and a decrease in CRP.[49] This guideline is supported by a series of studies by Peltola and associates[42,43,50] advocating for shorter regimens of intravenous antibiotics and shorter total duration of antibiotics. Additional studies have confirmed that outcomes are equivalent with early versus late conversion from intravenous to oral antibiotic therapy and shortened overall antibiotic regimens.[51,52]

Surgical Intervention

The recommended treatment of septic arthritis is urgent decompression of the joint via open arthrotomy, irrigation, and debridement. Timely surgical intervention is of particular interest in septic arthritis of the hip where the femoral head is at risk of avascular necrosis. Recently less invasive techniques have been described with some success, but an open procedure is necessary when there is concurrent infection or subperiosteal abscess to drain.

Arthroscopy

Arthroscopic irrigation and debridement of septic arthritis of the knee has become an accepted practice in the adult population, and the use of arthroscopy to treat septic arthritis in the pediatric population is gaining evidence to support its use. Single port (or double port when synovectomy indicated) arthroscopy was recently described as a successful treatment of septic arthritis of the hip, knee, ankle, and shoulder in children aged 3 weeks to 6 years.[53,54] A recent retrospective series comparing open versus arthroscopic debridement of septic arthritis of the knee demonstrated a decreased need for repeat irrigation and debridement.[55] However, hip arthroscopy as a treatment of hip septic arthritis is gaining traction in uncomplicated cases of hip septic arthritis in the hands of a skilled hip arthroscopist.[56]

Serial Aspiration

Serial aspiration of the hip under ultrasound guidance and sedation has been described with some success. In a series of 28 patients, the average number of aspirations was 3.6, with 4 patients eventually requiring an arthrotomy. There were no complications noted in long-term follow-up.[57] In addition, a single aspiration of the shoulder with a large dose of antimicrobials was described in one series of 9 patients, aged 3 months to 12 years, without any known negative sequelae. One patient in this series required open arthrotomy because of a lack of clinical improvement during their hospital course.[58] The indications for this approach are not clearly defined.

Outcomes and Complications

If neglected, acute bacterial septic arthritis can lead to chondral damage, joint space narrowing, and joint destruction. Avascular necrosis is a potential complication of septic arthritis of the hip.[59] Septic arthritis in the skeletally immature can lead to physeal injury and potentially growth arrest causing a leg-length discrepancy or angular deformity.[60] These patients do warrant some routine follow-up from the orthopedic surgeon after their septic arthritis is treated. In neonates there is a potential for a slip of the proximal femoral epiphysis following septic arthritis or osteomyelitis. If recognized early and reduced anatomically, the potential for recovery is excellent.[61]

SUMMARY

Acute septic arthritis is a condition with the potential for joint destruction, physeal damage, and osteonecrosis, which warrants urgent diagnosis and treatment. Currently the organism most likely responsible is S aureus; however, our understanding of pathogens continues to evolve as detection methods, such as targeted real-time PCR, continue to improve. MRI has improved our ability to detect concurrent infections and is a useful clinical adjunct. Treatment involves surgical drainage and intravenous antibiotics followed by transition to oral antibiotics when clinically appropriate. The standard for surgical treatment is open arthrotomy with decompression of the joint, irrigation, and debridement as well as treatment of any concurrent infections.

REFERENCES

1. Gafur OA, Copley LA, Hollmig ST, et al. The impact of the current epidemiology of pediatric musculoskeletal infection on evaluation and treatment guidelines. J Pediatr Orthop 2008;28(7):777–85.
2. Arnold JC, Bradley JS. Osteoarticular infections in children. Infect Dis Clin North Am 2015;29(3):557–74.
3. Baitch A. Recent observations of acute suppurative arthritis. Clin Orthop 1962;22:157–66.
4. Jackson MA, Burry VF, Olson LC. Pyogenic arthritis associated with adjacent osteomyelitis: identification of the sequela-prone child. Pediatr Infect Dis J 1992;11(1):9–13.
5. Nelson JD, Koontz WC. Septic arthritis in infants and children: a review of 117 cases. Pediatrics 1966;38(6):966–71.
6. Roy S, Bhawan J. Ultrastructure of articular cartilage in pyogenic arthritis. Arch Pathol 1975;99(1):44–7.
7. Smith RL, Schurman DJ, Kajiyama G, et al. The effect of antibiotics on the destruction of cartilage in experimental infectious arthritis. J Bone Joint Surg Am 1987;69(7):1063–8.
8. Moumile K, Merckx J, Glorion C, et al. Bacterial aetiology of acute osteoarticular infections in children. Acta Paediatr 2005;94(4):419–22.
9. Arnold SR, Elias D, Buckingham SC, et al. Changing patterns of acute hematogenous osteomyelitis and septic arthritis: emergence of community-associated methicillin-resistant Staphylococcus aureus. J Pediatr Orthop 2006;26(6):703–8.
10. Dohin B, Gillet Y, Kohler R, et al. Pediatric bone and joint infections caused by Panton-Valentine leukocidin-positive Staphylococcus aureus. Pediatr Infect Dis J 2007;26(11):1042–8.
11. de Groot R, Glover D, Clausen C, et al. Bone and joint infections caused by Kingella kingae: six cases and review of the literature. Rev Infect Dis 1988;10(5):998–1004.
12. Ceroni D, Cherkaoui A, Ferey S, et al. Kingella kingae osteoarticular infections in young children: clinical features and contribution of a new specific real-time PCR assay to the diagnosis. J Pediatr Orthop 2010;30(3):301–4.
13. Dubnov-Raz G, Scheuerman O, Chodick G, et al. Invasive Kingella kingae infections in children: clinical and laboratory characteristics. Pediatrics 2008;122(6):1305–9.
14. Dubnov-Raz G, Ephros M, Garty BZ, et al. Invasive pediatric Kingella kingae infections: a nationwide collaborative study. Pediatr Infect Dis J 2010;29(7):639–43.
15. Obletz BE. Acute suppurative arthritis of the hip in the neonatal period. J Bone Joint Surg Am 1960;42-A:23–30.
16. Luhmann JD, Luhmann SJ. Etiology of septic arthritis in children: an update for the 1990s. Pediatr Emerg Care 1999;15(1):40–2.
17. Kohen DP. Neonatal gonococcal arthritis: three cases and review of the literature. Pediatrics 1974;53(3):436–40.
18. Paakkonen M, Kallio MJ, Lankinen P, et al. Preceding trauma in childhood hematogenous bone and joint infections. J Pediatr Orthop B 2014;23(2):196–9.
19. Morrison MJ, Herman MJ. Hip septic arthritis and other pediatric musculoskeletal infections in the era of methicillin-resistant Staphylococcus aureus. Instr Course Lect 2013;62:405–14.
20. Jung ST, Rowe SM, Moon ES, et al. Significance of laboratory and radiologic findings for differentiating between septic arthritis and transient synovitis of the hip. J Pediatr Orthop 2003;23(3):368–72.
21. Levine MJ, McGuire KJ, McGowan KL, et al. Assessment of the test characteristics of C-reactive protein for septic arthritis in children. J Pediatr Orthop 2003;23(3):373–7.
22. Kan JH, Young RS, Yu C, et al. Clinical impact of gadolinium in the MRI diagnosis of musculoskeletal infection in children. Pediatr Radiol 2010;40(7):1197–205.
23. Laine JC, Denning JR, Riccio AI, et al. The use of ultrasound in the management of septic arthritis of the hip. J Pediatr Orthop B 2015;24(2):95–8.
24. Eich GF, Superti-Furga A, Umbricht FS, et al. The painful hip: evaluation of criteria for clinical decision-making. Eur J Pediatr 1999;158(11):923–8.
25. Chen WL, Chang WN, Chen YS, et al. Acute community-acquired osteoarticular infections in children: high incidence of concomitant bone and joint involvement. J Microbiol Immunol Infect 2010;43(4):332–8.
26. Mazur JM, Ross G, Cummings J, et al. Usefulness of magnetic resonance imaging for the diagnosis of acute musculoskeletal infections in children. J Pediatr Orthop 1995;15(2):144–7.
27. Rosenfeld S, Bernstein DT, Daram S, et al. Predicting the presence of adjacent infections in septic arthritis in children. J Pediatr Orthop 2016;36(1):70–4.
28. Nduaguba AM, Flynn JM, Sankar WN. Septic arthritis of the elbow in children: clinical

presentation and microbiological profile. J Pediatr Orthop 2016;36(1):75–9.

29. Ernat J, Riccio AI, Fitzpatrick K, et al. Osteomyelitis is commonly associated with septic arthritis of the shoulder in children. J Pediatr Orthop 2015. [Epub ahead of print].

30. Shmerling RH, Delbanco TL, Tosteson AN, et al. Synovial fluid tests. What should be ordered? JAMA 1990;264(8):1009–14.

31. Lyon RM, Evanich JD. Culture-negative septic arthritis in children. J Pediatr Orthop 1999;19(5): 655–9.

32. Choe H, Inaba Y, Kobayashi N, et al. Use of real-time polymerase chain reaction for the diagnosis of infection and differentiation between gram-positive and gram-negative septic arthritis in children. J Pediatr Orthop 2013;33(3):e28–33.

33. Carter K, Doern C, Jo CH, et al. The clinical usefulness of polymerase chain reaction as a supplemental diagnostic tool in the evaluation and the treatment of children with septic arthritis. J Pediatr Orthop 2016;36(2):167–72.

34. Ceroni D, Dubois-Ferriere V, Cherkaoui A, et al. Detection of Kingella kingae osteoarticular infections in children by oropharyngeal swab PCR. Pediatrics 2013;131(1):e230–5.

35. Kocher MS, Zurakowski D, Kasser JR. Differentiating between septic arthritis and transient synovitis of the hip in children: an evidence-based clinical prediction algorithm. J Bone Joint Surg Am 1999; 81(12):1662–70.

36. Kocher MS, Mandiga R, Murphy JM, et al. A clinical practice guideline for treatment of septic arthritis in children: efficacy in improving process of care and effect on outcome of septic arthritis of the hip. J Bone Joint Surg Am 2003;85-A(6): 994–9.

37. Kocher MS, Mandiga R, Zurakowski D, et al. Validation of a clinical prediction rule for the differentiation between septic arthritis and transient synovitis of the hip in children. J Bone Joint Surg Am 2004;86-A(8):1629–35.

38. Singhal R, Perry DC, Khan FN, et al. The use of CRP within a clinical prediction algorithm for the differentiation of septic arthritis and transient synovitis in children. J Bone Joint Surg Br 2011;93(11): 1556–61.

39. Willis AA, Widmann RF, Flynn JM, et al. Lyme arthritis presenting as acute septic arthritis in children. J Pediatr Orthop 2003;23(1):114–8.

40. Cristofaro RL, Appel MH, Gelb RI, et al. Musculoskeletal manifestations of Lyme disease in children. J Pediatr Orthop 1987;7(5):527–30.

41. Baldwin KD, Brusalis CM, Nduaguba AM, et al. Predictive factors for differentiating between septic arthritis and Lyme disease of the knee in children. J Bone Joint Surg Am 2016;98(9):721–8.

42. Peltola H, Paakkonen M, Kallio P, et al, Osteomyelitis-Septic Arthritis Study Group. Prospective, randomized trial of 10 days versus 30 days of antimicrobial treatment, including a short-term course of parenteral therapy, for childhood septic arthritis. Clin Infect Dis 2009;48(9):1201–10.

43. Peltola H, Paakkonen M, Kallio P, et al, Osteomyelitis-Septic Arthritis Study Group. Short- versus long-term antimicrobial treatment for acute hematogenous osteomyelitis of childhood: prospective, randomized trial on 131 culture-positive cases. Pediatr Infect Dis J 2010;29(12):1123–8.

44. Odio CM, Ramirez T, Arias G, et al. Double blind, randomized, placebo-controlled study of dexamethasone therapy for hematogenous septic arthritis in children. Pediatr Infect Dis J 2003;22(10):883–8.

45. Harel L, Prais D, Bar-On E, et al. Dexamethasone therapy for septic arthritis in children: results of a randomized double-blind placebo-controlled study. J Pediatr Orthop 2011;31(2):211–5.

46. Fogel I, Amir J, Bar-On E, et al. Dexamethasone therapy for septic arthritis in children. Pediatrics 2015;136(4):e776–82.

47. Nelson JD. Antibiotic concentrations in septic joint effusions. N Engl J Med 1971;284(7):349–53.

48. Peltola H, Kallio MJ, Unkila-Kallio L. Reduced incidence of septic arthritis in children by Haemophilus influenzae type-b vaccination. Implications for treatment. J Bone Joint Surg Br 1998;80(3): 471–3.

49. Jaberi FM, Shahcheraghi GH, Ahadzadeh M. Short-term intravenous antibiotic treatment of acute hematogenous bone and joint infection in children: a prospective randomized trial. J Pediatr Orthop 2002;22(3):317–20.

50. Paakkonen M, Peltola H. How short is long enough for treatment of bone and joint infection? Adv Exp Med Biol 2011;719:39–46.

51. Ballock RT, Newton PO, Evans SJ, et al. A comparison of early versus late conversion from intravenous to oral therapy in the treatment of septic arthritis. J Pediatr Orthop 2009;29(6):636–42.

52. Jagodzinski NA, Kanwar R, Graham K, et al. Prospective evaluation of a shortened regimen of treatment for acute osteomyelitis and septic arthritis in children. J Pediatr Orthop 2009;29(5):518–25.

53. Thompson RM, Gourineni P. Arthroscopic treatment of septic arthritis in very young children. J Pediatr Orthop 2017;37(1):e53–7.

54. Sanpera I, Raluy-Collado D, Sanpera-Iglesias J. Arthroscopy for hip septic arthritis in children. Orthop Traumatol Surg Res 2016;102(1):87–9.

55. Dave OH, Patel KA, Andersen CR, et al. Surgical procedures needed to eradicate infection in knee septic arthritis. Orthopedics 2016;39(1):50–4.

56. El-Sayed AM. Treatment of early septic arthritis of the hip in children: comparison of results of open

arthrotomy versus arthroscopic drainage. J Child Orthop 2008;2(3):229–37.

57. Givon U, Liberman B, Schindler A, et al. Treatment of septic arthritis of the hip joint by repeated ultrasound-guided aspirations. J Pediatr Orthop 2004;24(3):266–70.

58. Paakkonen M, Peltola H, Kallio M, et al. Pediatric septic shoulder arthritis. Is routine arthrotomy still necessary? Duodecim 2011;127(7):716–9 [in Finnish].

59. Vidigal Junior EC, Vidigal EC, Fernandes JL. Avascular necrosis as a complication of septic arthritis of the hip in children. Int Orthop 1997;21(6):389–92.

60. Ogden JA. Pediatric osteomyelitis and septic arthritis: the pathology of neonatal disease. Yale J Biol Med 1979;52(5):423–48.

61. Aroojis AJ, Johari AN. Epiphyseal separations after neonatal osteomyelitis and septic arthritis. J Pediatr Orthop 2000;20(4):544–9.

Upper Extremity

Flexor Tenosynovitis

Brad T. Hyatt, MD*, Mark R. Bagg, MD

KEYWORDS

- Pyogenic • Flexor tenosynovitis • Hand infection • Flexor sheath • Kanavel

---

KEY POINTS

- Physical examination, including evaluation of Kanavel's four cardinal signs, is the primary mode of diagnosis for flexor tenosynovitis (FTS).
- The mainstay treatment of FTS is the same as any other abscess: surgical debridement and irrigation, followed by IV antibiotics; occasionally early identified cases may be treated with IV antibiotics alone.
- Multiple approaches have been described for debridement and irrigation (eg, closed sheath irrigation, open midaxial incision); the surgeon must use judgment to balance adequate debridement and the size, location, and morbidity of incisions.
- Postoperative irrigation on the ward is not supported by evidence and the benefits rarely merit the increased burden for nurses and discomfort to patients.
- Diabetes mellitus and peripheral vascular disease place patients at higher risk of poor outcomes including stiffness and amputation; early administration of antibiotics is the intervention that most correlates with good outcomes.

INTRODUCTION

The potential diagnosis of flexor tenosynovitis (FTS) tends to provoke anxiety in primary evaluators and surgeons given the difficulty of diagnosis and treatment. The unique anatomy and function of the hand make prompt and appropriate surgical or nonsurgical treatment imperative.[1] The surgical treatment of FTS is considered an essential skill for graduating orthopedic surgery residents.[2] Postoperative rehabilitation must not be overlooked as a key component of functional recovery. This article demystifies FTS and provides the latest evidence available for diagnosis and treatment.

HISTORICAL PERSPECTIVE

The seminal work of Kanavel[3,4] describing the aggressive surgical treatment of pyogenic FTS dramatically improved the natural history of this infection, including the sequelae of finger stiffness, tendon necrosis and rupture, hand dysfunction, systemic infection, and even death.

The introduction of antibiotics further revolutionized management such that the mainstay of FTS treatment today is intravenous (IV) antibiotics coupled with surgical debridement and irrigation; occasionally, cases identified early may even be treated by IV antibiotics alone. More recent advances include efforts to decrease the morbidity of surgical access while adequately debriding the closed space of the flexor sheaths.

ANATOMY

The flexor tendon sheath provides nutrition and an optimal gliding and restraining interface to the extrinsic tendons to the digits. The sheath is formed of two layers, as a "double-walled 'tube'"[5]: the visceral layer, which is synonymous with the epitenon, and the parietal layer, which is confluent with the fibrous pulley system.[6] In the normal hand, these two layers coalesce to form a sealed synovial space. In the index, middle, and ring fingers, the sheath extends 1 to 3 mm proximal to the palmar aponeurosis pulley at the level of the metacarpal necks.[6] The small

---

Disclosure Statement: The authors have nothing to disclose.
The Hand Center of San Antonio, 21 Spurs Lane, San Antonio, TX 78240, USA
* Corresponding author.
E-mail address: bradhyatt@gmail.com

finger sheath is confluent with the ulnar bursa in a significant portion of hands (80% in earlier texts[7] and 30% in more recent studies[8]) and Parona space in the forearm. The sheaths of the fingers end proximal to the distal interphalangeal joint.[6] The thumb sheath extends from 2 cm proximal to the radial styloid to just distal to the interphalangeal joint.[9]

Multiple communicating patterns between the flexor sheaths, the ulnar and radial bursae, and Parona space have been identified[10]; furthermore, septic sheaths may develop abnormal connections given increased synovial pressure and tissue degradation.[5] During the initial evaluation and serial examinations, the surgeon must keep in mind that an infection starting in one digit may spread to the hand, forearm, and other digits. An infection involving the radial and ulnar flexor sheaths is thus termed a "horseshoe" abscess.

Once bacteria are inoculated into the space between the visceral and parietal layers, the synovial fluid that normally provides nutrition to the tendon becomes a medium for bacterial growth. Sheath interconnections in the palm and with Parona space in the forearm allow for spread, and the closed nature of the sheath limits the host's ability to combat the infection.[5]

The confined space within the dermis of the digits has been compared with the fascia of muscle compartments,[11–13] where increased pressure within the digit (or compartment) can limit perfusion and delivery of antibiotics and the host's innate immune system. In 14 digits taken to surgery for FTS, Schnall and colleagues[14] found all patients had increased subcutaneous pressures compared with contralateral control digits, with an average pressure of 33 mm Hg (range, 20–73). Eight of the patients had pressures greater than 30 mm Hg,[14] fitting an older definition of compartment syndrome.[15]

If surgery is required, an understanding of pertinent hand anatomy is paramount. Extra care must be taken because the edematous hand and digits may have displaced neurovascular structures that are under greater tension than usual. With Kaplan cardinal line drawn from "the apex of the interdigital fold between the thumb and the index finger to the hook of the hamate,"[16] the superficial palmar arch is found 18 ± 4 mm distal to the intersection of Kaplan cardinal line and a line extending from the ulnar border of the middle finger.

Common digital arteries branch from the superficial arch and course distally until branching into proper digital arteries. At the level of finger web spaces, the proper digital arteries and veins

flank the flexor tendons sheath. The arterial supply to the thumb is typically via the princeps pollicis (80%), a branch of the radial artery or deep palmar arch, or a branch of the superficial palmar arch (20%).[17]

Branches of the median and ulnar nerves typically pass between the superficial and deep transverse metacarpal ligaments, after which the nerve courses on the palmar aspect of the digital artery.[18] In the thumb, the radial digital nerve crosses over the flexor pollicis longus tendon 0.9 ± 2.3 mm proximal to a line extending along the radial border of the index finger.[19]

The pulley systems of the fingers and thumb have been extensively studied[8–10,20–22] and should be understood to perform safe and adequate debridement and irrigation. In addition to five annular pulleys, the index, middle, ring, and small fingers also have three cruciate pulleys; the palmar aponeurosis also has some pulley function (Table 1).[6] The thumb has 4 well-described variations of pulleys (Table 2).[9,21,23]

MICROBIOLOGY

Most cultures from FTS identify skin flora, specifically *Staphylococcus* and *Streptococcus*. In a recent large series with 71 consecutive patients, *Staphylococcus* and *Streptococcus* accounted for 70% of FTS infections, including 13% methicillin-resistant *Staphylococcus aureus* (MRSA). No growth was found in 18%, and the remaining 11% were caused by gram-negative organisms, *Mycobacterium*, and *Cryptococcus*.[24] Table 3 shows the culture results from representative studies from 1975 to 2012.

Atypical organisms should also be considered, especially for patients with diabetes

Table 1	
Pulleys of the index-small fingers	
Pulley Name	**Pulley Location**
PA	Metacarpal neck
A1	MP joint
A2	Proximal half of proximal phalanx
C1	Distal half of distal proximal phalanx
A3	PIP joint
C2	Proximal quarter of middle phalanx
A4	Middle quarter of middle phalanx
C3	Distal quarter of middle phalanx
A5	Distal most aspect of middle phalanx

Abbreviations: MP, metacarpophalangeal joint; PA, palmar aponeurosis; PIP, proximal interphalangeal joint.

Table 2 Pulleys of the thumb	
Pulley Name	**Pulley Location**
A1	MP joint
Av	Variable, proximal half of proximal phalanx
Type I	Absent
Type II	Transverse
Type III	Oblique
Type IV	Confluent with A1
Oblique	Third quartile of proximal phalanx
A2	Distal quartile of proximal phalanx

mellitus or who are immunocompromised.[32] Although less frequent, MRSA-induced FTS has shown a higher rate of complications including tissue necrosis, long-term stiffness, and amputation.[30,33,34] *Mycobacterium* species should be considered in cases of indolent infections.[35,36] *Mycobacterium marinum* should be suspected when a penetrating injury happens in a marine setting. *Mycobacterium tuberculosis*[36] and *Candida*[37] may be seen in immunocompromised hosts. *Neisseria gonorrhea* should be considered in sexually active patients, especially those without history of a puncture wound near the flexor sheath.[38]

PATIENT PRESENTATION
History
Certain aspects of the history should be emphasized when evaluating a patient with suspected FTS, specifically the details regarding the inciting injury and the patient's immune status. Patients typically present 2 to 5 days following an injury,[38] often after failing a course of outpatient antibiotics.[25,26] Although hematogenous spread may seed the flexor sheath in rare cases,[39,40] most are caused by a penetrating injury.[5,26,38]

Patients should be asked about associated symptoms including fever, chills, anorexia, and malaise. Additionally, the evaluator must ask about the proximal extent of pain and swelling in the upper extremity, and other sites of pain (Box 1).

Physical Examination
In the diagnosis of a patient with suspected FTS, consideration of Kanavel's four cardinal sign is necessary but not sufficient (Box 2). Kanavel originally described three cardinal signs in 1912. Although "uniform swelling" was mentioned in his original description, it was not codified as a

cardinal sign until later.[3,4,41] Close examination of Kanavel's exact words[3] is worthwhile (Box 3):

1. "Exquisite tenderness over the course of the sheath, limited to the sheath" refers to tenderness elicited by the examiner with palpation volarly, not dorsally or laterally. The adjacent digits should be used as controls to help the patient and examiner differentiate sheath tenderness from generalized hand tenderness. The proximal and distal extent of the tenderness should also be documented for comparison with serial examinations.
2. "Flexion of the finger": the affected digit should be compared at rest with the adjacent digits, and the thumb is compared with the resting posture of the contralateral thumb. The posture of the digit typically results from flexion of the metacarpophylangeal joint and the interphalangeal joints, with the proximal interphalangeal joint carrying the greatest degree of flexion.
3. "Exquisite pain on extending the finger, most marked at the proximal end" refers to pain elicited by the examiner passively extending the digit. Care must be taken to distinguish the pain of extension from the pain associated with the direct pressure of the examiner's fingers, especially in the vicinity of a laceration or abscess. Additionally, the patient should be asked to report the location of pain, because true FTS is unlikely to cause pain that is most pronounced dorsally. Again, adjacent digits are used as controls to help distinguish this sign.
4. "The whole of the involved digit is uniformly [sic] swollen" distinguishes FTS from lesions with localized edema, such as an abscess or a laceration. The authors prefer to avoid the word "fusiform" given the confusion and disagreement regarding the word's definition, especially across medical and surgical specialties.

Multiple studies have attempted to give more diagnostic value to specific signs, with conflicting results.[29,30,42] Importantly, up to 46% of patients with surgically proven FTS may not exhibit all four cardinal signs preoperatively.[30] Signs of FTS may be less apparent in the thumb and small finger, given the larger volume of the sheaths with connections to the ulnar and radial bursae.[41] The Kanavel signs may be even less reliable in the evaluation of children, as one report showed a case of surgically proven FTS in a 2.5-year-old child with none of the four signs exhibited preoperatively.[43]

Table 3
Cultures from surgically proven cases of flexor tenosynovitis

Microbes	Pollen,[25] 1974		Neviaser,[26] 1978		Maloon et al,[27] 1990		Juliano & Eglseder[28] 1991		Schnall et al,[14] 1996		Pang et al,[29] 2007		Dailiana et al,[30] 2008		Bishop et al,[24] 2013		Nikkhah,[31] 2012		Average[a]
Staphylococcus	11	36.7%	12	60.0%	26	56.5%	5	17.9%	2	14.3%	32	42.7%	9	22.0%	27	38.0%	4	25.0%	34.8%
MRSA	—	—	—	—	—	—	—	—	—	—	11	14.7%	10	24.4%	9	12.7%	1	6.3%	14.4%
Streptococcus	5	16.7%	—	—	7	15.2%	1	3.6%	1	7.1%	—	—	2	4.9%	14	19.7%	3	18.8%	12.6%
Gram negatives	—	—	4	20.0%	3	6.5%	2	7.1%	—	—	18	24.0%	4	9.8%	5	7.0%	1	6.3%	11.5%
Polymicrobial	1	3.3%	—	—	—	—	—	—	7	50.0%	—	—	3	7.3%	—	—	0	—	20.2%
No growth	13	43.3%	4	20.0%	10	21.7%	19	67.9%	4	28.6%	17	22.7%	13	31.7%	13	18.3%	6	37.5%	32.4%
Total number of cases	30	—	20	—	46	—	28	—	14	—	75	—	41	—	71	—	16	—	—

[a] Average percentages do not add to 100% given categorization of data and exclusion of rare and atypical organisms.
Data from Refs.[13,24–31]

Box 1
History focused on FTS

Injury factors

Was there a penetrating injury?

For example, knife, needle, thorn, animal bite

If no injury, then other sources of infection?

For example, *Neisseria gonorrhea*, *Clostridium difficile*

When was the injury?

What treatments have been tried?

For example, oral antibiotics, splinting

Patient factors

Handedness, occupation

Immunocompromise

For example, diabetes mellitus, human immunodeficiency virus, needle drug user

Drug allergies, specifically antibiotics

Although the sensitivity and specificity of each cardinal sign or combination of signs has not been studied,[41] many authors agree that tenderness along the flexor sheath is of greatest value in discriminating FTS from other infections of the hand.[5,25,38] The value of Kanavel's cardinal signs is to guide the examination as part of an appropriate history and examination, distinguish FTS from other hand infections, provide an efficient communication tool between providers, and provide a specific framework for performing and documenting serial examinations.

Box 2
Physical exam of FTS

- Kanavel's cardinal signs
  - Tenderness over flexor sheath
  - Digit resting in a flexed posture
  - Tenderness with passive extension
  - Uniform swelling of the entire digit
- Presence/absence of puncture wound
- Skin scaling/dryness/cracking
- Involvement of other digits
- Presence/absence of abscess
- Erythema extending proximally
- Lymphangitis
- Lymphadenopathy
- Web space maceration

Box 3
Kanavel's original examination description of flexor tenosynovitis

"The fingers are all slightly flexed. Now, how shall the differential diagnosis be made? Press deeply and firmly in all parts of the hand and fingers; the patient will volunteer the information that all points hurt; but if the tendon sheath is involved, pressure upon it throughout its course causes an immediate and involuntary expression of pain, and while before the patient has allowed his hand to remain passive in yours, he will now attempt to withdraw it voluntarily, and there is no doubt in your mind of the exquisite tenderness over this area. If this tenderness is outlined by the extent of the sheath, your diagnosis is nearly made. As a matter of fact, the greatest tenderness is generally complained of on deep pressure at the proximal end of the finger sheaths in the palm of the hand, just over the metacarpophalangeal articulation."

From Kanavel AB. The symptoms, signs, and diagnosis of tenosynovitis and fascial-space abscesses. In Infections of the Hand. 1st edition. Philadelphia: Lea & Febiger; 1912. p. 202.

Studies

FTS is a clinical diagnosis; plain films should be obtained to evaluate for retained foreign bodies and rule out fracture. Although MRI has been described in the diagnosis of FTS,[44,45] its sensitivity and specificity in diagnosis have not been studied. If used, the value of MRI is primarily to rule out other conditions, such as abscess, or in the evaluation of an obtunded patient. Ultrasound has been studied in the early detection of FTS,[46] but is not widely used in the diagnosis.[38]

Because of their lack of specificity, laboratory studies, such as white blood cell count, erythrocyte sedimentation rate, and C-reactive protein, are not definitive in distinguishing FTS from other infectious and inflammatory conditions of the hand.[24] They may have value in following response to treatment with serial tests.[38]

Differential Diagnosis

The differential diagnosis for patients presenting with suspected FTS includes infectious and inflammatory conditions (Table 4). The history can discern a penetrating inoculating injury from a recurrent inflammatory condition; in most but not all reported cases of gouty tenosynovitis, there is a history of gouty arthritis.[47–49] The examination aims to distinguish the origin of the patient's complaints as the entire hand, a discreet abscess, or localizing to the flexor sheath. As a generalization, non-FTS infections

Table 4	
Differential diagnosis of FTS	
Diagnosis	**Distinguishing Features**
Cellulitis	Diffuse edema not restricted to one digit, pain not restricted to digit, equal pain with flexion and extension
Paronychia	Purulence about nail fold
Felon	Abscess restricted to finger pulp
Deep space infection	Diffuse edema or palpable abscess
Herpetic whitlow	Clear, fluid-filled vesicles; history of herpes simplex virus; medical or dental occupation
Septic arthritis	Typically a dorsal penetrating wound, exquisite pain with passive and active joint motion
Extensor tenosynovitis	Tenderness over dorsal wrist and hand, pain with passive digit flexion
Gouty tenosynovitis	History of gouty arthritis, often multiple digits involved
Gouty arthritis	History of gout, pain with joint motion

of the hand do not initially exhibit Kanavel's cardinal signs, but left untreated may lead to secondary FTS.[5]

A related but distinct entity, extensor tenosynovitis (ETS), is worth discussion. The extensor tendons are enclosed by sheaths similar to the flexor tendons, and confined within the dorsal extensor compartments.[45] ETS is typically found in the nondominant hand of needle drug users[50] or immunocompromised patients.[51,52] ETS is diagnosed with tenderness along the *dorsal* tendon sheaths at the level of the carpus and pain with passive digit and wrist *flexion*. Although the natural history of ETS has not been specifically studied, surgical debridement is probably indicated when a large volume of purulence is evident on examination or advanced imaging (Fig. 1).

TREATMENT

The treatment options for FTS are broadly described by three categories: (1) IV antibiotics with serial examinations, (2) percutaneous or closed-sheath irrigation and drainage, and (3) open debridement and irrigation. The choice of treatment is based on several factors, including timing of presentation, severity of physical examination, host factors (eg, immunocompromised patient), and operating room availability. Although many authors have recommendations regarding the appropriate application of each treatment strategy,[5,25,53] no definitive guidelines exist. In the patient who fails to improve with initial treatment, prompt aggressive surgical intervention is indicated.[1,3,38,54]

Regardless of treatment option, most authors agree that IV antibiotics should be administered for a minimum of 48 hours.[5,38] With improvement, the patient is transitioned to oral antibiotics, ideally based on culture results.

Nonoperative Treatment

There are no comparative data for nonoperative versus operative treatment of FTS, although most authors support a trial of nonoperative treatment with inpatient IV antibiotics if the infection is identified within 48 hours of inoculation, the patient is otherwise healthy and immunocompetent, and there is no suspicion for associated abscess or necrosis.[5,26,38,42,55] For true FTS, this is the minority of patients. In addition to antibiotics, level V evidence recommends splinting and elevation.[38,42]

Antibiotic choice is based on the nature of inoculation (eg, animal bite, hematogenous spread), patient factors (eg, immunocompromise, antibiotic allergies), and local antibiotic resistance patterns.[38,53,56] As shown in Table 3, most FTS cases involve gram-positive organisms with an increasing rate of MRSA infections; gram-negative and polymicrobial infections make up a small but significant number of infections. Empiric antibiotics should cover S aureus and Streptococcus, with a low threshold to also cover MRSA and gram-negative organisms until culture sensitivities are available. A common initial choice is vancomycin and piperacillin/tazobactam.[53,56] Infectious disease consultation is recommended for patients with an immunocompromised status, antibiotic allergies, and those with atypical organisms or chronic infections.[38,53]

For the success of nonoperative treatment, definite improvement should be seen within 24 hours (recommendation range from 12–48 hours[38,42]) of initiation of antibiotics. Specifically, the patient needs to report an improvement in pain, and the Kanavel signs must be improved compared with previous examinations. Patients with worse symptoms and those

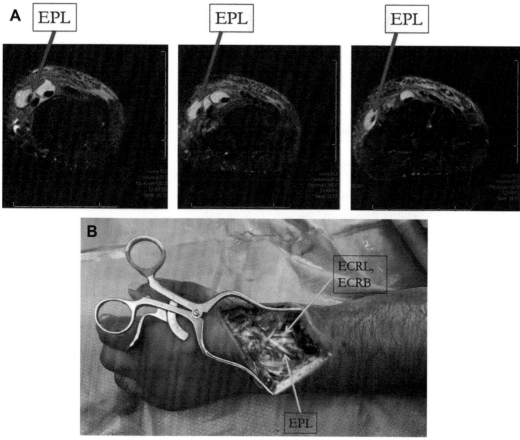

Fig. 1. (*A*) T2-weighted MRI showing extensor tenosynovitis. (*B*) Operative photograph showing extensor tendons during debridement and irrigation. ECRB, extensor carpi radialis brevis; ECRL, extensor carpi radialis longus; EPL, extensor pollicis longus.

with equivocal changes in examination should be taken to surgery promptly.

Operative Treatment

Multiple less-invasive methods of sheath irrigation have been described to adequately evacuate microbes and purulence without the morbidity of open debridement (**Table 5**).[25,26,28,57–60] The success of closed-sheath irrigation has been well established for early infections[26,61] and open debridement is clearly required for cases with necrosis or a chronic time course (eg, >1 week),[5,38] yet not all cases fall into these extremes. In an effort to guide treatment, Michon[62] created a classification system based on operative findings (**Table 6**). Although not validated or widely used, the Michon classification may be a valuable algorithm to consider when deciding how aggressive to be with the debridement component of FTS surgery.[5]

Closed sheath irrigation typically involves an approach to the A1 pulley using a zigzag Bruner-type incision,[5,26,57] a longitudinal or oblique incision,[60] or a transverse incision.[25] The sheath is entered just proximal to the A1 pulley or the A1 pulley is released completely or partially. Typically, purulence is found here, and cultures are obtained. A counterincision is made distally near the A5 pulley or at the base of the distal phalanx. This incision is made longitudinally over the midline[60] or in the midaxial plane with the neurovascular bundle remaining with the volar flap; alternatively, a limited zigzag incision is made for better visualization.[5]

Depending on the technique chosen, a plastic tube is passed into the sheath from proximal to distal. The plastic tube can be an 18-gauge angiocatheter advanced 1.5 to 2 cm into the sheath, a pain pump catheter,[60] or a 4F or 5F catheter pediatric feeding tube[59] advanced until it exits at the counterincision. The sheath is copiously irrigated with care to ensure fluid is flushing through the sheath rather than extravasating into surrounding tissue or exiting the

Table 5
Techniques for the treatment of FTS

Technique or Innovation	Originally Described by or Popularized by
Open debridement and irrigation	Kanavel,[3] 1912
Bruner or zigzag incisions	
Midaxial incision	
Intraoperative sheath irrigation with catheter (following open debridement)	Dickson-Wright,[63] 1943–1944
Irrigation continued postoperatively	Dickson-Wright,[63] 1943–1944
Limited proximal (typically near A1 pulley) and distal (typically near A5 pulley) incisions	
Continued postoperative through-and-through irrigation with	
Hydrogen peroxide followed by oxytetracycline solution	Carter et al,[57] 1966
Saline solution via syringe	Neviaser,[26] 1978
Commercially available Marcaine infusion pump	Gaston and Greenberg,[60] 2009
Continued postoperative intrasheath injection (without specific egress pathway)	
Benzyl penicillin	Pollen,[25] 1974
Antibiotic fluid	Besser,[58] 1976
Lactated Ringer solution	Juliano & Eglseder,[28] 1991
Closed continuous irrigation with fenestrated catheter tube	
Normal saline	Harris & Nanchahal,[59] 1999

Data from Refs.[3,25,26,28,57–60,63]

entry portal. Irrigation is continued until the outflowing fluid is clear of purulence, plus one song (authors' preference).

The wounds are either left open or only loosely closed. If an irrigating catheter is left in place, irrigation is continued on the postsurgical ward according to the protocol chosen. Typically, 100 to 1000 mL of fluid is incrementally irrigated through the catheter per day and the catheter is removed 24 to 48 hours postoperatively.[26,59–61]

Although postoperative irrigation has been advocated with various techniques,[25,26,28,57–61,63] the authors believe it is unnecessary for successful treatment and adds complexity for nurses and discomfort and possibly morbidity to patients.[64] For example, improper technique could lead to fluid extravasation, resulting in the aforementioned compartment-syndrome-like condition of the digit.[14] Furthermore, in one retrospective study, 20 patients with intraoperative irrigation only were compared with 55 patients with intraoperative and postoperative irrigation; there were no differences in final outcomes, including range of motion (ROM), complications, and need to return to the operating room.[65]

Table 6
Michon classification for severity of flexor tenosynovitis

Intraoperative Stage	Characteristic Findings	Treatment Recommendation
Stage I	Increased fluid in the sheath, primarily serous exudate	Minimal invasive drainage and catheter irrigation
Stage II	Cloudy/purulent fluid, granulomatous synovium	Minimal invasive drainage ± indwelling catheter irrigation
Stage III	Septic necrosis of tendon, pulleys, or tendon sheath	Extensile open debridement; possible amputation

From Michon J. Phlegmon of the tendon sheaths. Ann Chir 1974;28:277–80. [in French].

ROM exercises are initiated on the first or second postoperative day.[5,25,60] Once culture sensitivities are available and the examination is improving, the patient is transitioned to oral antibiotics and discharged to home.

For patients in whom a more aggressive approach is required, open debridement is performed via midaxial or zigzag Bruner incisions. Volar zigzag incisions have the advantage of excellent visualization and access to the tendon sheath, but also have a higher risk of flap necrosis and residual tendon exposure. For this reason, most authors recommend a midaxial incision, with the neurovascular bundle remaining with the volar flap.[5,53] The term "midlateral" is often erroneously used in the place of, or interchangeably with, "midaxial;" although the two approaches are anatomically close to each other, the distinction is important. The midaxial approach is formed by connecting the apices of the flexion creases, such that a straight line is created with the digit extended. This plane lies dorsal to the neurovascular bundle and is strategically in a tension-free zone. The midlateral approach is volar to the midaxial, is directly over the neurovascular bundle, and crosses the flexion crease at 90°, risking postoperative contracture.[66]

The midaxial incision is extended from the distal interphalangeal joint crease to the web space, with a separate counterincision overlying the A1 pulley.[5] Depending on the extent of debridement, the sheath is opened through small fenestrations, the cruciate pulleys are excised, or selected annular pulleys are vented. The A2 and A4 pulleys should be left intact if at all possible to avoid postoperative flexor tendon bowstringing. After copious irrigation, the incisions are loosely closed. A catheter is left in place if postoperative irrigation is desired.[63] The hand is elevated in a splint in the intrinsic plus position.[5] ROM exercises are initiated 1 to 2 days postoperatively and antibiotics transitioned as described previously.

OUTCOMES

Final ROM is the most common end point used to measure success in treating FTS; other end points include need for tenolysis and amputation. Multiple studies have correlated poor ROM with delayed treatment.[54,55] In a systematic review of 28 studies, treatment within 48 hours led to 80% excellent ROM.[55] Giladi and colleagues[55] further found that the use of antibiotics had the largest impact on final ROM. They found that 302 of 561 (54%) patients who received antibiotics had excellent ROM,

compared with 17 of 177 (15%) patients who had surgery without antibiotics. The timing of the antibiotics was not consistently reported for individual studies.

Among those patients treated with antibiotics and surgery, the authors further compared open debridement with a catheter irrigation technique. Final ROM was rated excellent in 57 of 218 (26%) patients treated open, compared with 245 of 343 (74%) patients treated with catheter irrigation (P<.001).[55] It should be noted that this difference is likely caused by severity of infection and surgical technique. Tenolysis may be indicated once inflammation and edema in the digit has resolved and "tissue equilibrium" is reached, as indicated by a greater passive than active ROM.[5]

In the review by Giladi and colleagues,[55] overall amputation rate was 4.5%. Risks factors for amputation included diabetes (39% amputation rate), peripheral vascular disease (71%), and renal failure (64%). Of the patients undergoing amputation, 15 of 37 (40.5%) had a delay in treatment of greater than 3 days. This delay in treatment is thought to be caused in part by peripheral neuropathy associated with the previously mentioned conditions.[5]

In a study with similar findings,[29] the authors proposed a three-tier clinical classification system to help predict FTS prognosis. Patients in group 1 had FTS at surgery, group 2 had FTS and subcutaneous purulence, and group 3 had FTS with ischemic changes. The amputation rate for each group was 0%, 8%, and 59%, respectively, and the percentage return of total active motion was 80%, 72%, and 49%, respectively. Risk factors associated with poor outcomes included age greater than 43 years; comorbidities including diabetes mellitus, peripheral vascular disease, and renal failure; subcutaneous purulence; digital ischemia; and polymicrobial infection.

SUMMARY

FTS results from inoculation of microbes in the unique environment of flexor sheath. An understanding of sheath and hand anatomy is required for evaluation and treatment. Antibiotic choice is based on patient and injury factors, with a low threshold to use broad-spectrum agents. Limited surgical approaches may be appropriate for early cases, but extensile approaches should be used if needed for adequate debridement. The best outcomes are found in healthy patients with prompt antibiotic administration and often surgical debridement.

REFERENCES

1. Stern PJ, Staneck JL, McDonough JJ, et al. Established hand infections: a controlled, prospective study. J Hand Surg Am 1983;8:553–9.
2. Noland SS, Fischer LH, Lee GK, et al. Essential hand surgery procedures for mastery by graduating orthopedic surgery residents: a survey of program directors. J Hand Surg Am 2013;38:760–5.
3. Kanavel AB. The symptoms, signs, and diagnosis of tenosynovitis and fascial-space abscesses. In: Infections of the hand. 1st edition. Philadelphia: Lea & Febiger; 1912. p. 201–26.
4. Kanavel AB. Infections of the hand: a guide to the surgical treatment of acute and chronic suppurative processes in the fingers, hand and forearm. 7th edition. Philadelphia: Lea & Febiger; 1939.
5. Boles SD, Schmidt CC. Pyogenic flexor tenosynovitis. Hand Clin 1998;14:567–78.
6. Doyle JR. Anatomy of the finger flexor tendon sheath and pulley system. J Hand Surg Am 1988; 13:473–84.
7. Gardner E, Gray DI, O'Rahilly R. Synovial flexor sheaths. In: Anatomy. 3rd edition. Philadelphia: WB Saunders; 1969. p. 151–3.
8. Phillips CS, Falender R, Mass DP. The flexor synovial sheath anatomy of the little finger: a macroscopic study. J Hand Surg Am 1995;20:636–41.
9. Doyle JR, Blythe WF. Anatomy of the flexor tendon sheath and pulleys of the thumb. J Hand Surg Am 1977;2:149–51.
10. Fussey JM, Chin KF, Gogi N, et al. An anatomic study of flexor tendon sheaths: a cadaveric study. J Hand Surg Eur Vol 2009;34:762–5.
11. Gaspard DJ, Kohl RD Jr. Compartmental syndromes in which the skin is the limiting boundary. Clin Orthop Relat Res 1975;113:65–8.
12. Matsen FA 3rd. Compartmental syndrome. An unified concept. Clin Orthop Relat Res 1975;113:8–14.
13. Schnall SB, Vu-Rose T, Holtom PD, et al. Tissue pressures in pyogenic flexor tenosynovitis of the finger. Compartment syndrome and its management. J Bone Joint Surg Br 1996;78:793–5.
14. Schnall SB, Holtom PD, Silva E. Compartment syndrome associated with infection of the upper extremity. Clin Orthop 1996;306:128–31.
15. Mubarak SJ, Owen CA, Hargens AR, et al. Acute compartment syndromes: diagnosis and treatment with the aid of the wick catheter. J Bone Joint Surg Am 1978;60:1091–5.
16. Vella JC, Hartigan BJ, Stern PJ. Kaplan's cardinal line. J Hand Surg Am 2006;31:912–8.
17. Parks BJ, Arbelaez J, Horner RL. Medical and surgical importance of the arterial blood supply of the thumb. J Hand Surg Am 1978;3:383–5.
18. Slutsky DJ. The management of digital nerve injuries. J Hand Surg Am 2014;39:1208–15.
19. Patel RM, Chilelli BJ, Ivy AD, et al. Hand surface landmarks and measurements in the treatment of trigger thumb. J Hand Surg Am 2013;38:1166–71.
20. Doyle DR. Anatomy of the flexor tendon sheath and pulley system: a current review. J Hand Surg Am 1989;14:349–51.
21. Schubert MF, Shah VS, Craig CL, et al. Varied anatomy of the thumb pulley system: implications for successful trigger thumb release. J Hand Surg Am 2012;37:2278–85.
22. Zafonte B, Rendulic D, Szabo RM. Flexor pulley system: anatomy, injury, and management. J Hand Surg Am 2014;39:2525–32.
23. Bayat A, Shaaban H, Giakas G, et al. The pulley system of the thumb: anatomic and biomechanical study. J Hand Surg Am 2002;27:628–35.
24. Bishop GB, Born T, Kakar S, et al. The diagnostic accuracy of inflammatory blood markers for purulent flexor tenosynovitis. J Hand Surg Am 2013;38:2208–11.
25. Pollen AG. Acute infection of the tendon sheaths. Hand 1974;6:21–5.
26. Neviaser RJ. Closed tendon sheath irrigation for pyogenic flexor tenosynovitis. J Hand Surg Am 1978;3:462–6.
27. Maloon S, de Beer JD, Opitz M, et al. Acute flexor tendon sheath infections. J Hand Surg 1990;15:474–7.
28. Juliano PJ, Eglseder WA. Limited open-tendon-sheath irrigation in the treatment of pyogenic flexor tenosynovitis. Orthop Rev 1991;20:1065.
29. Pang HN, Teoh LC, Yam AK, et al. Factors affecting the prognosis of pyogenic flexor tenosynovitis. J Bone Joint Surg Am 2007;89:1742–8.
30. Dailiana ZH, Rigopoulos N, Varitimidis S, et al. Purulent flexor tenosynovitis: factors influencing the functional outcome. J Hand Surg Eur Vol 2008;33:280–5.
31. Nikkhah D, Rodrigues J, Osman K, et al. Pyogenic flexor tenosynovitis: one year's experience at a UK hand unit and a review of the current literature. Hand Surg 2012;17:199–203.
32. Wynn SW, Elhassan BT, Gonzalez MH. Infections of the hand in the immunocompromised host. J Hand Surg Am 2004;4:121–7.
33. Katsoulis E, Bissell I, Hargreaves DG. MRSA pyogenic flexor tenosynovitis leading to digital ischaemic necrosis and amputation. J Hand Surg Br 2006;31:350–2.
34. Stevanovic MV, Sharpe F. Acute Infections of the Hand. In: Wolfe SW, Hotchkiss RN, Pederson WC, et al, editors. Green's operative hand surgery. 7th edition. Philadelphia: Elsevier; 2017. p. 17–61.
35. Pang HN, Lee JY, Puhaindran ME, et al. *Mycobacterium marinum* as a cause of chronic granulomatous tenosynovitis in the hand. J Infect 2007;54:584–8.

36. Kabakaş F, Uğurlar M, Turan DB, et al. Flexor teno-synovitis due to tuberculosis in hand and wrist: is tenosynovectomy imperative? Ann Plast Surg 2016;77:169–72.

37. Townsend DJ, Singer DI, Doyle JR. Candida teno-synovitis in an AIDS patient: a case report. J Hand Surg Am 1994;19:293–4.

38. Draeger RW, Bynum DK Jr. Flexor tendon sheath infections of the hand. J Am Acad Orthop Surg 2012;20:373–82.

39. Schaefer RA, Enzenauer RJ, Pruitt A, et al. Acute gonococcal flexor tenosynovitis in an adolescent male with pharyngitis. A case report and literature review. Clin Orthop Relat Res 1992;281:212–5.

40. Wright TW, Linscheid RL, O'Duffy JD. Acute flexor tenosynovitis in association with *Clostridium diffi-cile* infection: a case report. J Hand Surg Am 1996;21:304–6.

41. Kennedy CD, Huang JI, Hanel DP. In brief: Kana-vel's signs and pyogenic flexor tenosynovitis. Clin Orthop Relat Res 2016;474:280–4.

42. Neviaser RJ, Gunther SF. Tenosynovial infections in the hand: diagnosis and management. Instr Course Lect 1980;29:108–28.

43. Luria S, Haze A. Pyogenic flexor tenosynovitis in children. Pediatr Emerg Care 2011;27:740–1.

44. Ceroni D, Merlini L, Salvo D, et al. Pyogenic flexor tenosynovitis of the finger due to *Kingella kingae*. Pediatr Infect Dis J 2013;32:702–3.

45. Patel DB, Emmanuel NB, Stevanovic MV, et al. Hand infections: anatomy, types and spread of infection, imaging findings, and treatment options. Radiographics 2014;34:1968–86.

46. Schecter WP, Markison RE, Jeffrey RB, et al. Use of sonography in the early detection of suppurative flexor tenosynovitis. J Hand Surg Am 1989;14: 307–10.

47. Moore JR, Weiland AJ. Gouty tenosynovitis in the hand. J Hand Surg Am 1985;10:291–5.

48. Weniger FG, Davison SP, Risin M, et al. Gouty flexor tenosynovitis of the digits: report of three cases. J Hand Surg Am 2003;28:669–72.

49. Aslam N, Lo S, McNab I. Gouty flexor tenosynovitis of the digits: report of three cases. J Hand Surg Am 2004;29:526 [author reply 526].

50. Reinus WR, De Cotiis D, Schaffer A. Changing pat-terns of septic tenosynovitis of the distal extrem-ities. Emerg Radiol 2015;22:133–9.

51. Newman ED, Harrington TM, Torretti D, et al. Sup-purative extensor tenosynovitis caused by *Staphy-lococcus aureus*. J Hand Surg Am 1989;14:849–51.

52. Mason SJ, Keith PP. Chronic suppurative crypto-coccal extensor tenosynovitis in a patient with Cas-tleman's disease: a case report. Hand (N Y) 2011;6: 450–3.

53. Osterman M, Draeger R, Stern P. Acute hand infec-tions. J Hand Surg Am 2014;39:1628–35.

54. Glass KD. Factors related to the resolution of treated hand infections. J Hand Surg Am 1982;7: 388–94.

55. Giladi AM, Malay S, Chung KC. A systematic review of the management of acute pyogenic flexor teno-synovitis. J Hand Surg Eur Vol 2015;40:720–8.

56. Abrams RA, Botte MJ. Hand infections: treatment recommendations for specific types. J Am Acad Orthop Surg 1996;4:219–30.

57. Carter SJ, Burman SO, Mersheimer WL. Treatment of digital tenosynovitis by irrigation with peroxide and oxytetracycline: review of nine cases. Ann Surg 1966;163:645–50.

58. Besser MI. Digital flexor tendon irrigation. Hand 1976;8:72.

59. Harris PA, Nanchahal J. Closed continuous irriga-tion in the treatment of hand infections. J Hand Surg Br 1999;24:328–33.

60. Gaston RG, Greenberg JA. Use of continuous Mar-caine irrigation in the management of suppurative flexor tenosynovitis. Tech Hand Up Extrem Surg 2009;13:182–6.

61. Gutowski KA, Ochoa O, Adams WP Jr. Closed-catheter irrigation is as effective as open drainage for treatment of pyogenic flexor tenosynovitis. Ann Plast Surg 2002;49:350–4.

62. Michon J. Phlegmon of the tendon sheaths. Ann Chir 1974;28:277–80 [in French].

63. Dickson-Wright A. Tendon sheath infection. Proc R Soc Med 1943–1944;37:504.

64. Henry M. Septic flexor tenosynovitis. J Hand Surg Am 2011;36:322–3.

65. Lille S, Hayakawa T, Neumeister MW, et al. Contin-uous postoperative catheter irrigation is not necessary for the treatment of suppurative flexor tenosynovitis. J Hand Surg Br 2000;25:304–7.

66. Catalano LW, Zlotolow DA, Purcelli Lafer M, et al. Surgical exposures of the wrist and hand. J Am Acad Orthop Surg 2012;20:48–57.

Atypical Hand Infections

Edward Chan, MD*, Mark Bagg, MD

KEYWORDS

- Atypical • Hand • Infection • Fungal • Mycobacterial • Viral

KEY POINTS

- Atypical infections of the hand are caused by organisms such as *Mycobacterium*, fungi, and viruses, and often do not respond to conventional management.
- They exist within a wide spectrum of presentations, ranging from cutaneous lesions to deep infections such as tenosynovitis and osteomyelitis.
- Having a high clinical suspicion for atypical hand infections is vital because diagnosis often requires special tests and/or cultures. Obtaining a detailed medical, work, and travel history is extremely important. An indolent clinical course, late diagnosis, and delayed treatment are common.
- In addition to medical therapies, surgical debridement is often required to effectively treat these infections.

INTRODUCTION

Most hand infections are caused by common *Staphylococcus* and *Streptococcus* bacterial species; however, infections caused by atypical organisms, such as *Mycobacterium*, viruses, and fungi are becoming more common, especially among immunocompromised patients. Atypical hand infections exist within a wide spectrum of presentations, from superficial, cutaneous lesions to deep abscesses and, rarely, rapidly disseminating processes, which may be life-threatening and limb-threatening. They can manifest as either acute infections, with obvious swelling, erythema, and pain, or more indolent, chronic infections. Atypical hand infections are commonly misdiagnosed or diagnosed in a delayed fashion, and may not respond to the standard antibiotic therapy. Surgical debridement is often required to eliminate the offending organism or lower the disease burden. The purpose of this article is to provide an overview and update on atypical hand infections caused by mycobacterial, viral, and fungal organisms.

GENERAL WORKUP

Having a working knowledge about atypical hand infections and maintaining a high suspicion for them when clinically appropriate is essential to successful diagnosis and treatment. Workup begins with a careful history, focusing on information such as chronicity of symptoms, immune status, recent travel, and immigration history. Lesions with a history of poor response to previous treatment should raise a red flag. Unless the diagnosis can be made clinically, biopsy and cultures are often required to confirm the offending organism and guide treatment. Tissue specimens or synovial fluid samples are generally better than swabs. Intraoperatively, biopsy tissue should be divided into 2 parts: the first half is sent in formalin for histopathology, whereas the second half is sent without formalin and divided into a so-called 8-pack.[1] The first 3 packs are for immediate staining: gram stains for bacteria, acid-fast bacillus (Ziehl-Neelsen or Kinyoun) stains for mycobacteria, and potassium hydroxide (KOH) or calcofluor-white stains for fungi. The 5 remaining packs are sent for

Department of Hand Surgery, The Hand Center of San Antonio, 21 Spurs Lane, #310, San Antonio, TX 78240, USA
* Corresponding author.
E-mail address: edwardschan11@gmail.com

Orthop Clin N Am 48 (2017) 229–240
http://dx.doi.org/10.1016/j.ocl.2016.12.013
0030-5898/17/© 2016 Elsevier Inc. All rights reserved.

cultures: aerobic bacteria, anaerobic bacteria, mycobacteria at 37°C, mycobacteria at 30°C and 42°C, and fungi on mycotic culture media (Sabouraud dextrose agar or brain-heart infusion agar). The reason for culturing at different temperatures is that some mycobacteria grow better at a specific temperature versus another (Table 1). It is important to make sure the tissue sent for the 8-pack is in a sterile container without formalin, which kills organisms.

MYCOBACTERIAL INFECTIONS

Mycobacterial infections include tuberculous, non-tuberculous infections, and leprosy. Tuberculous infections, caused by Mycobacterium tuberculosis, used to be the most commonly reported mycobacterial hand infection. However, since 1960, nontuberculous hand infection cases have been more frequently reported.[2] There are 60 known nontuberculous mycobacteria that affect humans, and 19 have been implicated in causing hand infections. The clinical features of tuberculous and nontuberculous hand infections are indistinguishable. However, there are differences in histopathologic findings, as well as in the optimal temperature for tissue cultures (see Table 1). Leprosy, caused by M leprae, has a different clinical presentation, and mainly attacks the nerves and skin.

Tuberculosis of the Hand

Tuberculosis is a pulmonary disease primarily spread by inhalation, and is now commonly seen in immunocompromised patients, such as those with acquired immunodeficiency syndrome (AIDS). There also has been a recent increase in drug-resistant tuberculosis.[2] Extrapulmonary tuberculosis is rarely seen in the hand but when it does occur, M tuberculosis is the most common causative organism.[3] Often with tuberculosis infections of the hand, constitutional symptoms such as night sweats and weight loss are absent, and chest radiographs can be normal.[3]

The various clinical presentations include cutaneous infections, tenosynovitis, osteomyelitis, septic arthritis, and dactylitis. Tenosynovitis of the flexor or extensor tendon sheath is most common.[3] The tenosynovitis can extend into the carpal tunnel and cause a carpal tunnel syndrome.[4] In these cases, rice bodies (Fig. 1), which are tubercles in the synovial tissue that become detached and contain live mycobacteria that grow on culture, are seen coming from the tenosynovium walls intraoperatively. Tuberculosis can also invade the bones and joints of the hand. Distal radius osteomyelitis and radiocarpal arthritis via direct inoculation from adjacent tenosynovitis in the carpal tunnel have been reported.[2] Tuberculosis osteomyelitis can be unifocal or multifocal, and the appearance of bony involvement can vary from cystic lesions, to a honeycomb pattern, to sclerosis. Dactylitis has been mostly reported in children and presentations range from mild soft-tissue involvement to bony destruction. The osseous destruction can present as either a cystic lesion or a tubular expansion of the bone. Usually, appropriate antibiotic treatment leads to reformation

Table 1 Mycobacterial infections			
Organism	**Histopathology**	**Culture Medium**	**Drug Therapy**
M tuberculosis	Caseating granulomas	Lowenstein-Jensen at 37°C	Isoniazid + rifampin (×6 mo), ethambutol + pyrazinamide (×2 mo)
M leprae	Destroyed (enlarged, fibrosed, calcified) nerves, nerve abscesses, granulomas (+/− caseation)	Not appliciable	Paucibacillary: dapsone + rifampin Multibacillary: dapsone + rifampin + clofazimine
M marinum	Noncaseating granulomas	Lowenstein-Jensen at 30°C	Clarithromycin ± rifampin ± ethambutol (resistant to isoniazid)
M haemophilum, M chelonae, M ulcerans	Noncaseating granulomas	Lowenstein-Jensen at 30°C	Rifampin ± ethambutol ± isoniazid
M xenopi	Noncaseating granulomas	Lowenstein-Jensen at 42°C	Rifampin ± ethambutol ± isoniazid
Other mycobacteria	Noncaseating granulomas	Lowenstein-Jensen at 37°C	Rifampin ± ethambutol ± isoniazid

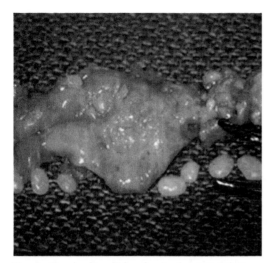

Fig. 1. Rice bodies. Tubercles in the synovial tissue that become detached and contain live mycobacteria that grow on culture. They are seen coming from the tenosynovium walls intraoperatively.

of the damaged bone.[2] Other less common presentations of tuberculous infections in the hand include cutaneous nodules, tuberculous bursitis, and a hypersensitivity-type of reaction with aseptic arthritis and soft tissue swelling.[3]

Pathologic specimens usually show caseating granulomas. Tzanck smears, Ziehl-Neelsen (acid-fast) staining, and cultures are frequently negative. Cultures can take up to 3 to 6 weeks to yield a positive diagnosis. Appropriate treatment of tuberculous infections of the hand consists of multidrug therapy with isoniazid, rifampin, and pyrazinamide, with or without ethambutol. A typical treatment course consists of 2 months of treatment with this regimen; after the 2 months, the isoniazid and rifampin are continued for 4 months. However, some investigators are now recommending a longer treatment course, up to 18 months. Initiating full treatment and completing the full course is essential to preventing recurrence, as well as the formation of resistant strains.

Mycobacterium leprae

M leprae causes leprosy, or Hansen disease, which is endemic in Africa and Asia. The organism is carried by Southwestern armadillos. It typically affects the skin and peripheral nerves. The main clinical types of the disease are tuberculoid, borderline, and lepromatous. Tuberculoid disease affects patients with more competent resistance, and typically presents with a single anesthetic skin lesion, and early nerve thickening and dysfunction. Nerve abscess is also common and lepromin skin tests are strongly positive. In contrast, the lepromatous form affects patients with incompetent resistance, and is associated with multiple skin lesions with relative preservation of skin sensation and delayed nerve thickening. Lepromin skin tests in these patients are usually negative. One common issue with the lepromatous type is secondary bacterial infection of ulcers.[3] Borderline tuberculoid disease affects those with intermediate resistance and their presentation fluctuates between tuberculoid and lepromatous types.

Diagnosis begins by recognizing 3 cardinal signs emphasized by the World Health Organization:

- An anesthetic skin patch
- Nerve thickening
- A hypopigmented skin lesion.[1]

A slit-skin smear, which uses a thin (~3 mm) sample of tissue taken with a scalpel, confirms the diagnosis and also helps to classify the disease as paucibacillary (negative smear) versus multibacillary (positive smear). When a slit-skin smear is negative, skin and nerve biopsies can also be considered if the diagnosis is in doubt.

In the upper extremity, the ulnar nerve is usually the first major nerve affected. Treatment includes systemic multidrug therapy with dapsone and rifampin, with the addition of clofazimine for multibacillary disease. Systemic steroids are also often used, especially in the setting of lepromatous reactions in which patients present with acute onset of skin, nerve, or synovial lesions.[3] The additional benefit of nerve decompression is a topic of controversy. A recent Cochrane review was unable to show a significant added benefit to steroid therapy.[3] However, nerve decompression and drainage of nerve abscesses are procedures commonly done that are thought to relieve pain and preserve nerve function. Other procedures that may be of benefit in patients with leprosy affecting the upper extremity include release of contractures after long-standing ulnar nerve palsy.[2] Tendon transfers may also be appropriate, depending on which nerves are affected and what alternative motors are available. For example, combined ulnar and median nerve paralysis is the second-most common deformity, behind the ulnar claw hand. Described tendon transfers to correct ulnar claw hand include the extensor-to-flexor 4-tailed tendon transfer and the palmaris longus 4-tailed tendon transfer.[5]

Mycobacterium marinum

M marinum is the most common mycobacteria causing hand infections.[2] It is seen in patients who have been injured by aquatic organisms, such as those cleaning aquarium tanks, fishing, and preparing seafood for consumption.[6–9] The presentation can vary and has been classified previously into 3 types: type I consists of self-limited verrucal lesions, type II presents with single or multiple subcutaneous granulomas with or without ulceration, and type III infections are deep-tissue infections involving either tenosynovium, bursa, bone, or joints. Hurst and colleagues[7] reported on 15 subjects with M marinum infections in the hand, and classified 6 of them as type II infections and 9 of them as type III, with most of these being tenosynovitis. Of the 27 lesions in their 14 subjects, 21 were in the fingers and 6 were in the wrist. Deep M marinum infections most commonly manifest as extensor or flexor tenosynovitis but can also present as joint infections. Flondell and colleagues[6] describe a case of invasive M marinum hand infection that spared the extensor tendons, but led to necrotic interosseous muscles and septic metacarpophalangeal joint arthritis.

M marinum infections often present in a delayed fashion. In a recent case series on 5 subjects with chronic flexor tenosynovitis, Pang and colleagues[8] reported an average delay of 32 days between injury and time of presentation. In the series by Hurst and colleagues,[7] the average time between symptom onset and initial consultation was 7.7 months. This delay is due to an indolent course of illness, nonspecific presentation, and long time to positive culture results. Initial diagnoses are often erroneous. There are no pathognomonic features of the disease. In some of the described cases of M marinum flexor tenosynovitis, the subjects were afebrile, with a normal white count, absent Kanavel signs, and were initially diagnosed with cellulitis and abscess.[8] Diffuse pain and swelling to the hand and/or digits is the most common presentation with M marinum infections, with some patients also having painful ulcers.[7,9]

At the time of surgery, the tenosynovium in M marinum flexor tenosynovitis is commonly described as chronic, granulomatous inflammatory tissue.[7–9] Histopathology from tissue taken intraoperatively from M marinum infections typically shows noncaseating granulomas, unlike M tuberculosis, which typically shows caseating granulomas.[3] Only 46% of patients have positive pathologic findings.[8] Although commonly performed, Ziehl-Neelsen staining (for acid-fast bacilli) is frequently negative. Cultures for M marinum must be performed on special medium, specifically Lowenstein-Jensen media at 30°C for at least

4 to 6 weeks. This temperature requirement explains why the organism usually infects cooler parts of the body.

Treatment depends on the type of infection and structures affected. Although verrucal lesions are typically superficial and self-limiting, deeper lesions are usually treated with a combination of surgery and antibiotics. Subcutaneous granulomas may be adequately treated with surgical excision of masses but infections that present as flexor tenosynovitis, deep abscesses, or septic arthritis require more extensive debridement (Fig. 2). The optimal antibiotic regimen for M marinum has not been defined but usually includes some combination of clarithromycin, rifampin, or ethambutol.[1,2] M marinum is almost always resistant to isoniazid and streptomycin.[8]

Other Mycobacterial Species

M avium intracellulare (MAI) is the second-most common mycobacteria to infect the upper extremity. In immunocompromised patients, it can cause systemic illness, but it can also affect immunocompetent hosts by causing infection of the deep tissues. In their series of atypical Mycobacterium infections of the upper extremity, Kozin and Bishop[10] found that MAC was responsible for the second-most infections overall, behind M marinum, but it accounted for the most deep infections. Granulomatous tenosynovitis is the typical presentation. As with other mycobacterial tenosynovitis, histopathology of the synovial tissue can show caseating granulomas. Ziehl-Neelsen staining is often performed but can commonly be negative.

Akahane and colleagues[11] described a case of chronic recurrent MAC granulomatous

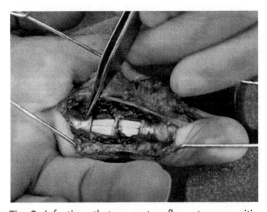

Fig. 2. Infections that present as flexor tenosynovitis, deep abscesses, or septic arthritis require extensive debridement.

tenosynovitis and emphasized that confirming the microbiological diagnosis can be difficult. In their case, the patient underwent an initial debridement for finger and wrist tenosynovitis, in which they noted cystic masses; synovial tissue cultures taken from these were negative. Four months later, the patient had a recurrence of swelling in the wrist and underwent another debridement. Again, tissue cultures were negative but this time synovial fluid from the cysts were positive for MAC on Lowenstein-Jensen culture at 37°C and with polymerase chain reaction (PCR).

Other nontuberculous mycobacterial organisms that have been implicated in upper extremity infections include *M kansasii*, *M malmoense*, *M chelonei*, *M terrae*, *M fortuitum*, and *M ulcerans*. Tenosynovitis of the fingers and wrist is a common presentation.[12–14] Chronic flexor tenosynovitis has been reported to present as carpal tunnel syndrome due to mass effect of the inflamed flexor tenosynovium in the carpal tunnel.[12] Other deep hand infections are possible as well, including bony involvement. *M kansasii* has been documented to cause osteomyelitis in the scaphoid, in an immunocompetent patient who sustained an injury from a meat hook.[15] This patient also presented initially with carpal tunnel syndrome, and had a carpal tunnel release and subsequent steroid injections before finally being diagnosed 3 years after the initial injury. This story of an indolent disease course, misdiagnosis, misguided treatment with steroid injections, and delayed diagnosis is common in mycobacterial infections. On presentation, disabling pain, fever, and elevated inflammatory markers are typically absent.[12]

Any suspicion for mycobacterial infection in the upper extremity should prompt an acid-fast stain of the involved tissues. Almost 30% of patients will have positive acid-fast stains.[12] Histologic examination of tissue is also important, often showing granulomas. Maximizing results of tissue cultures requires using the right culture media and temperature. Egg-based media (Lowenstein-Jensen) is most commonly used for mycobacteria and samples are incubated at both 37° and 30°C. Organisms such as *M marinum* and *M chelonae* may grow only at 30°C, whereas others such as *M tuberculosis* grow at 37°C. The rate of growth on cultures also varies between species because some will grow in 7 to 10 days on culture, whereas others such as *M malmoense* can take up to 12 weeks.

Treatment of these mycobacterial infections is similar to that mentioned previously for *M marinum*. When the infection is deep, most investigators believe that the combination of surgery and antibiotic therapy is warranted. Excision of infected tissue, such as tenosynovectomy, is thought to decrease the overall disease load, even if it does not remove all infected tissue. However, there is no absolute consensus in the literature on treatment protocols. Successful treatment with medications alone has been reported in infectious tenosynovitis caused by *M marinum*, *M kansasii*, and *M chelonae*.[12,13] Cases of mycobacterial tenosynovitis treated with tenosynovectomy alone, without medications, have also been documented. Antimicrobial therapy is typically with rifampin, isoniazid, and ethambutol, except for *M marinum*, which is less sensitive to isoniazid, as previously mentioned. Treatment should be for at least 9 months, with some investigators suggesting duration of up to 18 months.[12]

FUNGAL INFECTIONS
Cutaneous and Nail Fungal Infections
Cutaneous (superficial) fungal infections of the skin, hair, and nail of the hand are common but many of these are treated by primary care physicians and dermatologists.[2] These infections are generally caused by either *Candida albicans* or 1 of 3 dermatophyte genera: *Trichophyton*, *Microsporum*, and *Epidermophyton*. When the skin is infected, these infections are termed dermatomycoses. Some texts use the term tinea to refer to all dermatophyte infections, whereas others use it to specifically describe *Trichophyton* infections.[1–3] Dermatomycoses usually occur in the glabrous skin of the palm and the intertriginous skin. Treatment consists of topical imidazoles or tolnaftate for 2 to 3 weeks; oral agents are also available but rarely needed in immunocompetent patients.[2]

Nail infections caused by fungus are termed onychomycosis. Common in middle-aged women, the presentation can vary from superficial white lesions that can be scraped off, to subungual onychomycosis, in which the fungus is within the nail plate.[16] Diagnosis of onychomycosis is made from physical examination and/or histologic analysis. KOH preparation of a nail sample can help identify the presence of fungi under direct microscopic examination. Periodic acid-Schiff staining can also be helpful. Treatment of onychomycosis usually begins with topical antifungals, with ciclopirox the most commonly used agent in the United States.[16] Surgical removal of the nail followed by topical therapy can also be effective, with the nail usually regrowing between 5 and 10 months later. Nail ablation, either chemical or surgical, has also been described in conjunction with topical and/or oral antifungals, with high cure rates.[16] Systemic oral antifungals are also commonly used because topical medication alone has a low cure rate, up to just 36% in American studies.[2,16] Terbinafine and itraconazole are the most frequently used systemic agents and duration of treatment of 6 weeks is recommended. These medications are contraindicated in patients with liver disease, severe congestive heart failure, or gastric ulcers.

Histoplasmosis

Histoplasmosis is associated with bat and cat feces, and has also been found in acidic soils; it is endemic to the Ohio River and Mississippi River Valleys (Table 2). Usually, it is contracted via inhalation and is a pulmonary pathogen. In most hosts it is subclinical and self-limited but in immunocompromised patients it can lead to disseminated disease. Uncommonly, it has also been documented in musculoskeletal infections of the upper extremity. A characteristic

Table 2
Fungal infections

Organism	Risk Factors or Epidemiology	Diagnosis	Treatment
Histoplasmosis	Ohio and Mississippi River Valleys	Biopsy: Grocott silver stain, large round single-celled spores Serology: complement fixation test Culture: often negative	Surgical + medical (ketoconazole or itraconazole or IV amphotericin B)
Mucormycosis	Contaminated trauma, diabetes, immunocompromised	Clinical: enlarging black skin eschar, gangrene Biopsy: organisms scattered within areas of necrosis, 90° hyphae on KOH stain Culture: positive in less than half	Early, radical surgical debridement + high-dose IV amphotericin B
Sporotrichosis	Soil, rose thorn	Biopsy: cigar-shaped (narrow-based) budding yeasts Culture: growth can be delayed up to 8 weeks	Cutaneous: itraconazole Deep: surgery + IV amphotericin B
Coccidiomycosis	US Southwest, San Joaquin Valley	Biopsy: noncaseating granuloma, characteristic spherules and hyphae Serology: complement fixation	Surgical + medical (fluconazole or itraconazole or IV amphotericin B)
Blastomycosis	Ohio and Mississippi River Valleys	Biopsy: periodic acid-Schiff stain, silver stain, large broad-based buds	Medical (ketoconazole or itraconazole) +/− surgical
Cryptococcus	Pigeon droppings, immunocompromised	Biopsy: encapsulated, ovoid yeasts Serology: cryptococcal antigen titer Culture: growth within 48 hrs	Fluconazole or itraconazole or flucytosine or IV amphotericin
Aspergillosis	Immunocompromised (burns, wounds, IV sites)	Clinical: hemorrhagic vesicle or necrotic ulcer Biopsy: numerous fungal hyphae on KOH Culture: growth from tissue specimen (blood cultures often negative)	Early, radical surgical debridement + voriconazole

Abbreviation: IV, intravenous.

manifestation of this is tenosynovitis of the hand and wrist.[17–19] Both flexor and extensor tenosynovitis have been described. The mass effect of involved tenosynovium in the wrist can also lead to carpal tunnel syndrome as the initial presentation.[17] In their review of the literature, Vitale and colleagues[17] found that 4 out of 11 previously reported cases of histoplasmosis tenosynovitis occurred in immunocompetent patients.

Disseminated histoplasmosis may present with fever and weight loss. Mortality rate can be as high as 80% but is reduced to 20% with systemic antifungal therapy, so prompt recognition is important.[18] Fungal serologic tests for *Histoplasma*-yeast forms can be ordered. Intraoperative tissue cultures examined under the microscope with gomori methenamine silver stain can show *Histoplasma* organisms.[18] Serology evaluation via complement fixation test is another valuable diagnostic tool. Itraconazole and fluconazole have been described as being successful medical agents, used anywhere from 6 to 18 months. Oral ketoconazole and intravenous (IV) amphotericin B have also been used. A case of isolated *Histoplasma* tenosynovitis of the index finger that resolved with oral itraconazole alone has also been reported.[17] Specific treatment of deep hand infections involves the addition of surgical debridement; despite this, recurrences can still occur.

Mucormycosis

Mucormycosis includes 3 different fungi: *Rhizopus*, *Mucor*, and *Absidia*. It is typically found in soil, plants, and decaying material. The infection most commonly occurs in the sinuses and pulmonary system but also affects the cutaneous and subcutaneous tissues.[20] The cutaneous and subcutaneous forms of the infection are notoriously morbid, characterized by vascular thrombosis and gangrenous tissue necrosis. They constitute an acute, aggressive, rapidly developing infection that is often fatal if there is a delay in diagnosis or treatment. It has a higher rate of morbidity and mortality than other fungal infections; necrotizing fasciitis in mucormycosis has a mortality rate close to 80%.[1] Mucormycosis most commonly affects immunocompromised patients, with 1 study showing that 36% were diabetic.[21] Other populations that are susceptible include patients with hematological malignancies, IV drug use, deferoxamine therapy (for acute iron poisoning or hemochromatosis), renal failure, organ transplantation, long-term corticosteroid treatment, burns, and neonates.[20,21] Primary cases involving immunocompetent

patients are uncommon, although some recent papers have highlighted such cases and have cited an increase in *Mucor* infections.[20–22]

The initial signs of mucormycosis soft tissue infection include blisters, nodules, pustules, and necrotic ulcers. One classic early sign of invasive cutaneous mucormycosis is an enlarging black eschar in the wound, which eventually disseminates into the subcutaneous vasculature and the major arteries of the limb if left untreated.[20] Tissue biopsy confirms the diagnosis and characteristic 90° hyphae can be visualized with a 10% KOH stain. Early diagnosis and prompt, aggressive, radical surgical debridement is imperative for optimal treatment because mucormycosis has a high morbidity and mortality rate (**Figs. 3** and **4**). Antifungal therapy with IV liposomal amphotericin B is added in conjunction with surgery. Lineberry and colleagues[20] reported a case of cutaneous mucormycosis infection in the upper extremity of an immunocompetent patient following an arterial puncture. She was able to make a full recovery after undergoing surgical debridement, antifungal therapy, and hyperbaric oxygen wound therapy.

However, the clinical course can be more devastating, as illustrated by Moran and colleagues[22] in their series of mucormycosis upper extremity infections in immunocompetent patients who sustained trauma. They found 7 cases over 12 years, all stemming from injuries with significantly contaminated open wounds and considerable tissue damage. Three out of the 7 cases were associated with heavy soil contamination after motor vehicle accidents. The other 4 patients had sustained conveyor belt injuries at agricultural facilities. All of the patients had injuries described as having substantial soft-tissue loss, and 6 out of 7 had upper-extremity

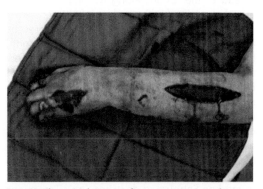

Fig. 3. The initial signs of mucormycosis soft tissue infection include blisters, nodules, pustules, and necrotic ulcers.

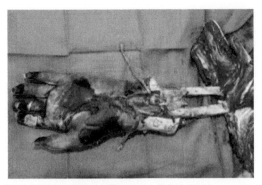

Fig. 4. One classic early sign of invasive cutaneous mucormycosis is an enlarging black eschar in the wound, which eventually disseminates into the subcutaneous vasculature and the major arteries of the limb if left untreated. Early diagnosis and prompt, aggressive, radical surgical debridement is imperative for optimal treatment.

fractures or dislocations. Fungal cultures were available at an average of 7 days and all patients were started on IV amphotericin. Despite an average of 10 surgical debridements per patient, 4 out of 7 required some sort of upper extremity amputation, with levels ranging from the fingers to the glenohumeral joint.

Sporotrichosis

Sporothrix schenckii is endemic throughout the world and is commonly associated with agricultural activities such as gardening (via thorn injury) or construction work (via exposure to subcutaneous tissues). The typical presentation is a wound of the upper extremity that becomes infected, followed by lymphocutaneous spread of the lesion. Milby and colleagues[23] described a case of sporotrichosis of the thumb that presented as a chronic, nonhealing ulcer. Diagnosis was not made until several months later when spread of the lesions along lymphatic channels raised suspicion for *Sporothrix* infection.

Although rare, sporotrichosis can also present as a deep infection in the upper extremity. Involvement of the wrist joint, hand bones, and olecranon bursa have been described.[23] Extensor tenosynovitis causing extensor tendon rupture has also been reported.[24] Similar to other atypical organisms, *S schenckii* can also cause carpal tunnel syndrome by way of a granulomatous flexor tenosynovitis in the wrist.[25] Pathologic findings on tissue culture can reveal granulomas and fungal cultures should be performed on Sabouraud dextrose agar. Treatment of lymphocutaneous sporotrichosis is with drug therapy, with itraconazole as the preferred

agent. For deep infections, surgery is often required, in concurrence with systemic antifungal therapy, such as amphotericin B, itraconazole, or ketoconazole.

Other Fungi

Several other fungi have also been reported to cause infection of the upper extremity. Coccidiomycosis is found in the southwestern United States, the San Joaquin Valley of California, and northern Mexico. Most patients have an asymptomatic course from the initial pulmonary infection, and disseminated disease occurs in less than 1% of those infected.[2] It has been reported to cause osteomyelitis of the hand, with 1 case describing the presentation as mimicking a metacarpal enchondroma.[26] Flexor and extensor tenosynovitis have also been reported, including 1 case that led to extensor tendon rupture.[27] Diagnosis is made by tissue culture and coccidioidal complement fixation, which is a serology test for antibodies against the organism. Treatment can be with ketoconazole, fluconazole, or itraconazole. In their case series and review of the literature, Campbell and colleagues[28] found that recurrence rate of coccidioidal tenosynovitis of the hand and wrist was high, at 50%, even after tenosynovectomy.

Blastomycosis is endemic to the Mississippi River and Ohio River Valleys. The route of infection is usually pulmonary but up to 80% develop cutaneous lesions and the dorsum of the hand is a common location. These skin lesions can often develop fistulae and drain to bone. Skeletal involvement is thus not uncommon and can be seen in up to 50% of patients.[2] Tissue culture and staining aids in the diagnosis. Itraconazole is the preferred antifungal agent used to treat blastomycosis.

Cryptococcus is a fungus that can be present on normal skin and is seen most commonly in immunocompromised hosts, such as AIDS patients. Reported infections caused by *Cryptococcus* include skin lesions, tenosynovitis, and necrotizing fasciitis.[2] Diagnosis is made with tissue biopsy and subsequent growth on culture. The recommended antifungal treatment regimen is amphotericin B with flucytosine, with fluconazole as an alternative.

Aspergillosis is found in decaying plant matter. It rarely affects immunocompetent individuals. Invasive aspergillosis commonly affects the pulmonary system but primary invasive aspergillosis of the hand has been documented in multiple cases involving immunocompromised children with hematological malignancy undergoing chemotherapy.[29–31] A typical presentation begins with a hemorrhagic blister around puncture wounds (ie, after IV infusion). The blister quickly develops into a necrotic ulcer with a black eschar in the center.[29] Tissue biopsy shows fungal hyphae. Early, aggressive debridement, antifungal therapy, and reversal of the hosts' immunodeficiency by reducing doses of immunosuppressive therapy are needed to prevent widespread dissemination, which can be fatal. Amphotericin B has been used as an antifungal in the past but voriconazole is now preferred because it is more potent and has fewer side effects.[1]

VIRAL INFECTIONS

Herpetic Whitlow

Herpetic whitlow is the commonly used term for hand infections caused by the herpes simplex virus (HSV). Whitlow is actually a misnomer because it is a synonym for felon, implying a purulent infection of the digital pulp. Both types of the virus, HSV-1 and HSV-2, can cause the infection and they are clinically indistinguishable. Herpetic whitlow in children is almost all caused by HSV-1, whereas adults can be infected by both types.[32]

The classic disease presentation begins as 1 or more clear vesicles that develop on a single digit about 3 to 4 days following skin irritation or minor trauma (Table 3). Vesicles may also be pale yellow and have an erythematous base. Commonly, they are distally located (ie, near the nail). The lesions are commonly preceded by throbbing pain, numbness, or tingling, and patients may also report an influenza-like prodromal syndrome.[32,33] Eventually, the vesicles may coalesce and appear similar to a felon or paronychia; however, they can be distinguished from felons by the lack of increased pressure in the pulp space. There is a 12-day period during which viral shedding can occur, leading to satellite lesions elsewhere and putting the patient in their most contagious state.[32]

Pain subsides after this period and the lesions evolve in appearance. The vesicles first become more turbid or hemorrhagic appearing. Then they begin to crust and eventually peel off to reveal the underlying healed skin. Diagnosis can be confirmed with Tzanck smear of a sample taken by scraping the base of the lesion and staining with toluidine blue. Serum antibody titers and rapid viral antigen detection techniques using lesion fluid specimens or scrapings are other available diagnostic tools.

Usually, no treatment is necessary because the natural history of herpetic whitlow is complete resolution within 3 weeks.[32] However, vigilance should be maintained with proper wound care to prevent secondary bacterial infection. For this reason, deep incisions as a treatment option should be avoided. Also, in immunosuppressed patients, oral or IV acyclovir, valacyclovir, famciclovir, or foscarnet may be required to help resolve the infection.[2]

Papillomavirus

Papillomavirus is responsible for cutaneous warts in the hand. It has been associated with poultry and meat handlers.[2] In immunocompetent patients, warts are mainly a cosmetic nuisance and will often disappear spontaneously in most children.[1] However, if they occur in the palm, they can cause pain with gripping. They also have the potential to multiply and affect

Table 3 Viral infections			
Organism	**Clinical Presentation**	**Diagnosis**	**Treatment**
Herpes simplex (herpetic whitlow)	Clear, vesicular lesions on erythematous base	Tzanck smear of scrapings, serum antibody titers, lesion-specific antigen detection, viral cultures	Observation, acyclovir (for immunocompromised)
Papillomavirus	Wart (cauliflower-like, raised, demarcated, grayish mass with irregular surface)	Clinical, biopsy (acanthosis, papillomatosis, hyperkeratosis, parakeratosis)	Observation, cryotherapy, electrosurgery, acid therapy, surgical excision
Parapoxvirus (orf)	Single erythematous macule or papule, progresses to red center and surrounding halo	Clinical, biopsy, PCR	Observation, imiquimod (for immunocompromised)

the surrounding skin or other hand. Periungual warts can extend into the nail bed and under the nail plate and can cause bone destruction of the distal phalanx. Diagnosis is mainly clinical but biopsy can provide confirmation when there is doubt.

Treatment of bothersome warts usually begins with nonsurgical modalities, including liquid nitrogen freezing, electrodiathermy, and acid preparations. However, recurrence can be high, according to some investigators.[2] If conservative treatment fails, surgical excision of the wart is an option. Typically, infectious disease and/or dermatology consultations are also recommended.[1] Caution should be exercised with treatment because excessive freezing can burn and damage the deep structures, and surgical excision can inadvertently spread and seed the incisional tract with satellite recurrent lesions.

Human papillomavirus (HPV) can also cause other rare diseases involving the upper extremities. A group of dermatologists reported on a case of epidermodysplasia verruciformis, a rare skin ailment caused by HPV, which severely affected the hands and feet. The patient had multiple wart-like lesions that were so large that they led to functional impairment of the hands. The patient was successfully treated by shaving off the lesions, with no recurrence after 2 years.[34] HPV infection of the nail bed has also been implicated as an inciting factor in the development of Bowen disease in the hand, which is a form of in situ squamous cell carcinoma.[35]

Parapoxvirus (Orf)

Parapoxvirus is the organism responsible for orf, a zoonotic infection that is transmitted to humans via contact with infected animals, most commonly sheep. It is thus most frequently seen in those with professional exposure, such as butchers, sheep shearers, and veterinarians. Most of these professionals do not seek medical attention because they know that the disease is self-limiting within a period of a few weeks and usually does not require treatment.[36] The patients who typically present to the hand surgeon with orf are nonprofessionals who are not as familiar with the condition. Annual outbreaks in countries with large Muslim populations have been documented during religious feasts when many sheep are slaughtered by nonprofessionals.[36]

In immunocompetent patients, the presentation usually begins with a single erythematous macule or papule. It then proceeds to the target stage, at which it develops a reddish center and is surrounded by a halo. The lesion then weeps and then dries up, forming a crust, and eventually resolves spontaneously with no residual scarring. The entire course lasts from 4 to 8 weeks on average.[2,36] The lesion can be associated with pain, pruritus, lymphangitis, and axillary adenitis. Systemic symptoms are rare but erythema multiforme and Steven-Johnsons syndrome have been documented in immunocompromised patients.[37] The diagnosis is typically made based on history and clinical examination but can be confirmed with electron microscopy of biopsied tissue from the lesion. PCR can also be used to identify the virus from serous fluid taken from the lesion.

Treatment consists of keeping the lesion clean to prevent secondary bacterial infection until the lesion resolves. Secondary bacterial infections should be treated accordingly with antibiotics. Prophylactic antibiotics are recommended if biopsy is to be performed because incision of the lesion is a common cause for infections.[36] Management of orf in immunocompromised individuals can be more difficult, especially those with multiple giant lesions. One recent study reported on the use of topical imiquimod, an imidazoquinoline that stimulates local proinflammatory cytokine production, to shorten the duration of orf to 5 to 10 days.[37] Imiquimod is recommended by most to treat immunocompromised patients.[36] Large lesions that are refractory to medical treatment in these patients may require wide excision and skin grafting. Even with this, recurrence is not uncommon. Excision of the lesion back to normal tissue, followed by hypochlorite dressings for 1 week before the application of skin grafting and coverage with systemic antiviral therapy, such as subcutaneous interferon, may help reduce recurrence.[38]

SUMMARY

Although most hand infections are caused by common bacteria, a multitude of other organisms can cause atypical infections in the upper extremity and it is important for hand surgeons to be aware and knowledgeable of their presentation and treatment. Various mycobacteria, fungi, and viruses can be responsible for a wide range of infections in the hand, from cutaneous lesions, to septic tenosynovitis, to osteomyelitis. These can affect both immunocompromised and immunocompetent individuals, although their presentation may vary.

Having a high clinical suspicion for atypical infections is essential because diagnosis often requires special tests and/or cultures. Even then, confirming the causative organism can be difficult. Obtaining details about the patient's medical, work, and travel history is thus extremely important. Previous case series have shown that an indolent clinical course, late diagnosis, and delayed treatment are common. In addition to medical therapies, surgical debridement is often required to effectively treat these infections.

REFERENCES

1. Patel MR. Chronic infections. In: Wolfe SW, editor. Green's operative hand surgery. 7th edition. Philadelphia: Elsevier; 2017. p. 62–127.

2. Elhassan BT, Wynn SW, Gonzalez MH. Atypical infections of the hand. J Am Soc Surg Hand 2004; 4(1):42–9.

3. Al-Qattan MM, Helmi AA. Chronic hand infections. J Hand Surg Am 2014;39(8):1636–45.

4. Suso S, Peidro L, Ramon R. Tuberculous synovitis with "rice bodies" presenting as carpal tunnel syndrome. J Hand Surg Am 1988;13(4):574–6.

5. Taylor NL, Raj AD, Dick HM, et al. The correction of ulnar claw fingers: a follow-up study comparing the extensor-to-flexor with the palmaris longus 4-tailed tendon transfer in patients with leprosy. J Hand Surg Am 2004;29(4):595–604.

6. Flondell M, Ornstein K, Björkman A. Invasive *Mycobacterium marinum* infection of the hand. J Plast Surg Hand Surg 2013;47:532–4.

7. Hurst LC, Amadio PC, Badalamente MA, et al. *Mycobacterium marinum* infections of the hand. J Hand Surg Am 1987;12A(3):428–35.

8. Pang HN, Yi-Liang Lee J, Puhaindran ME, et al. *Mycobacterium marinum* as a cause of chronic granulomatous tenosynovitis in the hand. J Infect 2007; 54(6):584–8.

9. Tsai H-C, Lee SS-J, Wann S-R, et al. *Mycobacterium marinum* tenosynovitis: three case reports and review of the literature. Jpn J Infect Dis 2006;59(5): 337–40.

10. Kozin S, Bishop AT. Atypical *Mycobacterium* infections of the upper extremity. J Hand Surg Am 1994; 19A(3):480–7.

11. Akahane T, Nakatsuchi Y, Tateiwa Y. Recurrent granulomatous tenosynovitis of the wrist and finger caused by *Mycobacterium intracellulare*: a case report. Diagn Microbiol Infect Dis 2006;56(1):99–101.

12. Zenone T, Boibieux A, Tigaud S, et al. Non-tuberculous mycobacterial tenosynovitis: a review. Scand J Infect Dis 1999;31:221–8.

13. Mateo L, Rufí G, Nolla JM, et al. *Mycobacterium chelonae* tenosynovitis of the hand. Semin Arthritis Rheum 2004;34:617–22.

14. Gabl M, Pechlaner S, Hausdorfer H, et al. Flexor tenosynovitis in the hand caused by *Mycobacterium malmoense*: a case report. J Hand Surg Am 1997;22(2):338–40.

15. Minkin BI, Bills CL, Bullock DW, et al. *Mycobacterium kansasii* osteomyelitis of the scaphoid. J Hand Surg Am 1987;12A(6):1092–4.

16. Coleman NW, Fleckman P, Huang JI. Fungal nail infections. J Hand Surg Am 2014;39(5):985–8.

17. Vitale MA, Roden AC, Rizzo M. Tenosynovitis of the wrist and thumb and carpal tunnel syndrome caused by *Histoplasma capsulatum*: case report and review of the literature. Hand (N Y) 2015;10:54–9.

18. Liang KV, Ryu JH, Matteson EL. Histoplasmosis with tenosynovitis of the hand and hypercalcemia mimicking sarcoidosis. J Clin Rheumatol 2004; 10(3):138–42.

19. Cucurull E, Sarwar H, Williams CS IV, et al. Localized tenosynovitis caused by *Histoplasma capsulatum*: case report and review of the literature. Arthritis Care Res 2005;53(1):129–32.

20. Lineberry KD, Boettcher AK, Blount AL, et al. Cutaneous Mucormycosis of the upper extremity in an immunocompetent host: case report. J Hand Surg Am 2012;37(4):787–91.

21. Fathi P, Vranis NM, Paryavi E. Diagnosis and treatment of upper extremity Mucormycosis Infections. J Hand Surg Am 2016;40(5):1032–4.

22. Moran SL, Strickland J, Shin AY. Upper-extremity Mucormycosis infections in immunocompetent patients. J Hand Surg Am 2006;31A(7):1201–5.

23. Milby AH, Pappas ND, O'Donnell J, et al. Sporotrichosis of the upper extremity. Orthopedics 2010; 33(4):273–5.

24. Hay EL, Collawn SS, Middleton FG. *Sporothrix schenckii* tenosynovitis: a case report. J Hand Surg Am 1986;11(3):431–4.

25. Stratton CW, Lichtenstein KA, Lowenstein SR, et al. Granulomatous tenosynovitis and carpal tunnel syndrome caused by *Sporothrix schenckii*. Am J Med 1981;71:161–3.

26. Huang JI, Seeger LL, Jones NF. Coccidioidomycosis fungal infection in the hand mimicking a metacarpal enchondroma. J Hand Surg Am 2000; 25(5):475–7.

27. Szabo RM, Lanzer WL, Gelberman RH, et al. Extensor tendon rupture due to *Coccidioides immitis*: report of a case. Clin Orthop Relat Res 1985;194: 176–80.

28. Campbell M, Kusne S, Renfree KJ, et al. Coccidioidal tenosynovitis of the hand and wrist: report of 9 cases and review of the literature. Clin Infect Dis 2015;61(10):1514–20.

29. Al-Qattan MM. Opportunistic mycotic infections of the upper limb. J Hand Surg Eur 1996;21B(2):148–50.

30. Goldberg B, Eversmann WW, Eitzen EM. Invasive aspergillosis of the hand. J Hand Surg Am 1982; 7(1):38–42.

31. Jones NF, Conklin WT, Albo VC. Primary invasive aspergillosis of the hand. J Hand Surg Am 1986; 11(3):425–8.

32. Rubright JH, Shafritz AB. The herpetic whitlow. J Hand Surg Am 2011;36(2):340–2.

33. Franko OI, Abrams RA. Hand Infections. Orthop Clin North Am 2013;44(4):625–34.

34. Fang F, Zhao L, Jiang MJ, et al. Epidermodysplasia verruciformis with severe hand and foot deformity successfully treated with surgical excision. J Plast Reconstr Aesthet Surg 2008;61(3):338–41.

35. Aguayo R, Soria X, Abal L, et al. Bowen's disease associated with human papillomavirus infection of the nail bed. Dermatol Surg 2011;37(1):116–8.

36. Al-Qattan MM. Orf infection of the hand. J Hand Surg Am 2011;36(11):1855–8.

37. Erbağci Z, Erbağci İ, Tuncel AA. Rapid improvement of human orf (ecthyma contagiosum) with topical imiquimod cream: report of four complicated cases. J Dermatolog Treat 2005;16(5–6):353–6.

38. Tan ST, Blake B, Chambers S. Recurrent orf in an immunocompromised host. Br J Plast Surg 1991;44:465–7.

Foot and Ankle

Charcot Arthropathy Versus Osteomyelitis
Evaluation and Management

John Womack, MD

KEYWORDS

- Charcot arthropathy • Osteomyelitis • Foot and ankle • Evaluation • Management

KEY POINTS

- Charcot arthropathy of the foot and ankle can be difficult to differentiate from osteomyelitis.
- Appropriate use of imaging studies, including plain radiographs, MRI, and nuclear medicine studies can aid greatly in diagnosis and treatment guidance of these conditions.
- Early identification and treatment of both Charcot arthropathy and osteomyelitis can lead to better outcomes and patient satisfaction.

J.M. Charcot first described arthropathy associated with tabes dorsalis in the foot and ankle 140 years ago.[1] Despite the passage of 140 years, Charcot disease of the foot and ankle remains a poorly understood condition with little consensus on evaluation or management. Although Charcot and colleagues[2] first described this condition in relation to tertiary syphilis, it was not until 1936 that W.R. Jordan first established the association between neuro-arthropathy and diabetes mellitus, which is the leading cause in the developed world today.

The economic impact of diabetes mellitus and its complications are staggering. It is estimated that the prevalence of Charcot arthropathy in the general diabetic population is 0.08%, but in high-risk patients can range as high as 13%.[3] When encountered in the presence of severe infection, the morbidity and mortality rates from complications can exceed 35% even if the infection is managed well.[3] Early and correct diagnosis and management are key factors in successful treatment.

Diabetes and peripheral neuropathy may contribute to the formation of Charcot arthropathy through a variety of mechanisms. Osteopenia, reactive oxygen species, and oxidized lipids may all upregulate RANKL expression in diabetic patients. Still other causes may be hypervascularity of the bones and local inflammation caused by trauma, ulceration, or recent infection.[4] Whatever the cause, the end result is fragmentation and destruction of joint architecture leading to collapse of the foot or ankle and ulceration, which then results in osteomyelitis.

CLINICAL PRESENTATION

Charcot arthropathy typically presents with a warm, swollen foot and ankle that cannot be differentiated easily from infection. Many times the patient has been evaluated for a deep venous thrombosis and undergone oral or parenteral antibiotic therapy for cellulitis before a clinician obtains a radiograph or MRI that suggests the presence of Charcot arthropathy or osteomyelitis. A study by Chanteleau[5] showed that 19 (80%) of 24 patients with Charcot arthropathy were initially misdiagnosed with gout, deep venous thrombosis, or cellulitis. Patients with Charcot arthropathy may have a history of antecedent trauma, but typically present before ulceration of the foot or ankle. By contrast, osteomyelitis is typically caused by exposure of the bone to the environment, although it may more rarely be spread to bone

---

Disclosure Statement: The author has nothing to disclose.
Piedmont Orthopaedic Associates, 35 International Drive, Greenville, SC 29615, USA
E-mail address: womackjw@gmail.com

by traveling through the bloodstream from another source. Twenty percent of diabetic patients will develop osteomyelitis and many of these will succumb to amputation as a result.[6] The diagnostic challenge is made even harder by cases in which both Charcot and arthropathy are present concomitantly due to a history of infection or surgery to the affected joints. A systematic approach to evaluation and management of the patient, although not perfect, can help the clinician identify the correct diagnosis and treatment in most cases.

HISTORY AND PHYSICAL EXAMINATION

Diabetic foot infections are almost always caused by bacteria from infections in the adjacent soft tissues. A history of a local ulceration or a "sausage toe" is characteristic of infection.[7] Patients with osteomyelitis of the foot and ankle are largely afebrile and the wounds may not show any local signs of inflammation, particularly as the wounds are often present chronically. Ertugrul and colleagues[7] found that ulcer size greater than 2 cm^2 carries a 56% sensitivity and a 96% specificity for the presence of osteomyelitis. Some investigators have described the "probe-to-bone" test for ulcers, in which a blunt metal probe is introduced into the wound to see if bone is palpable. The sensitivity and specificity of this test are widely variable in studies, but it is perhaps reasonable that if you can probe bone, then so can a colonizing bacteria.[8–10] Indeed, Lavery and colleagues[9] demonstrated in their study of 1666 patients that a positive probe-to-bone test increases the probability of osteomyelitis greater than 50%, whereas a negative test is a strong predictor of absence of infection. The use of a "dependent rubor" test also has been suggested. With this test, if the erythema in an affected foot and ankle resolves with elevation, this suggests Charcot arthropathy, whereas persistence of erythema with elevation of the leg suggests an infection is present.

HEMATOLOGIC STUDIES

Routine laboratory testing for infection markers should be a part of the initial infection workup for any patient with a foot wound that is suspicious for osteomyelitis. Routine complete blood count with differential, a C-reactive protein, and an erythrocyte sedimentation rate (ESR) can all yield clues in the workup. Many investigators have concluded that an ESR that is substantially elevated (>70 mm/h) strongly supports a diagnosis of osteomyelitis and tends to slowly decline with appropriate therapy.[11,12] It should be noted, however, that many patients with histologically proven osteomyelitis may be afebrile and have a normal white blood cell count, so that using hematologic studies without other correlating factors may not be a useful tool to aid in differentiating Charcot arthropathy from osteomyelitis.

BONE BIOPSY

Butalia and colleagues[13] have suggested that surgical percutaneous bone biopsy after a 14-day antibiotic-free period represents the gold standard for diagnosis and management of osteomyelitis of the foot. Other studies have shown that an antibiotic holiday of as little as 48 hours is sufficient before biopsy, however.[14] The importance of histologic analysis in addition to microbiology is important, as several studies have shown that 40% to 60% of histologically proven cases of osteomyelitis at surgery or biopsy of the foot and ankle are negative at culture.[15] Many patients with a diabetic foot wound and suspected osteomyelitis will have undergone swab cultures of the wound before consultation with an orthopedic surgeon. Although these cultures are often used to guide treatment, their actual utility is quite suspect. Senneville and colleagues[16] compared the diagnostic value of swab cultures to percutaneous bone biopsy for diabetic foot osteomyelitis. Their study showed only 17.4% of patients had both biopsy and swab cultures that were identical and that the overall concordance of isolates was only 22.5%.[16] The use of ulcer swab cultures alone should therefore be treated with caution in guiding diagnosis and treatment. Additionally, patients with suspected osteomyelitis who have a negative percutaneous bone biopsy have a 25% chance of developing osteomyelitis within 2 years of biopsy.[17] Whether or not biopsy can be considered the gold standard to diagnose osteomyelitis of the foot and ankle remains unclear. The data obtained from this procedure can clearly have utility, however, when guiding decisions of antimicrobial therapy or internal versus external fixation of a Charcot foot and ankle deformity.

IMAGING STUDIES

Plain radiography of the involved area should be requisite in the investigation of Charcot arthropathy and osteomyelitis of the foot and ankle. The accuracy of plain radiography itself in correctly differentiating osteomyelitis from Charcot arthropathy is only approximately 50% to 60%, with the findings of demineralization, periosteal reaction, and cortical destruction being most diagnostic. Problematically, however, these findings may not appear until 2 to 3 weeks after onset of clinical symptoms and require a loss of 40% to 50% of bone mass to see a difference.[18] Despite these limitations, the information gained from standing plain radiographs can be invaluable when taken in the context of the patient's clinical presentation when making diagnostic or treatment decisions (Table 1).

MRI with contrast has become a useful tool in the evaluation of diabetic foot infections and helpful in differentiating from Charcot arthropathy. Evidence now shows that proper application of this imaging modality can be superior to nuclear imaging tests in aiding diagnosis.[19] The mere presence of bone marrow edema in both of these conditions is a very nonspecific finding. The pattern of bone marrow edema, clinical correlation, and other factors must be taken into account for an MRI to be of maximal value. Osteomyelitis of the foot and ankle tends to have a focal involvement of one weight-bearing joint, whereas Charcot arthropathy tends to involve several joints or bones.[20] The presence of an adjacent fluid collection, sinus tract, or soft tissue infection strongly suggests osteomyelitis is present and can improve diagnostic accuracy.[21] MRI has limitations in patients with recent surgery, retained hardware, presence of a pacemaker, or aneurysm clips or renal insufficiency that does not allow contrasted studies to be completed safely. A recent meta-analysis has shown that the sensitivity of MRI to diagnose osteomyelitis in the foot and ankle stands at 90% with a specificity of 79%, but that its ability to differentiate infection from Charcot arthropathy may not be superior to nuclear imaging studies (Table 2).[18]

The use of nuclear imaging studies to evaluate bone infections is well established. Three-phase bone scintigraphy has a high sensitivity for the diagnosis of osteomyelitis (80%–100%) but very poor specificity.[22] False positives can be caused by trauma, arthritis, recent surgery, or Charcot arthropathy. A negative bone scan virtually excludes infection.[23]

Labeled leukocyte scans (commonly called tagged white blood cell scans) are similarly sensitive but more specific than scintigraphy.

The 2 most common substances used in these studies are [99]Technetium and [111]Indium. The [99]Technetium methylene diphosphonate (MDP) labels hydroxyapatite, which is used to measure bone turnover. Because Charcot disease involves bone reparative activity, this method may not be able to accurately differentiate

Table 1
Characteristic features of plain radiographs in osteomyelitis and Charcot arthropathy

Osteomyelitis	Charcot Arthropathy
Periosteal reaction or elevation	Nonspecific changes: Periosteal reaction
Loss of cortex with bony erosion	Traumatic fractures
New bone formation	Bone destruction
Sequestrum: devitalized bone with radiodense appearance that has become separated from normal bone	Joint fragmentation and dislocation
Involucrum: layer of new bone growth outside existing bone	

Data from Cavanagh PR, Young MJ, Adams JE, et al. Radiographic abnormalities in the feet of patients with diabetic neuropathy. Diabetes Care 1994;17(3):201–9.

Table 2
Characteristic features of MRI studies in osteomyelitis and Charcot arthropathy

Osteomyelitis	Charcot Arthropathy
Low focal intensity on T1-weighted images	Altered bone marrow signal with low intensity on both T1-weighted and T2-weighted images
High focal signal on T2-weighted images	Signal intensity changes with osteosclerosis and cystlike lesions
High bone marrow signal in short tau inversion recovery images	Cortical fragmentation
Less specific or secondary changes:	Joint deformity or subluxation
Cortical disruption	Bone marrow edema pattern: periarticular and subchondral
Adjacent cutaneous ulcer	Predominant midfoot involvement
Soft tissue mass	Deformity is common along with bony debris
Adjacent soft tissue inflammation or edema	Overlying skin usually intact but may be edematous

Data from Marcus CD, Ladam-Marcus VJ, Leone J, et al. MR imaging of osteomyelitis and neuropathic osteoarthropathy in the feet of diabetics. Radiographics 1996;16(6):1337–48.

bone infection from trauma or other reparative processes. Indeed, [99]Technetium MDP scans are only 67% positive in patients with positive bone cultures for osteomyelitis.[24] [111]Indium-labeled leukocytes localize in neutrophil-mediated inflammatory processes, such as bacterial infections in bone. These scans in theory do not accumulate in areas of bone turnover (such as a fracture or Charcot) and should not appear in the absence of infection.[25] However, these 2 tests are not without error. A meta-analysis of both scans shows a positive predictive value of 90% with a sensitivity of 74% to 86% and a specificity of 68% to 85% depending on which scan was selected.[26]

One of the biggest challenges to the specificity of nuclear imaging studies is the risk of false positives from the increased marrow turnover in conditions like Charcot arthropathy. Indeed, studies have shown that although it is very sensitive, 3-phase bone scintigraphy cannot reliably distinguish osteomyelitis from a neuropathic joint because bone remodeling is high in both conditions. In fact, 50% of uninfected Charcot joints show uptake of labeled leukocytes.[27] A combined [99]Technetium MDP with [111]Indium bone scan technique has been suggested to combat this weakness, commonly referred to as a dual bone scan. This combined technique results in a test that is 50% sensitive, 100% specific, and 81% accurate for the diagnosis of osteomyelitis.[28]

Another combination that has been described is to combine an [111]Indium scan with a [99]Technetium sulfur colloid scan. The ^{99}Tc sulfa colloid scan is used to image areas of reticuloendothelial cells found in liver, spleen, and bone marrow. In ^{99}Tc sulfa colloid scans, areas of bone infection have no uptake, as the marrow elements in that area infarct and reduce accumulation. [111]Indium-labeled white cells by contrast will gather in areas of infection. With this combined technique, areas with low sulfur colloid and high indium uptake are likely to have osteomyelitis, whereas areas with relative uptake of both indicate low probability for osteomyelitis. This concept, called "spatial congruence," has a positive predictive value of 88% to 92%.[28] This technique can greatly improve accuracy in differentiating between bone marrow infection and inflammation.

The use of PET scans and single-photon emission computed tomography/computed tomography scans has also been explored and these scans have shown promise in helping to differentiate osteomyelitis from Charcot arthropathy. Some studies have shown that the sensitivity and specificity of PET with fludeoxyglucose F18

scans to be 100% and 93%, respectively, versus 76% and 75% with MRI.[29] This technique is not widely available, however, and its clinical usefulness remains to be seen.

TREATMENT

The best treatment for osteomyelitis of the foot and ankle remains unclear. The standard recommendation for treating chronic osteomyelitis with 6 weeks of parenteral antibiotics is widely accepted, but lacks definitive clinical data as the definitive length of treatment or that parenteral antibiotics are superior to oral antibiotics in many cases.[30] Some investigators have suggested that surgical debridement of the infected area may not be necessary, as antibiotics alone may eliminate bone infection in many cases.[31]

In cases of chronic osteomyelitis, most investigators advocate surgical debridement and antibiotics, but note that the best route of antibiotic administration or length of treatment is not well known. The long-term recurrence rate even with good treatment is 20% to 30%.[32] Peters and colleagues[33] published an article reviewing the accepted evidence for diabetic foot osteomyelitis. The investigators concluded that there was no evidence that surgical debridement was routinely necessary. They also concluded that the superior route of antibiotic administration was not known, and that the use of local antibiotics, hyperbaric oxygen, and other adjunctive factors was not well supported either.[33]

Treatment for Charcot arthropathy without osteomyelitis is largely nonoperative. Use of total contact casting or a Charcot restraint orthotic walker is well supported in the literature with 60% success rates and a low rate of complications.[34] Surgical treatment and its timing are not universally accepted. In this author's opinion, surgery is reserved for the patient with an impending ulceration or unbraceable and unstable foot. The use of bisphosphonate therapy also has been advocated by some investigators, but the data are not strong enough to support routine use of this therapy.[35]

Treatment for Charcot arthropathy with concomitant osteomyelitis may include debridement, antibiotic therapy, and the use of limited internal or external fixation. Despite the 25% risk of major amputation that a diabetic foot infection carries,[36] successful reconstruction of Charcot feet with concomitant osteomyelitis has resulted in 95.7% limb salvage rates as reported by Pinzur and colleagues.[37]

Table 3 Criteria for diagnosing osteomyelitis in the diabetic foot			
Category	**Criteria**	**Posttest Probability of Osteomyelitis, %**	**Management Recommendation**
Definite (beyond any reasonable doubt)	Bone sample with positive culture AND positive histology Purulence in bone found at surgery OR in bone removed at surgery OR Intraosseous abscess found on MRI OR Any 2 probable criteria OR 1 probable and 2 possible criteria OR any 4 possible criteria below	>90	Treat for osteomyelitis
Probable (more likely than not)	Visible cancellous bone in ulcer OR MRI showing bone edema with other signs of osteomyelitis OR Bone sample with positive histology but negative or absent culture OR any 2 possible criteria below	51–90	Consider treating, but further investigation may be needed
Possible (less rather than more likely)	Plain radiograph with cortical destruction OR MRI with edema OR Probe-to-bone positive OR Visible cortical bone OR Erythrocyte sedimentation rate >70 mm/h with no other source OR nonhealing wound despite adequate blood flow and offloading >6 wk OR ulcer >2 wk with clinical sign of infection	10–50	Treatment may be needed, but further investigation usually needed
Unlikely	No signs or symptoms of inflammation AND normal radiographs AND ulcer present <2 wk or absent AND any superficial ulcer OR normal MRI OR Normal bone scan	<10	Usually no need for further investigation

Data from Berendt AR, Peters EJ, Bakker K, et al. Diabetic foot osteomyelitis: a progress report on diagnosis and a systematic review of treatment. Diabetes Metab Res Rev 2008;24(Suppl 1):S145–61; and Ertugrul BM, Lipsky BA, Savk O. Osteomyelitis or Charcot neuro-osteoarthropathy? Differentiating these disorders in diabetic patients with a foot problem. Diabet Foot Ankle 2013;4:21855.

SUMMARY

No definitive single method exists to consistently differentiate Charcot arthropathy from osteomyelitis of the foot and ankle in "tough-to-call" cases with ulceration or wounds. A combination of physical examination features, laboratory studies, and properly applied imaging tests can be used to guide diagnosis and treatment, however. **Table 3** is a clinical algorithm developed by Berendt and colleagues.[38] and outlined by Ertugrul and colleagues[39] that may guide the clinician in a stepwise approach to identifying cases of diabetic foot osteomyelitis. In cases in which the data are not clear, a bone biopsy may be of value, but whether or not this represents the "gold standard" remains unclear. Although successful treatments for both Charcot arthropathy and osteomyelitis have been outlined in the literature, the best course of treatment for these conditions will require more research. As the obesity epidemic worsens worldwide, solutions will be needed to address these issues sooner than later.

REFERENCES

1. Chisholm KA, Gilchrist JM. The Charcot joint: a modern neurological perspective. J Clin Neuromuscul Dis 2011;13:1–13.
2. Sanders LJ. The Charcot foot: historical perspective 1827-2003. Diabetes Metab Res Rev 2004;20:S4–8.
3. Jeffcoate W, Lima J, Norbega L. The Charcot foot. Diabet Med 2000;17:253–8.
4. Chihara S, Segreti J. Osteomyelitis. Dis Mon 2010; 56:5–31.
5. Chanteleau E. The perils of procrastination: effects of early vs. delayed detection and treatment of incipient Charcot fracture. Diabet Med 2005;22:1707–12.
6. Byren I, Peters EJ, Hoey C, et al. Pharmacotherapy of diabetic foot osteomyelitis. Expert Opin Pharmacother 2009;10:3033–47.
7. Ertugrul BM, Oncul O, Tulek N, et al. A prospective multi-center study: factors related to the management of diabetic foot infections. Eur J Clin Microbiol Infect Dis 2012;31:2345–52.
8. Grayson ML, Gibbons GW, Bolgh K, et al. Probing to bone to find infected pedal ulcers. A clinical sign of underlying osteomyelitis in diabetic patients. JAMA 1995;273:721–3.
9. Aragon-Sanchez J, Lispky BA, Lazaro-Martinez JL. Diagnosing diabetic foot osteomyelitis: is the combination of a probe to bone test and plain radiography sufficient for high risk inpatients? Diabet Med 2011;28:191–4.
10. Lavery LA, Armstrong DG, Peters EJ, et al. Probe-to-bone test for diagnosing diabetic foot osteomyelitis: reliable or relic? Diabetes Care 2007;30:270–4.
11. Ertugrul BM, Savk O, Ozturk B, et al. The diagnosis of diabetic foot osteomyelitis: examination findings and laboratory values. Med Sci Monit 2009;15: CR307–12.
12. Newman LG, Waller J, Palestro CJ, et al. Unsuspected osteomyelitis in diabetic foot ulcers. Diagnosis and monitoring by leukocyte scanning with Indium 111 oxyquinolone. JAMA 1991;266:1246–51.
13. Butalia S, Palda VA, Sargeant RJ, et al. Does this patient with diabetes have osteomyelitis of the lower extremity? JAMA 2008;299:806–13.
14. Crim BE, Wukich DK. Osteomyelitis of the foot and ankle in the diabetic population: diagnosis and treatment. J Diabet Foot Complications 2010;1:1.
15. Wu JS, Gorbachova T, Morrison WB, et al. Imaging-guided bone biopsy for osteomyelitis: are there factors associated with positive or negative cultures? Am J Roentgenol 2007;188:1529–34.
16. Senneville E, Lelliez H, Beltrand E, et al. Culture of percutaneous bone biopsy specimens for diagnosis of diabetic foot osteomyelitis: concordance with ulcer swab cultures. Clin Infect Dis 2006;42: 57–62.
17. Senneville E, Morant H, Descamps D, et al. Outcome of patients with diabetes with negative percutaneous biopsy performed for suspicion of osteomyelitis of the foot. Diabet Med 2012;29:56–61.
18. Hartemann-Huertier A, Senneville E. Diabetic foot osteomyelitis. Diabetes Metab 2008;34:87–95.
19. Tan PL, Teh J. MRI of the diabetic foot: differentiation of infection from neuropathic change. Br J Radiol 2007;80:939–48.
20. Ledermann HP, Morrison WB, Schweitzer ME. MR image analysis of pedal osteomyelitis distribution, patterns of spread, and frequency of associated ulceration and septic arthritis. Radiology 2002;223: 747–55.
21. Morrison WB, Schweitzer ME, Batte WG, et al. Osteomyelitis of the foot: relative importance of primary and secondary MR imaging signs. Radiology 1998;207:625–32.
22. Wang GL, Zhao K, Lie ZF, et al. A meta-analysis of fluorodeoxyglucose-positron emission tomography versus scintigraphy in the evaluation of suspected osteomyelitis. Nucl Med Commun 2011;32:1134–42.
23. Knight D, Gray HW, McKillop JH, et al. Imaging for infection: caution required with the Charcot joint. Eur J Nucl Med 1988;13:523–6.
24. Shults DW, Hunter GC, McIntyre KE, et al. Value of radiographs and bone scans in determining the need for therapy in diabetic patients with foot ulcers. Am J Surg 1989;158:525–9.
25. Lipman B, Collier BD, Carrera GF, et al. Detection of osteomyelitis in the neuropathic foot: nuclear medicine, MRI, and conventional radiography. Clin Nucl Med 1998;23:77–82.
26. Dinh MT, Abad CL, Safdar N. Diagnostic accuracy of the physical examination and imaging tests for osteomyelitis underlying diabetic foot ulcers: meta-analysis. Clin Infect Dis 2008;47:519–27.
27. Seabold JE, Flickinger FW, Kao SCS, et al. Indium-111-leukocyte/technetium 99m-MDP bone and magnetic resonance imaging: difficulty of diagnosing osteomyelitis in patients with neuropathic osteoarthropathy. J Nucl Med 1990;31:549–56.

28. Palestro CJ, Mehta HH, Patel M, et al. Marrow versus infection in the Charcot joint: Indium-111 leukocyte and technetium-99 sulfur colloid scintigraphy. J Nucl Med 1998;39:346–50.

29. Basu S, Chryssikos T, Houseni M, et al. Potential role of FDG PET in the setting of diabetic neuro-osteoarthropathy: can it differentiate uncomplicated Charcot's neuroarthropathy from osteomyelitis and soft tissue infection? Nucl Med Commun 2007;28:465–72.

30. Spellberg B, Lipsky BA. Controversies in diagnosing and managing osteomyelitis of the foot in diabetes. Clin Infect Dis 2012;54:393–407.

31. Jeffcoate WJ, Lipsky BA. Controversies in diagnosing and managing osteomyelitis of the foot in diabetes. Clin Infect Dis 2004;39(Suppl 2):S115–22.

32. Conterno LO, da Silva Filjo CR. Antibiotics for treatment chronic osteomyelitis in adults. Cochrane Database Syst Rev 2009;(3):CD004439.

33. Peters EJ, Lipsky BA, Berendt AR, et al. A systematic review of the effectiveness of interventions in the management of infection in the diabetic foot. Diabetes Metab Res Rev 2012;28:142–62.

34. Guyton GP. An analysis of iatrogenic complications from the total contact cast. Foot Ankle Int 2005;26:903–7.

35. Pakarinen TK, Laine HJ, Maenpaa K, et al. Effect of immobilization, off-loading and zoledronic acid on bone mineral density in patients with acute Charcot neuroarthropathy: a prospective randomized trial. Foot Ankle Surg 2013;19:121–4.

36. Zgonis T, Stapleton JJ, Roukis TS. A stepwise approach to the surgical management of severe diabetic foot infections. Foot Ankle Spec 2008;1:46–53.

37. Pinzur MS, Gil J, Belmares J. Deformity and maintenance with ring fixation treatment of osteomyelitis in Charcot foot with single stage resection of infection, correction of deformity, and maintenance with ring fixation. Foot Ankle Int 2012;33:1069.

38. Berendt AR, Peters EJ, Bakker K, et al. Diabetic foot osteomyelitis: a progress report on diagnosis and a systematic review of treatment. Diabetes Metab Res Rev 2008;24(Suppl 1):S145–61.

39. Ertugrul BM, Lipsky BA, Savk O. Osteomyelitis or Charcot neuro-osteoarthropathy? Differentiating these disorders in diabetic patients with a foot problem. Diabet Foot Ankle 2013;4:21855.

Posttraumatic Reconstruction of the Foot and Ankle in the Face of Active Infection

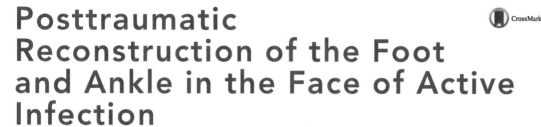

Brandon Jonard, MD[a], Erin Dean, MD[a,b],*

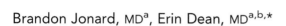

KEYWORDS

• Posttraumatic • Reconstruction • Osteomyelitis • Antibiotic spacer • External fixator

KEY POINTS

- Many options exist in the treatment of posttraumatic infection in the foot and ankle.
- Making the diagnosis often requires combining laboratory and radiologic testing, patient examination, and history.
- Antibiotic and surgical treatments should be tailored to individual patients based on the nature of their injury, extent of infection, comorbidities, and overall functional expectations.

INTRODUCTION

Posttraumatic infection of the foot and ankle is a challenging issue for orthopedic surgeons. Whether infection sets in as a result of the initial severe soft tissue injury or as a postoperative complication, clearing infection to allow successful reconstruction can be frustrating. Patient factors must be taken into account to determine the best approach for treatment. Thorough debridement is paramount followed by appropriate antibiotic treatment to clear the infection. Reconstruction can then be individualized based on host factors, type of injury, extent of bone or soft tissue loss, and patient expectations. Despite appropriate surgical and antibiotic treatment, the long-term recurrence rate for chronic osteomyelitis is about 20%.[1]

PATIENT EVALUATION: MAKING THE DIAGNOSIS

Often the presence of infection is clear with draining sinuses or wounds, erythema, or radiographic evidence of osteomyelitis. Other times the diagnosis may be more elusive. Imaging and laboratory studies as well as tissue cultures are included in the standard workup for infection.

Laboratory Testing

Laboratory values can be helpful but are nonspecific. Erythrocyte sedimentation rate (ESR), C-reactive protein (CRP), and white blood cell (WBC) levels should be obtained first. These tests are nonspecific but have been reported to have a sensitivity and specificity greater than 90% for the diagnosis of osteomyelitis, especially when used in combination.[2] Serum procalcintonin is a newer additional test with a high specificity for bacterial infection, which can be helpful for both diagnosing infection and monitoring treatment. Procalcitonin has been studied in acute osteomyelitis and septic arthritis in all age ranges and has been found to be a sensitive and specific marker at a cutoff of greater than 0.4 mg/mL.[3]

Imaging Studies
Radiographs
Plain radiographs are generally obtained first. In the presence of acute osteomyelitis, radiographs

---

Disclosure statement: The authors have nothing to disclose.
[a] Summa Health System, Department of Orthopedic Surgery, 444 North Main Street, Akron, OH 44309, USA;
[b] Crystal Clinic Orthopedic Center, 1310 Corporate Drive, Hudson, OH 44236, USA
* Corresponding author.
E-mail address: erindean@crystalclinic.com

may be negative because radiographic signs of infection are not visible for about 2 weeks after the onset of infection.[4] With more chronic infection, sclerotic bone may be present surrounding an infectious sequestrum.[4] Cortical destruction may also be present.[4] In the setting of posttraumatic infection, radiographs can be helpful to evaluate the traumatic bone injury, presence of nonunion, and extent of bone resorption to plan for surgical debridement and reconstruction. Comparing current radiographs to past and future radiographs can help to follow the progression of treatment as well.

Computed tomography

Computed tomography (CT) scans best demonstrate cortical destruction, periosteal reactions, and sequestrum.[4,5] Limitations include image degradation by streak artifact when metallic hardware is present and poor soft tissue and bone marrow resolution.[5,6] CT scans can be helpful when planning reconstruction, however, due to their 2- and 3-dimensional imaging capabilities that allow for better defining bone injury, presence of nonunion, and spatial relationships.

MRI

MRI is often the imaging option of choice for diagnosing osteomyelitis due to its early diagnostic capability. MRI can show bone marrow edema after only 1 to 2 days of onset of bone infection.[7] MRI has a sensitivity in diagnosing osteomyelitis of 82% to 100% and a specificity of 75% to 96%.[5] MRI can be helpful in showing abscess formation, sinus tracts, and soft tissue inflammation as well. MRI, however, is less helpful in the posttraumatic patient due to signal changes from the injury itself and susceptibility artifact from hardware.

Nuclear imaging

Nuclear imaging can provide a more specific evaluation for osteomyelitis without being compromised by the presence of hardware. The standard triple phase bone scan has a high sensitivity for identifying osteomyelitis in nonviolated bone.[4] However, increased osseous tracer uptake is noted in trauma or previous surgery, which decreases the usefulness of this test in the posttraumatic setting.[4,5] The nuclear medicine test of choice for these patients is a white cell scan in which the patient's WBCs are labeled with either Indium-111 or Tc^{99m}-HMPAO, before being intravenously returned to the patient.[4,5] These labeled white cells have increased uptake in infected bone. The WBC scan is combined with a standard bone marrow scan to differentiate from normal physiologic marrow uptake.[8]

When a WBC tagged scan is combined with a bone scan, the specificity is 80% to 90%.[5] Chronic or partially treated osteomyelitis can have false negative results.[5]

Deep Tissue or Bone Culture

The best way to diagnose osteomyelitis remains a deep bone biopsy. A positive culture provides a high level of specificity in the diagnosis of osteomyelitis. However, cultures have a low sensitivity with only 40% to 60% of patients with infection showing positive culture results.[9] Multiple intraoperative tissue samples encompassing the entire zone of infection should be obtained at debridement.[10]

INITIAL TREATMENT

1. Thorough debridement(s) to remove all nonviable tissue
2. Effective antibiotic treatment
3. Address patient-specific factors that may impede healing

Debridement

Upon diagnosis of infection, the patient should undergo thorough debridement to remove all evidence of necrotic tissue. Bone should be debrided until healthy-appearing bleeding bone remains and all sequestrum is removed. Multiple debridements may be required until no macroscopic sign of infection is present.[10] If hardware is present in the infected area, it should be removed if loose or unstable or if the bone is well healed. If the hardware is stable and the bone is nonunited, then the hardware may be left in place until the bone is healed.[11] Retaining hardware can reduce cure rates, however, due to biofilm formation.[12] In the presence of retained hardware, greater treatment success can be expected for patients infected with a single, less virulent organism compared with a more aggressive or multiple organisms[13] (Fig. 1).

Antibiotic Treatment

With extensive deep infection or osteomyelitis, obtaining the assistance of an infectious disease specialist can be very helpful for optimizing antibiotic treatment. Antibiotic treatment options and duration should be patient specific and culture directed. Polymicrobial infections are common in the foot and ankle, especially in those with diabetes, vascular disease, or immunocompromised patients.[10] *Staphylococcus aureus* is a very common pathogen in the foot and ankle, occurring in around 80% of infected patients in

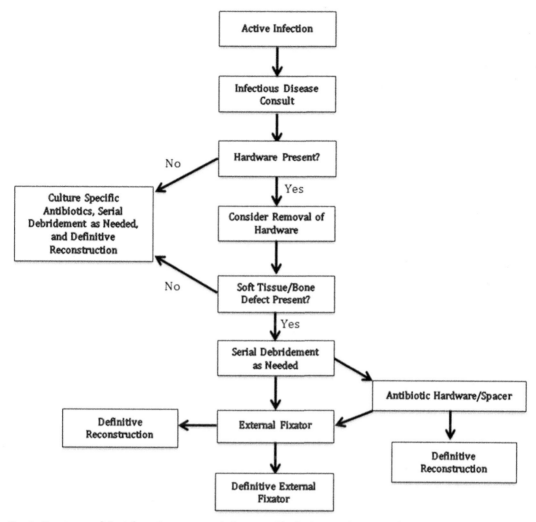

Fig. 1. Treatment of the infected posttraumatic foot or ankle. Patients with active infection require serial debridements and appropriate antibiotic therapy. Hardware that may be present from previous surgeries may be removed. External fixators as well as antibiotic spacers may be used on a case-by-case basis.

one study.[10] In this same study, *Pseudomonas aeruginosa* was a common primary or second infectious agent in 75% of patients, most commonly affecting diabetics.[10] This information should be taken into account when initial empiric antibiotics are chosen. ESR levels can be used to guide the duration of antibiotic treatment.[2] Once normalized, consideration is turned to definitive operative treatment.

Patient-Specific Factors Affecting Healing/ Treatment

Often, patient factors are out of the control of the treating orthopedic surgeon but can have a profound effect on treatment outcome. These factors should be part of the decision-making

algorithm and should be optimized at the onset of treatment when possible (Box 1, Fig. 2).

Diabetes

Diabetic patients have a known higher risk of postoperative complications, including infection and impaired wound healing. Patients with poor glycemic control should be counseled regarding their risk. Foot and ankle patients with a glycosylated hemoglobin (HgbA1c) level greater than 8% have a 2.5 times increased risk of developing infection.[14] Tight glucose control is imperative in improving outcomes in these patients. Patients with a fasting glucose level of greater than 140 mg/dL on the morning of surgery are 3 times more likely to develop that indicate higher potential for wound healing in patients with vascular disease.[15] In patients who do not meet these criteria, vascular surgery consultation is recommended. If the patient is a candidate, revascularization can aid in healing the reconstruction or offering a more distal amputation level if this route is chosen.

Tobacco use
Active tobacco users are twice as likely to develop postoperative infections after foot or ankle surgery when compared with non-tobacco users.[14,16] Tobacco use can impede skin healing and bone union. Counseling on smoking cessation should be done early in the treatment process to improve healing capability.[16] Smoking cessation options include oral medications or nicotine replacement products, referral to smoking cessation support networks such as 1-800-quit-now, or referral to a primary care provider.

infection than those with glucose levels less than 140 mg/dL.[14]

The presence of neuropathy also complicates the postoperative period by increasing the rate of infection and prolonging healing times. Post-operative infection is greater than 5 times more likely in patients with neuropathy.[14]

Peripheral Vascular Disease
When peripheral pulses are diminished, blood flow may not be adequate to allow for healing of the tissues or clearance of the infection. Patients with peripheral arterial disease are 3 times more likely to develop postoperative infections after foot or ankle surgery than those without vascular disease.[14] Box 2 lists vascular factors

Malnutrition
Malnutrition poses a serious risk to primary wound healing as well as any potential flap procedure that may be required for soft tissue or bone coverage. An albumin level less than 3.0 g/dL is a poor prognostic indicator for potential wound healing.[15] Consider checking protein, albumin, and prealbumin levels in patients with evidence of poor healing or suspected

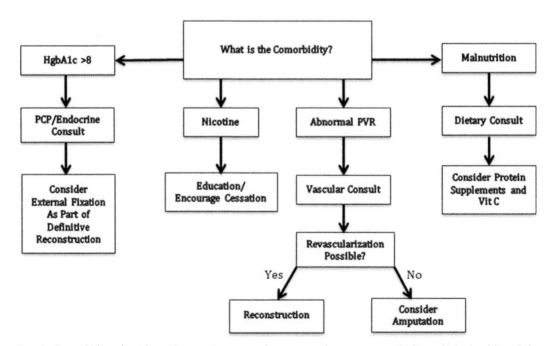

Fig. 2. Comorbidity algorithm. Many patients may have more than one comorbidity, which should each be addressed individually to better account for all patient risk factors.

Box 2
Factors favoring wound healing

Ischemic index greater than 0.5

Transcutaneous oxygen tension greater than 30 mm Hg

Toe pressure greater than 40 mm Hg

Ankle-brachial index greater than 0.45

---

malnutrition. Improving protein levels can aid in soft tissue and bone healing. Vitamin C (500 mg daily) and a multivitamin are helpful as well.[17]

Soft tissue loss/wounds

Wound management is essential in any traumatic situation, but becomes ever more important in the face of concomitant infection. The soft tissue envelop must provide adequate coverage over bone and hardware with potential to heal. Ultimately, the size and depth of the defect, type and volume of deficient tissue, availability of anastomosing vessels, and donor site condition determine options available for soft tissue reconstruction[10,18] (**Fig. 3**).

Investigations regarding negative pressure wound therapy have been increasingly popular in recent decades. Although there is still debate as to whether negative pressure therapy decreases bacterial loads, it has been proven to provide an active intermediate dressing for traumatic wounds until definitive closure can be performed. One report found that traumatic IIIB wounds were eventually been able to be closed primarily, using skin grafts, or secondarily after the use of negative pressure wound therapy.[19]

Closed incision negative pressure treatment (ciNPT) can aid in incisional healing as well by decreasing edema, improving perfusion to the area, and decreasing incisional tension.[20] ciNPT is recommended for high-risk incisions including reopened or high-tension incisions, especially in light of patient risk factors. The patient factors correlating with the highest risk of wound complication include obesity, diabetes, tobacco use, and prolonged surgical time.[20]

SURGICAL RECONSTRUCTION OPTIONS

After initial treatment with irrigation and debridement along with antibiotics, focus will

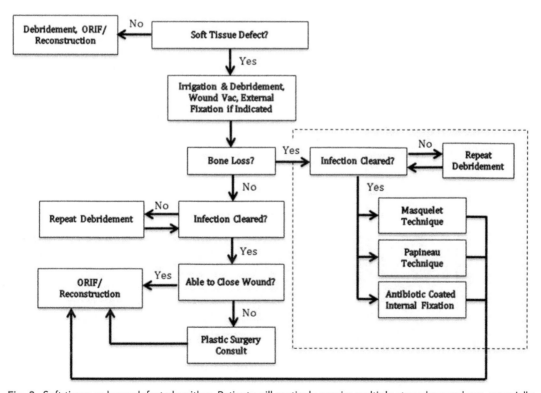

Fig. 3. Soft tissue or bone defect algorithm. Patients will routinely require multiple staged procedures, especially when soft tissue or bone defects are present. Bone defects should be cleared of infection and then treated with spacers and/or bone grafting. Soft tissue defects can be treated with negative pressure therapy and may require plastic surgery consultation.

transition to definitive reconstruction options. This process can often be multidisciplinary involving orthopedics, plastic surgery, and infectious disease services. It is also not uncommon for patients to benefit from psychiatric counseling, especially if long-term frames or amputation is a possibility. Primary reconstruction can be performed at the time of last debridement. Alternatively, a 2-staged approach can be taken allowing continued antibiotic treatment and wound maturation before definitive fixation (Fig. 4).

Primary Reconstruction

If the level of wound contamination is thought to be minimal, a primary reconstruction at the time of final irrigation and debridement may be considered. Given the risk of deep hardware infection, the surgeon should be confident that the benefit of definitive fixation outweighs the risks of potential continued postoperative infection. A well-timed treatment plan should be coordinated with plastic surgery colleagues in the setting of severe soft tissue loss before placing definitive hardware. However, if the soft tissues are adequately debrided and the tissue bed is mature enough for closure, definitive fixation may be used based on the presenting injury.[21]

Some scenarios may have a higher than normal risk of continued infection (ie, farm injuries, water injuries). In these scenarios, consultation with an infectious disease specialist should be considered for extended-term antibiotic treatment or for chronic suppressive antibiotics.

Secondary Reconstruction

In cases where there is significant contamination or bacterial load, infection with more virulent or multiple organisms, or complicating patient comorbidities, 2-staged reconstruction may be the best treatment option. Options include the Masquelet technique, Papineau technique, or antibiotic impregnated internal fixation techniques (see Fig. 3).

Masquelet technique

Thorough debridement of osteomyelitis can lead to large bone defects that make reconstruction more challenging. The Masquelet technique can be used in this setting by filling these bone defects with antibiotic impregnated cement beads or solid molded spacers.[22,23] Solid spacers afford more stability, whereas the beads allow higher surface area–to-volume ratio, theoretically improving antibiotic spread to the surrounding tissues. Local antibiotic treatment in

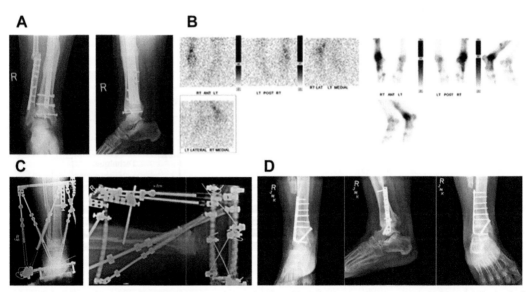

Fig. 4. Case example. A 33-year-old woman presented with ankle pain 1 year after sustaining tibia and fibula shaft fractures treated with percutaneous distal tibial fixation and IMN. She also reported a prior ankle fracture treated surgically. Radiographs showed lucency around the distal metaphyseal hardware (*A*). Laboratory values were elevated and nuclear imaging, including a bone scan and WBC scan, was suggestive of distal tibia osteomyelitis (*B*). The patient underwent staged treatment with initial debridement, placement of antibiotic cement spacer, and circular external fixator (*C*). Following 6 weeks of intravenous antibiotics and normalization of laboratory values, the frame was removed and blade plate fixation was used for ankle arthrodesis (*D*).

this fashion can decrease the systemic side effects of the antibiotics.[23] When left in place for 4 to 8 weeks, a nicely vascularized bed is created to accept the bone graft. Once free of infection, the spacer is removed and bone graft is placed. Often these patients will also require external fixation concomitantly for stabilization of the limb until the spacer is removed and definitive fixation can be placed.

Papineau technique

An alternative option for critical size bone defects in the face of an open wound is the Papineau technique. In this technique, the open defect is packed with cancellous bone graft, and the wound, with exposed graft, is covered with a moist-to-dry dressing or negative pressure wound dressing. Stabilization is usually obtained via an external fixator. When thorough debridement is performed and all infected bone has been removed, the Papineau technique has afforded very positive results.[24,25]

Antibiotic coated internal fixation devices

Antibiotic-coated internal fixation devices offer an alternative approach to the stabilization of the infected limb. Intramedullary devices coated in antibiotic cement can provide both stabilization and local antibiotic delivery, negating the need for external fixation. Similar techniques have reported favorable results when using antibiotic-coated locking plates for local delivery of antibiotics to infected periprosthetic hip fracture sites.[26] Data for these techniques, however, are largely limited to case reports.

OPTIONS FOR DEFINITIVE TREATMENT

Multiple options exist for definitive fixation once the infection has been cleared and the wound bed is healthy. Internal fixation, external fixation, or a combination of both, can be used. The final decision is based on patient factors and the location and character of the presenting bone injury.

Primary Open Reduction Internal Fixation

Standard methods of open reduction internal fixation (ORIF) may be used even in the most contaminated wounds as long as the treating surgeon is confident the initial posttraumatic infection has been cleared or, alternatively, if long-term antibiotics are planned. The decision for fixation technique depends on fracture pattern and surgeon preference. When planning for primary ORIF, adequate evidence should be obtained that the infection is cleared before proceeding. Common methods that may be used include the following:

- Laboratory findings (ie, WBC count, ESR, CRP, HgbA1c, albumin)
- Imaging (radiographs, CT scan, MRI, nuclear medicine)
- Patient factors/comorbidities
- Skin or wound appearance

Internal fixation may be used for the purposes of fracture reduction as well as for potential arthrodesis. Internal fixation has been compared with external fixation in posttraumatic patients with infection during arthrodesis.[27] Although their results suggest that limb salvage, fusion rate, and infection recurrence were similar between the 2 groups, they also recommend that internal fixation should be used whenever infection is deemed to be cleared.

External Fixation

Commonly used external fixation devices include spatial frames, Ilizarov devices, or traditional bar-clamp external fixators. External fixation can be used for temporary fixation while clearing deep infection, or can be used as part of the definitive fixation plan.

External fixation with limited internal fixation

External fixation can be used in combination with internal fixation acutely or as definitive treatment. This idea has been used in pilon management with external fixation and ORIF of the fibula to add additional stability to external fixation constructs while being forgiving for soft tissues.[28]

In addition, limited internal fixation can be added to a frame construct, once soft tissues allow and infection has been cleared, to create a definitive combined construct. Adding limited internal fixation can decrease the impact on the soft tissues compared with standard ORIF treatment. This approach can be helpful in the patient with comorbidities or tenuous soft tissues when additional stability beyond just the external fixator is desired. Limited internal fixation can include percutaneous or open lag screw fixation or short-segment or small-diameter plate fixation. This technique has been used in distal tibial pilon fractures with good results.[29] When compared with ORIF or intramedullary nailing (IMN) in distal tibia fractures, external fixation with limited internal fixation reduced operative and radiation times, postoperative complications, and reoperation rates.[30]

Definitive external fixation

Box 3 outlines which patients may benefit from definitive treatment in an external fixator. However, patients without these factors can also be

Box 3
Factors suggesting external fixation

Severe wound contamination

Severe soft tissue injury

Multiple medical comorbidities

Medically unstable

Soft tissue/bone loss

treated with a frame when desired. The decision to proceed with external fixation as a definitive plan depends on patient factors and surgeon preference. Good results can be expected with definitive frame treatment.[31,32] Shahid and colleagues[31] reported a 100% union rate with good to excellent results in 83% of patients treated with an Ilizarov fixator for infected tibial nonunions. Definitive external fixation can be helpful in treating segmental bone loss as well through distraction osteogenesis. Good results have been reported with this technique using bone transport through an Ilizarov frame.[33]

External fixation can also be used when arthrodesis is planned following treatment of infection in the posttraumatic patient. One review reports successful fusion of the ankle joint with Ilizarov treatment in 76 of 91 posttraumatic patients.[34] In addition, arthrodesis through the Ilizarov fixator has shown excellent results when used for treatment of infected nonunions around the ankle joint.[35] An additional study found a fusion rate of 89% in low-energy trauma patients and 85% in high-energy trauma patients using external fixation, although those who were considered high energy required a second operation more frequently.[36] Most patients were still able to achieve fusion through one operation.

Temporary Frame with Delayed Fracture Specific Open Reduction Internal Fixation

External fixation frames can be used for initial stability until the extremity has been adequately cleared of infection and definitive internal fixation can be performed. Once soft tissues are mature enough for definitive internal fixation, the external fixation device can be removed and the second stage of reconstruction may be initiated based on the injury type. Internal fixation can then be used for either fracture reduction or joint fusion. Studies have compared the results of internal versus external devices for foot and ankle fusion with results that indicate internal fixation was favorable.[27] If the treating surgeon is able to effectively transition to

internal fixation devices without significant risk of continued infection or risk to soft tissue, it is commonly favorable to do so.

COMPLICATIONS AND ALTERNATIVES

Patients with comorbidities have higher complication and recurrence rates leading to higher risk of requiring amputation.[10] Patients should be counseled regarding their risks at the onset of treatment to assure that patient expectations are reasonable. Even with appropriate surgical and antibiotic treatment, the long-term recurrence rate for chronic osteomyelitis is about 20%.[1]

For limb salvage to be successful, the patient must have a functional limb with acceptable residual pain levels and a soft tissue envelop capable of healing and clearing infection. Should patient factors limit reconstruction options, or should the patient wish to avoid long-term or multistaged reconstruction, amputation is an option. An early and open discussion regarding the possibility of amputation should be undertaken with patients, even if the patient does wish to proceed with the most aggressive treatment modality in an effort to save the limb. If infection recurs or patient factors prohibit reconstruction, amputation may be the only reliable option despite the best efforts from the treating orthopedic surgeon.

SUMMARY

Posttraumatic infections pose a difficult problem for orthopedic surgeons and patients alike. A multidisciplinary approach is required with high levels of coordination between specialties. Given the complexity and uniqueness of each individual case, multiple factors, including patient comorbidities, injury type, soft tissue or bone defects, as well as chronicity of the infection must be taken into account. Because of these factors, there is no single solution for any case. Individualized treatment regimens must be considered. Treatment will likely include multiple procedures for debridement and stabilization, wound coverage, and definitive reconstruction. Extended-term antibiotics are also frequently required. Because of the long and difficult course commonly seen with posttraumatic infections, honest and frank discussions of options should be undertaken with patients before the initiation of treatment. Ultimately, regardless of the end outcome, patient satisfaction will likely be incumbent on realistic expectations and inclusion during the decision-making process.

REFERENCES

1. Conterno LO, Filho CRDS. Antibiotics for treating chronic osteomyelitis in adults. Cochrane Database Syst Rev 2009;(3):CD004439.

2. Lin Z, Vasudevan A, Tambyah PA. Use of erythrocyte sedimentation rate and C-reactive protein to predict osteomyelitis recurrence. J Orthop Surg (Hong Kong) 2016;24(1):77–83.

3. Maharajan K, Patro D, Menon J, et al. Serum procalcitonin is a sensitive and specific marker in the diagnosis of septic arthritis and acute osteomyelitis. J Orthop Surg Res 2013;8(1):19.

4. Lee YJ, Sadegh S, Mankad K, et al. The imaging of osteomyelitis. Quant Imaging Med Surg 2016;6(2):184–98.

5. Restrepo C, Giménez CR, Mccarthy K. Imaging of osteomyelitis and musculoskeletal soft tissue infections. Rheum Dis Clin North Am 2003;29(1):89–109.

6. Pineda C, Espinosa R, Pena A. Radiographic imaging in osteomyelitis: the role of plain radiography, computed tomography, ultrasonography, magnetic resonance imaging, and scintigraphy. Semin Plast Surg 2009;23(02):080–9.

7. Jaramillo D. Infection: musculoskeletal. Pediatr Radiol 2011;41(S1):127–34.

8. Mettler FA, Guiberteau MJ. Essentials of nuclear medicine imaging. Philadelphia: Saunders/Elsevier; 2006.

9. Mathews CJ, Weston VC, Jones A, et al. Bacterial septic arthritis in adults. Lancet 2010;375(9717):846–55.

10. Malizos KN, Gougoulias NE, Dailiana ZH, et al. Ankle and foot osteomyelitis: treatment protocol and clinical results. Injury 2010;41(3):285–93.

11. Dunbar RP. OPINION: retain stable implant and suppress infection until union. J Orthop Trauma 2007;21(7):503–5.

12. Morgenstern M, Post V, Erichsen C, et al. Biofilm formation increases treatment failure in Staphylococcus epidermidis device-related osteomyelitis of the lower extremity in human patients. J Orthop Res 2016;34(11):1905–13.

13. Cook GE, Markel DC, Ren W, et al. Infection in orthopedics. J Orthop Trauma 2015;(Suppl 12):19–23.

14. Wukich DK, Crim BE, Frykberg RG, et al. Neuropathy and poorly controlled diabetes increase the rate of surgical site infection after foot and ankle surgery. J Bone Joint Surg Am 2014;96(10):832–9.

15. Pinzur MS, Stuck RM, Sage R, et al. Syme ankle disarticulation in patients with diabetes. J Bone Joint Surg Am 2003;85-A(9):1667–72.

16. Lindström D, Azodi OS, Wladis A, et al. Effects of a perioperative smoking cessation intervention on postoperative complications. Ann Surg 2008;248(5):739–45.

17. Mohammed BM, Fisher BJ, Kraskauskas D, et al. Vitamin C promotes wound healing through novel pleiotropic mechanisms. Int Wound 2016;13(4):572–84.

18. Levin L. Soft tissue coverage options for ankle wounds. Foot Ankle Clin 2001;6(4):853–66.

19. Schlatterer D, Hirshorn K. Negative pressure wound therapy with reticulated open cell foam-adjunctive treatment in the management of traumatic wounds of the leg: a review of the literature. J Orthop Trauma 2008;22(Suppl 10):S152–60.

20. Willy C, Agarwal A, Andersen CA, et al. Closed incision negative pressure therapy: international multidisciplinary consensus recommendations. Int Wound J 2016. [Epub ahead of print].

21. Tarkin IS, Sop A, Pape H-C. High-energy foot and ankle trauma: principles for formulating an individualized care plan. Foot Ankle Clin 2008;13(4):705–23.

22. Azi M, Teixeira A, Cotias R, et al. Membrane induced osteogenesis in the management of post-traumatic bone defects. J Orthop Trauma 2016;30(10):545–50.

23. Wang X, Luo F, Huang K, et al. Induced membrane technique for the treatment of bone defects due to post-traumatic osteomyelitis. Bone Joint Res 2016;5(3):101–5.

24. Polyzois VD, Galanakos SP, Tsiampa VA, et al. The use of Papineau technique for the treatment of diabetic and non-diabetic lower extremity pseudoarthrosis and chronic osteomyelitis. Diabet Foot Ankle 2011;2.

25. Deng Z, Cai L, Jin W, et al. One-stage reconstruction with open bone grafting and vacuum-assisted closure for infected tibial non-union. Arch Med Sci 2014;10(4):764–72.

26. Liporace FA, Yoon RS, Frank MA, et al. Use of an "antibiotic plate" for infected periprosthetic fracture in total hip arthroplasty. J Orthop Trauma 2012;26(3):18–23.

27. Moore J, Berberian WS, Lee M. An analysis of 2 fusion methods for the treatment of osteomyelitis following fractures about the ankle. Foot Ankle Int 2014;36(5):547–55.

28. Tong D, Ji F, Zhang H, et al. Two-stage procedure protocol for minimally invasive plate osteosynthesis technique in the treatment of the complex pilon fracture. Int Orthop 2011;36(4):833–7.

29. Zhao L, Li Y, Chen A, et al. Treatment of type C pilon fractures by external fixator combined with limited open reduction and absorbable internal fixation. Foot Ankle Int 2013;34(4):534–42.

30. Fang JH, Wu YS, Guo XS, et al. Comparison of 3 minimally invasive methods for distal tibia fractures. Orthopedics 2016;39(4):e627–33.

31. Shahid M, Hussain A, Bridgeman P, et al. Clinical outcomes of the Ilizarov method after an infected tibial nonunion. Arch Trauma Res 2013;2(2):71–5.

32. Eralp İL, Kocaoğlu M, Dikmen G, et al. Treatment of infected nonunion of the juxta-articular region of the distal tibia. Acta Orthop Traumatol Turc 2016; 50(2):139–46.

33. Yin P, Zhang L, Zhang L, et al. Ilizarov bone transport for the treatment of fibular osteomyelitis: a report of five cases. BMC Musculoskelet Disord 2015;16:242.

34. Fragomen AT, Borst E, Schachter L, et al. Complex ankle arthrodesis using the Ilizarov method yields high rate of fusion. Clin Orthop Relat Res 2012; 470(10):2864–73.

35. Rochman R, Hutson JJ, Alade O. Tibiocalcaneal arthrodesis using the Ilizarov technique in the presence of bone loss and infection of the talus. Foot Ankle Int 2008;29(10):1001–8.

36. Kenzora JE, Simmons SC, Burgess AR, et al. External fixation arthrodesis of the ankle joint following trauma. Foot Ankle Int 1986;7(1): 49–61.

Index

Note: Page numbers of article titles are in **boldface** type.

A

Acute hematogenous osteomyelitis (AHO)
  in children, **199–208**
    classification of, 203–204
    clinical presentation of, 201–202
    complications of, 205
    diagnosis of, 202–204
      advanced imaging in, 202–203
      convention radiography in, 202
      laboratory studies in, 203
      radiology in, 202
    discussion, 205–206
    epidemiology of, 200
    introduction, 199–200
    pathogenesis of, 200–201
    prognosis of, 203
    treatment of, 204–205
Acute phase reactants
  in acute phase response in children provoked by
    musculoskeletal infection, 187–190
Acute phase response
  in children
    musculoskeletal infection and, **181–197** See
      also Musculoskeletal infection, acute phase
      response in children provoked by
    described, 182–186
AHO. See Acute hematogenous osteomyelitis
  (AHO)
Aminoglycosides
  nephrotoxicity with, 140–141
Ankle
  posttraumatic infection of, **249–258**
    evaluation of, 249–250
    introduction, 249
    treatment of, 250–256
      complications of, 256
      definitive, 255–256
      factors affecting, 251–253
      initial, 250–253
      surgical, 253–255
Antibiotic(s)
  in children
    for AHO, 204–205
    for septic arthritis, 213
  in open fracture management, **137–153**
    introduction, 137

local antibiotics, 143–148
  advantages of, 143
  calcium sulfate, 147–148
  chitosan sponge, 146–147
  collagen sponge, 145–146
  gels, 145
  history of, 143
  PMMA, 143–144
  without carrier, 144–145
systemic antibiotics, 137–143
  body weight in dosing of, 141
  contemporary options, 141
  established guidelines for, 139–140
  history, incidence, and infecting organisms,
    137–139
  implications of changing wound care on
    infecting organisms, 142
  nephrotoxicity with, 140–141
  recommendations in 2017, 142–143
  timing of administration of, 139
  in posttraumatic infection of foot and ankle
    management, 250–251
Antibiotic-coated internal fixation devices
  in management of posttraumatic infection of foot
    and ankle, 255
Antibiotic nail
  in long bone infection management, **155–165**
    contraindications to, 156
    indications for, 156
    introduction, 155
    methodology of, 156–160
      debridement in, 157
      diagnosis in, 156–157
      placement in, 157–160
    outcomes of, 163–164
    pearls and pitfalls in, 160–163
    rationale for, 155–156
    senior author's preferred technique, 160
Anticoagulant(s)
  DVT and PE in patients on
    management of, 130–133
Arthritis
  septic
    in children, **209–216** See also Septic arthritis,
      in children
Arthrocentesis
  in septic arthritis diagnosis in children, 211–212

Arthropathy
    Charcot
        vs. osteomyelitis, **241–247** See also Charcot
            arthropathy, osteomyelitis vs.
Arthroplasty
    total joint See Total joint arthroplasty (TJA)
    total knee See Total knee arthroplasty (TKA)
Arthroscopy
    for septic arthritis in children, 213

B

Bone and implant-related infection
    longstanding
        management of
            TNP wound therapy in, 176–178

C

Calcium sulfate
    in open fracture management, 147–148
Charcot arthropathy
    causes of, 241
    osteomyelitis vs., **241–247**
        clinical presentation of, 241–242
        evaluation of
            bone biopsy in, 242
            hematologic studies in, 242
            history and physical examination in, 242
            imaging studies in, 242–244
        introduction, 241
        treatment of, 244
Children
    acute phase response in
        musculoskeletal infection and, **181–197** See
            also Musculoskeletal infection, acute phase
            response in children provoked by
    AHO in, **199–208** See also Acute hematogenous
        osteomyelitis (AHO), in children
    septic arthritis in, **209–216** See also Septic
        arthritis, in children
Chitosan sponge
    in open fracture management, 146–147
Coagulopathy
    acute phase response in children provoked by
        musculoskeletal infection and, 191–192
Collagen sponge
    in open fracture management, 145–146
Computed tomography (CT)
    in AHO diagnosis in children, 202–203
    in posttraumatic infection of foot and ankle
        evaluation, 250
Corticosteroids
    in modulation of acute phase response in children
        provoked by musculoskeletal infection, 192
C-reactive protein (CRP)
    in acute phase response in children provoked by
        musculoskeletal infection, 187–188

CRP. See C-reactive protein (CRP)
CT. See Computed tomography (CT)
Cutaneous fungal infections
    of hand, 233–234

D

Deep vein thrombosis (DVT)
    in orthopedic surgery, **127–135**
        diagnosis of, 128–129
        introduction, 127–128
        management of
            in acute phase, 129–130
            perioperative, 130–133
        risk factors for, 128
Diabetes
    as factor in management of posttraumatic
        infection of foot and ankle, 251–252
DVT. See Deep vein thrombosis (DVT)

E

Embolism
    pulmonary See Pulmonary embolism (PE)
Erythrocyte sedimentation rate (ESR)/fibrinogen
    in acute phase response in children provoked by
        musculoskeletal infection, 188
ESR. See Erythrocyte sedimentation rate (ESR)
External fixation
    for posttraumatic infection of foot and ankle,
        255–256

F

Fibrinogen
    in acute phase response in children provoked by
        musculoskeletal infection, 188
Flexor tenosynovitis (FTS), **217–227**
    anatomy related to, 217–218
    differential diagnosis of, 221–222
    evaluation of
        patient presentation in, 219–221
        physical examination in, 219–221
        studies in, 221
    historical perspective on, 217
    introduction, 217
    microbiology of, 218–219
    treatment of, 222–225
        outcomes of, 225
Foot
    posttraumatic infection of, **249–258**
        evaluation of, 249–250
        introduction, 249
        treatment of, 250–256
            complications of, 256
            definitive, 255–256
            factors affecting, 251–253
            initial, 250–253

surgical, 253–255
Fracture(s)
  open
    IIIB
      TNP wound therapy in, 171–172
    treatment of
      antibiotics in, **137–153** *See also*
        Antibiotic(s), in open fracture
        management
FTS. *See* Flexor tenosynovitis (FTS)
Fungal infections
  of hand, 233–237
    cutaneous, 233–234
    histoplasmosis, 234–235
    mucormycosis, 235–236
    nail, 233–234
    sporotrichosis, 236

G

Gels
  in open fracture management, 145

H

Hand infections
  atypical, **229–240** *See also specific infections*
    fungal infections, 233–237
    general workup for, 229–230
    introduction, 229
    mycobacterial infections, 230–233
    viral infections, 237–238
Hansen disease
  of hand, 231
Herpetic whitlow
  of hand, 237
Histoplasmosis
  of hand, 234–235

I

IL-6. *See* Interleukin-6 (IL-6)
Implant-related infections
  longstanding
    management of
      TNP wound therapy in, 176–178
Infection(s)
  active
    posttraumatic reconstruction of foot and ankle
      related to, **249–258** *See also* Ankle; Foot
  bone
    management of
      TNP wound therapy in, 176–178
  hand
    atypical, **229–240** *See also specific types and*
      Hand infections, atypical
  implant-related
    management of
      TNP wound therapy in, 176–178

long bone
  treatment of
    antibiotic nail in, **155–165** *See also*
      Antibiotic nail, in long bone infection
      management
Interleukin-6 (IL-6)
  in acute phase response in children provoked by
    musculoskeletal infection, 187
Internal fixation
  primary open reduction
    for posttraumatic infection of foot and ankle,
      255, 256

L

Leprosy
  of hand, 231
Local antibiotics. *See* Antibiotic(s)
Long bone infection
  treatment of
    antibiotic nail in, **155–165** *See also* Antibiotic
      nail, in long bone infection management
Lyme disease
  in children
    vs. septic arthritis, 212

M

Magnetic resonance imaging (MRI)
  in AHO diagnosis in children, 203
  in Charcot arthropathy *vs.* osteomyelitis
    determination, 243
  in posttraumatic infection of foot and ankle
    evaluation, 250
MAI. *See* Mycobacterium spp.
Malnutrition
  as factor in management of posttraumatic
    infection of foot and ankle, 252–253
Masquelet technique
  in management of posttraumatic infection of foot
    and ankle, 254–255
MRI. *See* Magnetic resonance imaging (MRI)
Mucormycosis
  of hand, 235–236
Musculoskeletal infection
  acute phase response in children provoked by,
    181–197
  bacterial hijacking of, 187
  coagulopathy, 191–192
  described, 182–186
  dysregulation of, 190–192
  future directions in, 192
  introduction, 181–182
  modulation of, 192
  patient evaluation overview, 187–192
    acute phase reactants, 187–190
  septic and toxin-mediated shock related to,
    190–191

Mycobacterial infections
  of hand, 230–233
    leprosy, 231
    MAI–related, 232–233
    tuberculosis, 230–231
Mycobacterium spp.
  hand infections due to
    M. leprae, 231
    M. marinum, 231–232
    MAI, 232–233

N

Nail fungal infections
  of hand, 233–234
Nuclear imaging studies
  in Charcot arthropathy vs. osteomyelitis
    determination, 243–244
  in posttraumatic infection of foot and ankle
    evaluation, 250

O

Obese patients
  physical function and physical activity in
    after TKA, 117–125
      introduction, 117–118
      study discussion, 121–124
      study materials and methods, 118–120
      study results, 120–121
Open fractures
  treatment of
    antibiotics in, 137–153 See also Antibiotic(s),
      in open fracture management
Orthopedic surgery
  DVT and PE in, 127–135 See also Deep vein
    thrombosis (DVT); Pulmonary embolism (PE)
  TNP wound therapy impact on, 167–179 See also
    Total negative pressure (TNP) wound therapy,
    impact on orthopedic infection
Osteomyelitis
  acute hematogenous
    in children, 199–208 See also Acute
      hematogenous osteomyelitis (AHO), in
      children
  causes of, 241
  Charcot arthropathy vs., 241–247 See also
    Charcot arthropathy, osteomyelitis vs.

P

Papillomavirus
  of hand, 237–238
Papineau technique
  in management of posttraumatic infection of foot
    and ankle, 255
Parapoxvirus
  of hand, 238
PE. See Pulmonary embolism (PE)
Peripheral vascular disease

as factor in management of posttraumatic
  infection of foot and ankle, 252
PET. See Positron emission tomography (PET)
PMMA. See Polymethylmethacrylate (PMMA)
Polymethylmethacrylate (PMMA)
  in open fracture management, 143–144
Positron emission tomography (PET)
  in Charcot arthropathy vs. osteomyelitis
    determination, 244
Primary open reduction internal fixation
  for posttraumatic infection of foot and ankle, 255
Procalcitonin
  in acute phase response in children provoked by
    musculoskeletal infection, 188–189
Protein C
  in modulation of acute phase response in children
    provoked by musculoskeletal infection, 192
Pulmonary embolism (PE)
  in orthopedic surgery, 127–135
    diagnosis of, 128–129
    introduction, 127–128
    management of
      in acute phase, 129–130
      perioperative, 130–133
    risk factors for, 128

R

Radiography
  in AHO, 202
  in Charcot arthropathy vs. osteomyelitis
    determination, 242–243
  in posttraumatic infection of foot and ankle
    evaluation, 249–250
Radiology
  in AHO, 202

S

Septic arthritis
  in children, 209–216
    bacteriology of, 209–210
    complications of, 213
    diagnosis of, 210–212
      arthrocentesis in, 211–212
      history and physical examination in, 210
      imaging in, 210–211
      laboratory studies in, 210
    introduction, 209
    outcomes of, 213
    pathophysiology of, 209
    treatment of, 212–213
    vs. Lyme disease, 212
    vs. transient synovitis, 212
  defined, 209
Septic shock
  acute phase response in children provoked by
    musculoskeletal infection and, 190–191

Serial aspiration
  for septic arthritis in children, 213
Shock
  septic
    acute phase response in children provoked by
      musculoskeletal infection and, 190–191
  toxin-mediated
    acute phase response in children provoked by
      musculoskeletal infection and, 190–191
Soft tissue wounds
  as factor in management of posttraumatic
    infection of foot and ankle, 253
Sporotrichosis
  of hand, 236
Synovitis
  transient
    vs. septic arthritis
      in children, 212
Systemic antibiotics. See Antibiotic(s)

T

Tenosynovitis
  flexor, **217–227** See also Flexor tenosynovitis
    (FTS)
IIIB open fracture
  management of
    TNP wound therapy in, 171–172
TJA. See Total joint arthroplasty (TJA)
TKA. See Total knee arthroplasty (TKA)
TNP wound therapy. See Total negative pressure
    (TNP) wound therapy
Tobacco use
  as factor in management of posttraumatic
    infection of foot and ankle, 252
Total joint arthroplasty (TJA)
  transfusion rates after
    TXA effects on, **109–115** See also Tranexamic
      acid (TXA), effects on transfusion rates
      after TJA
Total knee arthroplasty (TKA)
  physical function and physical activity in obese
    patients after, **117–125** See also Obese
    patients, physical function and physical activity
    in, after TKA
Total negative pressure (TNP) wound therapy
  in IIIB open fracture management, 171–172
  impact on orthopedic infection, **167–179**
    artificial skin, 170–171
    case examples, 175–176
    closed surgical incisions, 172–174

    in closed wound setting, 174
    commonalities of, 176
    coverage, 170
    debridement, 167–170
    introduction, 167
    longstanding bone and implant-related
      infection, 176–178
    rationale for, 176
Toxin-mediated shock
  acute phase response in children provoked by
    musculoskeletal infection and, 190–191
Tranexamic acid (TXA)
  effects on transfusion rates after TJA, **109–115**
    introduction, 109
    study of, 110–115
      discussion, 112–114
      follow-up routine, 110
      methods, 110
      outcome variables and measures, 110
      participants in, 110
      results, 110–112
      statistical analysis, 110
Transfusion rates
  after TJA
    TXA effects on, **109–115** See also Tranexamic
      acid (TXA), effects on transfusion rates after
      TJA
Transient synovitis
  in children
    vs. septic arthritis, 212
Tuberculosis
  of hand, 230–231
TXA. See Tranexamic acid (TXA)

V

Viral infections
  of hand, 237–238
    herpetic whitlow, 237
    papillomavirus, 237–238
    parapoxvirus, 238
Vitamin K replacement
  in modulation of acute phase response in children
    provoked by musculoskeletal infection, 192

W

Wound(s)
  soft tissue
    as factor in management of posttraumatic
      infection of foot and ankle, 253

Printed and bound by CPI Group (UK) Ltd, Croydon, CR0 4YY

13/05/2025

01869712-0003